AIDS/HIV

ISSN 1532-2718

AIDS/HIV

Barbara Wexler

INFORMATION PLUS® REFERENCE SERIES
Formerly Published by Information Plus, Wylie, Texas

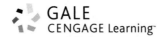

GALE
CENGAGE Learning·

Detroit • New York • San Francisco • New Haven, Conn • Waterville, Maine • London

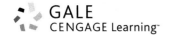

AIDS/HIV

Barbara Wexler
**Kepos Media, Inc.: Paula Kepos and
Janice Jorgensen, Series Editors**

Project Editors: Elizabeth Manar,
  Kathleen J. Edgar

Rights Acquisition and Management: Jacqueline
  Flowers, Barb McNeil, Robyn Young

Composition: Evi Abou-El-Seoud, Mary Beth
  Trimper

Manufacturing: Cynde Lentz

For product information and technology assistance, contact us at
Gale Customer Support, 1-800-877-4253.
For permission to use material from this text or product,
submit all requests online at **www.cengage.com/permissions.**
Further permissions questions can be e-mailed to
permissionrequest@cengage.com

Cover photograph: Image copyright Sebastian Kaulitzki, 2009. Used under license from Shutterstock.com.

While every effort has been made to ensure the reliability of the information presented in this publication, Gale, a part of Cengage Learning, does not guarantee the accuracy of the data contained herein. Gale accepts no payment for listing; and inclusion in the publication of any organization, agency, institution, publication, service, or individual does not imply endorsement of the editors or publisher. Errors brought to the attention of the publisher and verified to the satisfaction of the publisher will be corrected in future editions.

Gale
27500 Drake Rd.
Farmington Hills, MI 48331-3535

ISBN-13: 978-0-7876-5103-9 (set)   ISBN-10: 0-7876-5103-6 (set)
ISBN-13: 978-1-4144-4113-9   ISBN-10: 1-4144-4113-4

ISSN 1532-2718

This title is also available as an e-book.
ISBN-13: 978-1-4144-7002-3 (set)
ISBN-10: 1-4144-7002-9 (set)
Contact your Gale sales representative for ordering information.

Printed in the United States of America
1 2 3 4 5 6 7 14 13 12 11 10

TABLE OF CONTENTS

PREFACE

AIDS/HIV is part of the *Information Plus Reference Series*. The purpose of each volume of the series is to present the latest facts on a topic of pressing concern in modern American life. These topics include the most controversial and studied social issues in the 21st century: abortion, capital punishment, care of senior citizens, crime, the environment, health care, immigration, minorities, national security, social welfare, sports, women, youth, and many more. Even though this series is written especially for high school and undergraduate students, it is an excellent resource for anyone in need of factual information on current affairs.

By presenting the facts, it is the intention of Gale, Cengage Learning, to provide its readers with everything they need to reach an informed opinion on current issues. To that end, there is a particular emphasis in this series on the presentation of scientific studies, surveys, and statistics. These data are generally presented in the form of tables, charts, and other graphics placed within the text of each book. Every graphic is directly referred to and carefully explained in the text. The source of each graphic is presented within the graphic itself. The data used in these graphics are drawn from the most reputable and reliable sources, such as from the various branches of the U.S. government and from major organizations and associations. Every effort has been made to secure the most recent information available. Readers should bear in mind that many major studies take years to conduct and that additional years often pass before the data from these studies are made available to the public. Therefore, in many cases the most recent information available in 2010 is dated from 2007 or 2008. Older statistics are sometimes presented as well if they are of particular interest and no more-recent information exists.

Even though statistics are a major focus of the *Information Plus Reference Series*, they are by no means its only content. Each book also presents the widely held positions and important ideas that shape how the book's subject is discussed in the United States. These positions are explained in detail and, where possible, in the words of their proponents. Some of the other material to be found in these books includes historical background, descriptions of major events related to the subject, relevant laws and court cases, and examples of how these issues play out in American life. Some books also feature primary documents or have pro and con debate sections that provide the words and opinions of prominent Americans on both sides of a controversial topic. All material is presented in an even-handed and unbiased manner; readers will never be encouraged to accept one view of an issue over another.

HOW TO USE THIS BOOK

The spread of acquired immunodeficiency syndrome (AIDS) has become a global epidemic. As of 2007, an estimated 33 million people worldwide were living with human immunodeficiency virus (HIV), according to the Joint United Nations Program on AIDS/HIV. That same year there were 2.7 million new HIV cases diagnosed and 2 million HIV-related deaths. This book includes information on the nature of AIDS/HIV and the AIDS epidemic; symptoms and transmittal; patterns and trends in AIDS/HIV surveillance; populations at risk; children, adolescents, and AIDS/HIV; AIDS/HIV cost and treatment; people living with AIDS/HIV; testing, prevention, and education; HIV and AIDS worldwide; and knowledge, awareness, behavior, and opinion of those affected by AIDS/HIV.

AIDS/HIV consists of 10 chapters and 3 appendixes. Each chapter is devoted to a particular aspect of AIDS/HIV. For a summary of the information covered in each chapter, please see the synopses provided in the Table of Contents. Chapters generally begin with an overview of the basic facts and background information on the chapter's topic, then proceed to examine subtopics of particular interest. For example, Chapter 10: Knowledge, Awareness, Behavior, and Opinion begins with the observation that by the start of the 21st century Americans appeared less concerned about HIV/AIDS than in previous years. The chapter then goes on to provide the findings of public opinion polls and surveys to present a snapshot of Americans' views about the most pressing health problems facing the United States, their assessments of the risk of acquiring the virus, and their attitudes about HIV testing. The chapter also considers knowledge about HIV/AIDS and the relationship between knowledge, misconceptions, stigma, and discrimination. It offers examples of public awareness and education initiatives as well as organizations involved in funding these programs. Readers can find their way through a chapter by looking for the section and subsection headings, which are clearly set off from the text. They can also refer to the book's extensive index if they already know what they are looking for.

Statistical Information

The tables and figures featured throughout *AIDS/HIV* will be of particular use to readers in learning about this issue. These tables and figures represent an extensive collection of the most recent and important statistics on AIDS/HIV and related issues—for example, graphics cover clinical categories of AIDS infection; adult and adolescent HIV infection and AIDS cases; pediatric AIDS cases; office visits, by diagnostic and screening services ordered or provided; syringe exchange statistics; states with confidential HIV reporting; and teens' concerns about becoming infected with AIDS/HIV. Gale, Cengage Learning, believes that making this information available to readers is the most important way to fulfill the goal of this book: to help readers understand the issues and controversies surrounding AIDS/HIV in the United States and to reach their own conclusions.

Each table or figure has a unique identifier appearing above it, for ease of identification and reference. Titles for the tables and figures explain their purpose. At the end of each table or figure, the original source of the data is provided.

To help readers understand these often complicated statistics, all tables and figures are explained in the text. References in the text direct readers to the relevant statistics. Furthermore, the contents of all tables and figures are fully indexed. Please see the opening section of the index at the back of this volume for a description of how to find tables and figures within it.

Appendixes

Besides the main body text and images, *AIDS/HIV* has three appendixes. The first is the Important Names and Addresses directory. Here, readers will find contact information for a number of government and private organizations that can provide further information on AIDS/HIV. The second appendix is the Resources section, which can also assist readers in conducting their own research. In this section, the author and editors of *AIDS/HIV* describe some of the sources that were most useful during the compilation of this book. The final appendix is the detailed index, which facilitates reader access to specific topics in this book.

ADVISORY BOARD CONTRIBUTIONS

The staff of Information Plus would like to extend its heartfelt appreciation to the Information Plus Advisory Board. This dedicated group of media professionals provides feedback on the series on an ongoing basis. Their comments allow the editorial staff who work on the project to make the series better and more user-friendly. The staff's top priority is to produce the highest-quality and most useful books possible, and the Information Plus Advisory Board's contributions to this process are invaluable.

The members of the Information Plus Advisory Board are:

- Kathleen R. Bonn, Librarian, Newbury Park High School, Newbury Park, California
- Madelyn Garner, Librarian, San Jacinto College, North Campus, Houston, Texas
- Anne Oxenrider, Media Specialist, Dundee High School, Dundee, Michigan
- Charles R. Rodgers, Director of Libraries, Pasco-Hernando Community College, Dade City, Florida
- James N. Zitzelsberger, Library Media Department Chairman, Oshkosh West High School, Oshkosh, Wisconsin

COMMENTS AND SUGGESTIONS

The editors of the *Information Plus Reference Series* welcome your feedback on *AIDS/HIV*. Please direct all correspondence to:

Editors
Information Plus Reference Series
27500 Drake Rd.
Farmington Hills, MI 48331-3535

CHAPTER 1
THE NATURE OF HIV/AIDS

The acquired immunodeficiency syndrome (AIDS) is the late stage of an infection that is caused by the human immunodeficiency virus (HIV). HIV is a retrovirus that attacks and destroys certain white blood cells. The targeted destruction weakens the body's immune system and makes the infected person susceptible to infections and diseases that ordinarily would not be life threatening. AIDS is considered a bloodborne, sexually transmitted disease because HIV is spread through contact with blood, semen, or vaginal fluids from an infected person.

Before 1981 AIDS was virtually unknown in the United States. In that year, testing of blood and other samples for HIV began, and reporting of the disease became mandatory. Awareness grew as the annual number of diagnosed cases and deaths steadily increased. In "First 500,000 AIDS Cases—United States, 1995" (*Morbidity and Mortality Weekly Report*, vol. 44, no. 46, November 24, 1995), the Centers for Disease Control and Prevention (CDC) stated that the number of U.S. AIDS cases reported since 1981 reached the half-million mark in 1995. Indeed, in 1995 HIV infection was the leading cause of death among Americans aged 25 to 44.

By 1998, however, HIV/AIDS deaths among this age group had fallen dramatically, and HIV infection was the fifth most common cause of death among people in the United States between 25 and 44 years old. HIV/AIDS deaths fell to sixth place in the 2001 summary. This rank was the same in 2006, the most recent year for which data were available as of September 2009, with the disease claiming a reported 5,150 lives. (See Table 1.1.)

By contrast, in people aged 15 to 24, HIV rose from the ninth leading cause of death in 2004 to the eighth leading cause of death in 2006 and was responsible for 198 deaths. (See Table 1.1.)

Overall, HIV mortality (death) rates began to decline in 1996, even before the widespread use of new and effective drug treatments such as protease inhibitors. In 1997 HIV infection was the 14th leading cause of death overall in the United States. By 1999 HIV infection no longer ranked among the 15 leading causes of death in the United States. Figure 1.1 shows the sharp decline in deaths from HIV disease since the mid-1990s and the subsequent stabilization in the number of deaths attributable to HIV/AIDS from 1999 to 2005.

When examined at a general level, the overall decline in HIV/AIDS deaths between 1995 and 2000 was a positive trend for people infected with HIV and those suffering from AIDS. Nonetheless, the reality is that the actual number of people living with HIV/AIDS increased during this time span. In other words, even though not as many people were dying from HIV/AIDS, more people were living with the disease due to the success of new therapies. These people require ongoing treatment and care.

The observed decline in HIV/AIDS deaths is no reassurance to the estimated 40,000 people diagnosed with an HIV infection each year in the United States. The CDC reports in *HIV/AIDS Surveillance Report, 2007* (2009, http://www.cdc.gov/hiv/topics/surveillance/resources/reports/2007report/pdf/2007SurveillanceReport.pdf) that in 2007 there were 42,655 new cases of HIV/AIDS in adults, adolescents, and children in the 34 states with long-term, confidential name-based HIV reporting. Because not all states report HIV/AIDS cases, the CDC developed a method for estimating the incidence (the number of newly diagnosed cases during a specific time period) of HIV infection in the United States each year. Using this method, H. Irene Hall et al. note in "Estimation of HIV Incidence in the United States" (*Journal of the American Medical Association*, vol. 300, no. 5, August 2008) that there were 55,400 new infections each year from 2003 to 2006. The researchers estimate that approximately 56,300 people were newly infected with HIV in 2006.

TABLE 1.1

Deaths and death rates for the 10 leading causes of death by age groups, preliminary 2006

[Data are based on a continuous file of records received from the states. Rates are per 100,000 population in specified group. Figures are based on weighted data rounded to the nearest individual, so categories may not add to totals or subtotals]

Rank[a]	Cause of death (based on the International Classification of Diseases, tenth revision, second edition, 2004) and age	Number	Rate
	All ages[b]		
...	All causes	2,425,901	810.3
1	Diseases of heart	629,191	210.2
2	Malignant neoplasms	560,102	187.1
3	Cerebrovascular diseases	137,265	45.8
4	Chronic lower respiratory diseases	124,614	41.6
5	Accidents (unintentional injuries)	117,748	39.3
...	Motor vehicle accidents	44,572	14.9
...	All other accidents	73,177	24.4
6	Alzheimer's disease	72,914	24.4
7	Diabetes mellitus	72,507	24.2
8	Influenza and pneumonia	56,247	18.8
9	Nephritis, nephrotic syndrome and nephrosis	44,791	15.0
10	Septicemia	34,031	11.4
...	All other causes (residual)	576,491	192.5
	1–4 years		
...	All causes	4,636	28.5
1	Accidents (unintentional injuries)	1,591	9.8
...	Motor vehicle accidents	586	3.6
...	All other accidents	1,005	6.2
2	Congenital malformations, deformations and chromosomal abnormalities	501	3.1
3	Malignant neoplasms	372	2.3
4	Assault (homicide)	350	2.1
5	Diseases of heart	160	1.0
6	Influenza and pneumonia	114	0.7
7	Septicemia	88	0.5
8	Certain conditions originating in the perinatal period	67	0.4
9	In situ neoplasms, benign neoplasms and neoplasms of uncertain or unknown behavior	63	0.4
10	Cerebrovascular diseases	53	0.3
...	All other causes (residual)	1,277	7.8
	5–14 years		
...	All causes	6,136	15.2
1	Accidents (unintentional injuries)	2,228	5.5
...	Motor vehicle accidents	1,323	3.3
...	All other accidents	905	2.2
2	Malignant neoplasms	916	2.3
3	Assault (homicide)	387	1.0
4	Congenital malformations, deformations and chromosomal abnormalities	330	0.8
5	Diseases of heart	242	0.6
6	Intentional self-harm (suicide)	213	0.5
7	Chronic lower respiratory diseases	113	0.3
8	Cerebrovascular diseases	93	0.2
9	Septicemia	78	0.2
10	In situ neoplasms, benign neoplasms and neoplasms of uncertain or unknown behavior	76	0.2
...	All other causes (residual)	1,460	3.6

TABLE 1.1

Deaths and death rates for the 10 leading causes of death by age groups, preliminary 2006 [CONTINUED]

[Data are based on a continuous file of records received from the states. Rates are per 100,000 population in specified group. Figures are based on weighted data rounded to the nearest individual, so categories may not add to totals or subtotals]

Rank[a]	Cause of death (based on the International Classification of Diseases, tenth revision, second edition, 2004) and age	Number	Rate
	15–24 years		
...	All causes	34,632	81.6
1	Accidents (unintentional injuries)	15,859	37.4
...	Motor vehicle accidents	10,845	25.6
...	All other accidents	5,014	11.8
2	Assault (homicide)	5,596	13.2
3	Intentional self-harm (suicide)	4,097	9.7
4	Malignant neoplasms	1,643	3.9
5	Diseases of heart	1,021	2.4
6	Congenital malformations, deformations and chromosomal abnormalities	456	1.1
7	Cerebrovascular diseases	206	0.5
8	Human immunodeficiency virus (HIV) disease	198	0.5
9	Influenza and pneumonia	180	0.4
10	Pregnancy, childbirth and the puerperium	172	0.4
...	All other causes (residual)	5,204	12.3
	25–44 years		
...	All causes	125,173	148.9
1	Accidents (unintentional injuries)	30,949	36.8
...	Motor vehicle accidents	13,779	16.4
...	All other accidents	17,170	20.4
2	Malignant neoplasms	17,604	20.9
3	Diseases of heart	14,873	17.7
4	Intentional self-harm (suicide)	11,240	13.4
5	Assault (homicide)	7,525	8.9
6	Human immunodeficiency virus (HIV) disease	5,150	6.1
7	Chronic liver disease and cirrhosis	2,805	3.3
8	Diabetes mellitus	2,705	3.2
9	Cerebrovascular diseases	2,703	3.2
10	Septicemia	1,131	1.3
...	All other causes (residual)	28,488	33.9
	45–64 years		
...	All causes	464,463	620.4
1	Malignant neoplasms	151,654	202.6
2	Diseases of heart	101,588	135.7
3	Accidents (unintentional injuries)	29,505	39.4
...	Motor vehicle accidents	10,939	14.6
...	All other accidents	18,566	24.8
4	Diabetes mellitus	17,012	22.7
5	Cerebrovascular diseases	16,779	22.4
6	Chronic lower respiratory diseases	16,181	21.6
7	Chronic liver disease and cirrhosis	14,725	19.7
8	Intentional self-harm (suicide)	11,492	15.4
9	Nephritis, nephrotic syndrome and nephrosis	6,495	8.7
10	Septicemia	6,184	8.3
...	All other causes (residual)	92,848	124.0

...Category not applicable.
[a]Rank based on number of deaths.
[b]Includes deaths under 1 year of age.
Notes: For certain causes of death such as unintentional injuries, homicides, and suicides, preliminary and final data may differ because of the truncated nature of the preliminary file. Data are subject to sampling or random variation.

SOURCE: Melonie P. Heron et al., "Table 7. Deaths and Death Rates for the 10 Leading Causes of Death in Specified Age Groups: United States, Preliminary 2006," in "Deaths: Preliminary Data for 2006," *National Vital Statistics Reports*, vol. 56, no. 16, June 11, 2008, http://www.cdc.gov/nchs/data/nvsr/nvsr56/nvsr56_16.pdf (accessed June 11, 2009)

In "HIV Prevalence Estimates—United States, 2006" (*Morbidity and Mortality Weekly Report*, vol. 57, no. 39, October 3, 2008), Michael L. Campsmith et al. of the CDC indicate that the prevalence of HIV infection (an estimate of the number of people living with an HIV infection) was 1.1 million people in the United States in 2006. About one-fifth (21%) of these cases were undiagnosed.

Between 1996 and 1997 the number of AIDS deaths declined by 42%. This dramatic decrease was the result of the introduction and use of effective antiretroviral

FIGURE 1.1

Deaths in which HIV disease was named as the underlying cause, 1987–2005

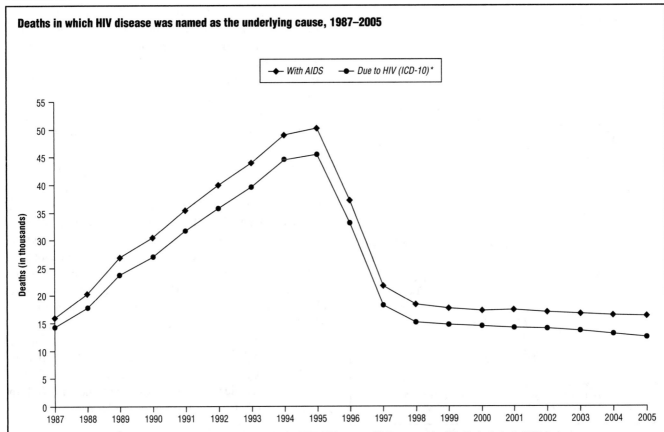

◆— With AIDS   ●— Due to HIV (ICD-10)*

*For comparison with data for 1999 and later years, data in the bottom line for 1987–1998 were modified to account for *ICD-10* rules instead of *ICD-9* rules.

SOURCE: "Slide 3. Comparison of Mortality Data from AIDS Case Reports and Death Certificates in Which HIV Disease Was Selected As the Underlying Cause of Death, United States, 1987–2005," in *HIV Mortality (through 2005)*, Centers for Disease Control and Prevention, August 5, 2008, http://www.cdc.gov/hiv/topics/surveillance/resources/slides/mortality/slides/mortality3.pdf (accessed June 11, 2009)

drugs that slow the progression of an HIV infection. This decline continued but slowed to 20% between 1997 and 1998, and to 8% between 1998 and 1999. This may be due to a combination of several factors: resistance to the drug treatments developed in some patients, complicated drug treatment regimens that are difficult for patients to maintain, and a possible lack of access to prompt testing or treatment. The CDC reports in "Basic Statistics" (February 26, 2009, http://www.cdc.gov/hiv/topics/surveillance/basic.htm) that a cumulative estimate of 1,051,875 people in the United States and dependent areas had been diagnosed with AIDS through 2007. Of these, 583,298 had died.

The AIDS epidemic is by no means strictly a U.S. phenomenon. According to the Joint United Nations Program on HIV/AIDS, in *Report on the Global AIDS Epidemic 2008* (August 2008, http://www.unaids.org/en/Knowledge Centre/HIVData/GlobalReport/2008/2008_Global_report .asp), an estimated 33 million people worldwide were living with HIV/AIDS in 2007. In that year alone, an estimated 2.7 million people became infected and 2 million people worldwide died of AIDS. In 2007 the countries of

sub-Saharan Africa continued to have the world's highest annual rates of HIV infection and deaths.

THE HUMAN IMMUNODEFICIENCY VIRUS

A virus is a tiny infectious agent composed of genes surrounded by a protective coating. Until a virus contacts a host cell, it is essentially an inert bag of genetic material. Viruses are parasites. They must invade other cells and commandeer the host cell's replication machinery to reproduce. A frequent outcome of viral infection is the destruction of the host cell, as the newly made virus particles burst out of the cell. The host cell destruction can harm the host (in the case of HIV, a human). The common cold, influenza (flu), and some forms of pneumonia are also caused by specific, non-HIV viruses.

HIV belongs to a group of viruses known as retroviruses. The name arises from the presence of a special enzyme—reverse transcriptase—that reverses the usual pattern of translating the genetic message. (See Figure 1.2.) In animals the genetic units of information that are called genes consist of deoxyribonucleic acid (DNA). DNA is the

FIGURE 1.2

Schematic of HIV

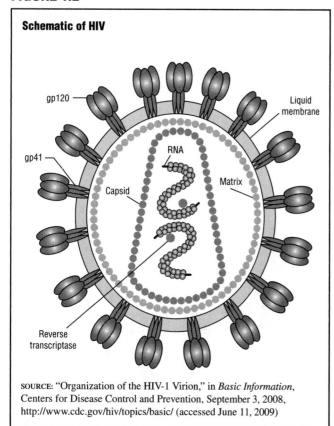

SOURCE: "Organization of the HIV-1 Virion," in *Basic Information*, Centers for Disease Control and Prevention, September 3, 2008, http://www.cdc.gov/hiv/topics/basic/ (accessed June 11, 2009)

blueprint from which another type of genetic material called ribonucleic acid (RNA) is made, in a process called transcription. In turn, the RNA serves as the blueprint for the various proteins that are the structural building blocks of the virus. In contrast to animals, retroviruses have their genes stored in RNA. After HIV infects a human cell, the viral reverse transcriptase works to transcribe HIV RNA into DNA. The viral DNA then becomes part of the host DNA—a process called integration—and is replicated along with the host DNA to produce new HIV particles.

Before 1980 retroviruses had been found in some animals. Indeed, as far back as 1911 Francis Peyton Rous (1879–1970) isolated an infectious and debilitating virus from a chicken. The Rous sarcoma virus was later shown to be both an oncogenic (cancer-causing) virus and the first known retrovirus. The first known human retroviruses, human T cell leukemia virus (HTLV-I) and the closely related human T cell lymphotropic virus (HTLV-II), were discovered in 1980 by Robert C. Gallo (1937–) and his colleagues at the U.S. National Cancer Institute (NCI). This breakthrough provided the groundwork for the discovery of the virus that would eventually be known as HIV.

Identifying the Virus

In September 1983 Luc Montagnier (1932–) and researchers at the Pasteur Institute took a sample from a

lymph node biopsy of a hospitalized patient in Paris and identified a retrovirus they named lymphadenopathy-associated virus (LAV). Eight months later Gallo's group at NCI isolated the same virus in AIDS patients, which they called HTLV-III. LAV and HTLV-III were found to be identical and are now referred to as HIV. A conflict arose about which researcher should be credited with the discovery. In 1991, in an intense, politically charged atmosphere, Gallo dropped his claim to the discovery of HIV.

The original HIV is now known as HIV-1. This is due to the 1986 discovery by scientists at the Pasteur Institute of a new AIDS-causing virus in West Africans, which was labeled as HIV-2. Even though the two forms of HIV have similar modes of transmission, the symptoms of HIV-2 were found to be milder than those of HIV-1. Furthermore, HIV-2 was shown to differ in molecular structure from HIV-1 in a way that ties it more closely to a virus that causes AIDS in macaque monkeys. The CDC estimates in the fact sheet "Human Immuno-deficiency Virus Type 2" (March 8, 2007, http://www.cdc.gov/hiv/resources/Factsheets/hiv2.htm) that by 1998, 79 people in the United States had been infected with HIV-2. (Unless otherwise specified, the term *HIV* in the remainder of this edition refers to HIV-1.)

The Origins of the Virus

Montagnier and Gallo, along with other investigators, believed that HIV had been present in Central Africa and other regions for some time, and at some point the virus crossed the species barrier from primates to humans. The rural nature of these societies and the limited access to the outside world by those infected with the virus may have confined the spread of HIV for many decades. However, once the migration of tribal Central Africans to urban areas began, the more liberated sexual practices there promoted the spread of HIV. Within a comparatively short time, the once rare and remote disease was spread by globe-trotting HIV-infected people.

It was long speculated that HIV evolved from simian immunodeficiency virus (SIV), a retrovirus that infects monkeys. The theory was that HIV evolved from a human infection with a mutated form of SIV that was infectious to humans. Consistent with this theory was the finding that HIV is a part of the lentivirus family, which includes SIV.

In 1982 Isao Miyoshi (1932–) of Kochi University identified an HTLV-related virus in Japanese macaque monkeys. Genetically similar to HTLV, it was designated as the simian T-lymphotropic virus (STLV). Further studies identified STLV in both Asian and African monkeys and in apes, with an infection rate ranging from 1% to 40%.

In 1988 Myron Essex (1939–) and Phyllis Jean Kanki (1956–) of the Harvard School of Public Health discovered that the simian virus found in African chimpanzees and African green monkeys was more homologous (related in primitive origin) to the human virus than to the simian virus in Asian macaques. This discovery provided strong support for an evolved version of African STLV as being the origin of human HTLV.

In 1999 an international team of researchers working at the University of Alabama announced its determination that the genetic sequence of a simian virus isolated from a tissue sample obtained from a chimpanzee was virtually identical to the HIV discovered by Montagnier. Interestingly, chimpanzees are only rarely infected with SIV. This implies that the chimpanzee may be a temporary carrier of the virus, which normally resides in some other, as yet unidentified, primate species. A common chimpanzee subspecies, *Pan troglodytes troglodytes*, which along with the bonobo is the closest living species to humans, naturally harbors HIV-1, and there have been documented occurrences of cross-species transmission from them to humans. Because these chimpanzees are still poached for bushmeat, humans may be at risk for continued exposure. A complete understanding of the mechanisms of cross-species transmission and the ability of these chimpanzees to resist infection may help researchers develop strategies to protect humans from HIV as well as from other viruses such as H1N1, SARS coronavirus, hantaviruses, and the Ebola and Marburg viruses that originate in animals.

ATTACKING THE IMMUNE SYSTEM

As with other infections, HIV must evade the immune system, which functions to detect and destroy invaders. To learn how HIV first attacks healthy cells while evading attack by the immune system, it is important to understand the complex structure of HIV and how normal white blood cells work.

Healthy White Blood Cells at Work

White blood cells are major components of the complicated, coordinated system of organs and cells that make up the human immune system. These organs and cells work together to prevent invasion by foreign substances. There are five types of white blood cells: macrophages (scavenger cells of the immune system), T4 or helper T cells, T8 or killer T cells, plasma B cells, and memory B cells. T and B white blood cells are also called lymphocytes. It is these lymphocytes that bear the major responsibility for carrying out immune system activities. Figure 1.3 shows how the virus attaches to an immune cell and reproduces.

Each type of white blood cell has a specific function. The macrophage, which begins as a smaller monocyte (single cell), readies the T4 cells to respond to particular invaders such as viruses. At the time of viral attack, the macrophage, which is sometimes referred to as the vacuum cleaner of the immune system, swallows the virus, but leaves a portion displayed so that the T4 cell can make contact. The macrophage also stimulates the production of thousands of T4 cells, which are all programmed to battle the invader.

When T4 lymphocytes attack an invading virus, they also send out chemical messages that cause the multiplication of B cells and T8 killer cells. These cells, along with the help of some T4 cells, destroy the infected cell. Other T4 cells, which are not actively involved in destroying the infected cells, send chemical messages to B cells, causing them to reproduce and divide into groups of either plasma cells or memory cells. Plasma cells make antibodies that cripple the invading virus, whereas memory cells increase the immune response if the invader ever attacks again.

HIV's Molecular Structure

HIV has nine genes. Three of these—designated env, gag, and pol code—form the structural components of the virus, such as the coats that surround the genetic material and form the outer surface of the virus particle. The remaining genes—tat, nef, rev, vpr, vpu, and vif—are involved in regulating the genetic activities that are necessary to create copies of the infecting virus.

HIV's complement of nine genes is minuscule when compared with the 30,000 genes that are in human DNA. Nevertheless, HIV is more complex than most other retroviruses, which have only three or four genes. Scientists believe these genes direct the production of proteins that make up parts of the virus and regulate its reproduction. The HIV core contains genes that are protected by a protein shell, whereas the entire virus is surrounded by a fatty membrane dotted with glycoproteins (proteins with sugar units attached), adding to its protection. Figure 1.4 shows the steps in the replication cycle of HIV.

Once HIV enters the human body, its primary target is a subset of immune cells that contain a molecule called CD4. In particular, the virus attaches itself to CD4+ T cells and, to a lesser extent, to macrophages. Figure 1.5 shows cell-to-cell spread of HIV through the CD4-mediated fusion of an infected cell with an uninfected cell.

Another Discovery

In November 1995 Ute-Christiane Meier et al. proposed in "Cytotoxic T Lymphocyte Lysis Inhibited by Viable HIV Mutants" (*Science*, vol. 270, no. 5240) that HIV defuses the killer cells that are supposed to destroy virus-stricken cells. The researchers isolated HIV from AIDS patients and demonstrated that the virus had undergone a mutation, or change, in its genetic structure. When killer T cells approached cells infected with the mutated virus, the T cells failed to kill the stricken cells, perhaps

FIGURE 1.3

How HIV attaches to an immune cell and reproduces

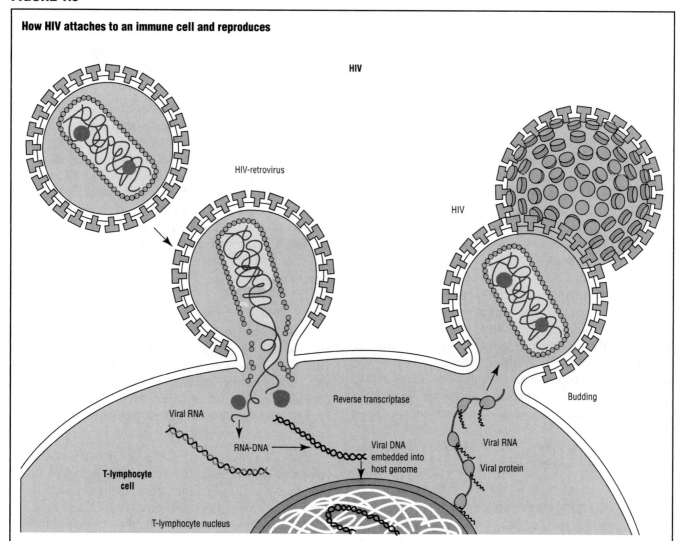

SOURCE: "Scientists Found out How the Virus Attaches to an Immune Cell and Reproduces; the Challenge Was to Prevent That Process," in *In Their Own Words... NIH Researchers Recall the Early Years of AIDS*, National Institutes of Health, June 2001, http://aidshistory.nih.gov/discovery_of_HIV/index.html (accessed June 11, 2009)

because they no longer recognized them. In fact, the T cells were unable to kill even cells infected with the original, unmutated virus. The mutations not only allowed the altered strains to multiply but also allowed unaltered strains to flourish.

AN ALTERNATE THEORY: "FRIENDLY FIRE." Not all researchers agree that the alteration of killer T cells is the underlying basis for the establishment of an HIV infection. Some believe that other cells in the immune system attack and kill CD4-containing cells in what has been called an autoimmune response. The CD4-containing cells that have not been invaded by the virus, but that display fragments of it, become targets for other cells—besides the killer cells—which see the infected cells as a camouflaged virus and kill them. In addition, HIV-infected cells may send out protein signals that weaken or destroy other healthy cells in the immune system.

Whatever the basis of the beginning of an HIV infection, it is agreed that HIV subsequently exhibits various behaviors, depending on the kind of cell it has invaded and how the cell behaves. The virus can remain dormant in T cells for two to 20 years, hidden from the immune system. When the cells are stimulated, however, the viral genes that have been incorporated into the DNA of the T4 cells can be replicated and the gene products assembled into new virus particles that then break free of the T4 cells and attack other cells. Once a T4 cell has been infected, it cannot respond adequately and may reproduce to form as few as 10 cells. An uninfected T4 cell usually reproduces 1,000 or more times to form the army needed to fight the HIV invader. When these crippled T4 cells do encounter the invader, the virus inside them reproduces and the cells are destroyed. To make the situation even worse, HIV reproduces itself at a rate far greater than any other known virus. The T4 cells

FIGURE 1.4

HIV replication cycle

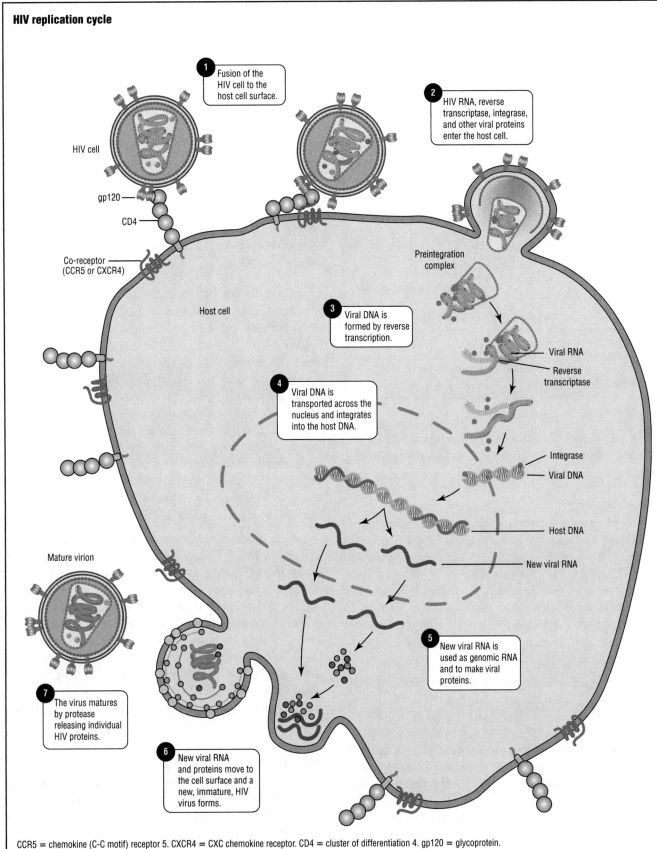

CCR5 = chemokine (C-C motif) receptor 5. CXCR4 = CXC chemokine receptor. CD4 = cluster of differentiation 4. gp120 = glycoprotein.

SOURCE: "HIV Replication Cycle," in *Biology of HIV*, National Institute of Allergy and Infectious Diseases, May 12, 2009, http://www3.niaid.nih.gov/topics/HIVAIDS/Understanding/Biology/hivReplicationCycle.htm (accessed June 11, 2009)

FIGURE 1.5

Cell-to-cell spread of HIV through the CD4-mediated fusion of an infected cell with an uninfected cell

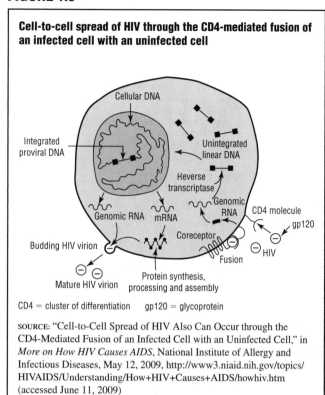

CD4 = cluster of differentiation   gp120 = glycoprotein

SOURCE: "Cell-to-Cell Spread of HIV Also Can Occur through the CD4-Mediated Fusion of an Infected Cell with an Uninfected Cell," in *More on How HIV Causes AIDS*, National Institute of Allergy and Infectious Diseases, May 12, 2009, http://www3.niaid.nih.gov/topics/HIVAIDS/Understanding/How+HIV+Causes+AIDS/howhiv.htm (accessed June 11, 2009)

essentially become factories for the invading enemy soldiers, ultimately producing them in overwhelming numbers.

The Attack

The immune system is unable to produce sufficient antibodies to fight off the complex HIV. The battle between HIV and the immune system begins when the virus slips into the bloodstream via a CD4 receptor enzyme on a T4 cell, to which it preferentially attaches itself. A CD4 receptor alone, however, is not enough to cause infection, and for years scientists searched for some other protein on the cell surface that HIV can exploit to gain entry.

This protein was discovered in May 1996 by a team of scientists at the National Institute of Allergy and Infectious Diseases (NIAID). The scientists named the protein fusin because it helps the virus fuse with a healthy cell membrane and inject genetic material into the cell. The CD4-containing cell signals to killer T cells that it is infected by displaying fragments of HIV proteins on its surface. This triggers the killer cells to spring into action, which multiply and seek out the infected CD4-containing cells to pierce them open and destroy them.

CONFIRMING A HIDING PLACE

Typically, an HIV infection begins with a sudden, flulike illness. Shortly after this first episode, the virus

virtually disappears and symptoms may not materialize for as long as 20 years. Over time, the immune system eventually collapses and the virus appears in ever-increasing amounts of CD4-containing cells floating free in the patient's blood. Even though previous studies focused on the presence of the virus in the blood, two independently conducted studies in 1993—Anthony S. Fauci et al.'s "Multifactorial Nature of Human Immuno-deficiency Virus Disease: Implications for Therapy" (*Science*, vol. 262, no. 5136, November 12, 1993) and Janet Embretson et al.'s "Massive Covert Infection of Helper T Lymphocytes and Macrophages by HIV during the Incubation Period of AIDS" (*Nature*, vol. 362, no. 6418, March 25, 1993)—confirmed suspicions long held by scientists that HIV hides in a patient's lymph nodes and similar tissue during the quiescent (first or early) stage of infection.

Searching for an Active Virus

Research by Fauci et al. focused on the search for the virus in the blood and lymphoid tissue (the lymph nodes, spleen, tonsils, and adenoids) of 12 HIV-infected patients whose infections had progressed to varying severities. Initially, the virus is concentrated almost entirely in the lymphoid tissues. Fauci et al. believe the virus infiltrates the lymph nodes within weeks of the initial infection. Particles of the virus, which are coated with antibodies, adhere to the follicular dendritic cells, a group of filtering cells that trap foreign material. CD4-containing cells nearby "see" the trapped material and are stimulated to attack the invaders. The stronger virus counterattacks and reproduces itself on some of these CD4-containing cells.

After this infiltration, the performance of the immune system declines. This decline, which ultimately is dramatically debilitating, occurs over an extended period—up to 20 years in some AIDS sufferers. During this decline the follicular dendritic cells also begin to deteriorate, and the quantity of HIV in the CD4-containing cells floating free in the blood increases significantly. In the final stage of the disease, there is an almost complete dissolution of the follicular dendritic cell network. At this point the amount of HIV in the blood and in the CD4-containing cells has grown to equal the amount in the lymph nodes.

NOT JUST THE IMMUNE SYSTEM

For some time scientists and researchers believed HIV attacked and affected only the immune system. Many early AIDS cases that provided evidence of the involvement of other regions of the body were not counted due to the narrower definitions of AIDS that existed before 1993. However, after 1993 clear evidence showed that the free virus (not attached to any other cells) could appear in the fluid surrounding the brain and the spinal cord and in the bloodstream. HIV can be found not only in T4 lymphocytes but also in other immune system cells, as well as in cells in the nervous system, intestine, and bone marrow.

CDC researchers proposed another reason HIV infections are so difficult to eliminate and why the immune system appears to be so susceptible to them. Their research shows that HIV can infect and grow in immature bone marrow cells, offering no clues about what the mature HIV-infected cells will become. The virus reproduces without revealing itself to the immune system, which under normal circumstances would destroy it. By developing in immature bone marrow cells, a great quantity of virus can be produced before the body ever attempts to resist it.

As they mature, the cells change, becoming infected monocytes and macrophages that may not only fail to fight infections but may also spread the virus to other immune system cells. Infected marrow cells may seed the virus into other parts of the body, including the brain. The infected cells that develop in the marrow are carried through the bloodstream to the rest of the body.

SEARCHING FOR ANSWERS

Researchers have long been puzzled by the fact that AIDS is virtually always fatal, even though relatively small amounts of the virus are found in patients, compared with other lethal viral infections. How the virus acts to kill the cells has been hotly debated. Certainly, this behavior is inconsistent with other retroviruses, which do not kill all the infected host cells. Even though HIV is considered a slow virus (a virus that exerts its effect over a long period), some AIDS activity occurs more quickly and may be associated with the coincidental presence of infectious mycoplasma (bacteria that lack a cell wall).

Restoring Immune Response

In December 1993 the NCI reported that the immune function had been restored to HIV-infected cells grown in a laboratory through the addition of interleukin-12 (IL-12). IL-12 is a member of a group of natural blood proteins called cytokines that were discovered in 1991 by scientists at the Wistar Institute and Hoffmann-La Roche Inc. Despite this promising result, the U.S. Food and Drug Administration (FDA) halted human testing of IL-12 in June 1995, after two patients died. After testing the protein on animals, researchers concluded that the problem was not in IL-12 itself, but in the timing of the doses. Consequently, human testing resumed in November 1995.

In December 1995 a new class of drugs called protease inhibitors received FDA approval. These drugs block the ability of HIV to mature and to infect new cells by suppressing the protein-degrading activity of a viral enzyme. Enzymes with this activity are classified as proteases, hence the designation of the enzyme blocker

as a protease inhibitor. If protease inhibitors can block the spread of HIV in the immune system, then AIDS will not develop. Though patients may be HIV positive the rest of their life, they may never die from an HIV infection.

Theories of HIV/AIDS Progression

Even after nearly three decades of research, there is still no consensus among HIV experts as to the pathogenesis (the origination and development) of AIDS. Despite this, there is agreement that the latent period between the establishment of an HIV infection and the appearance of the symptoms of AIDS averages from about two to 11 years. However, some people remain symptom free for as long as 20 years. Furthermore, a select group of between 5% and 10% of all HIV-infected people does not appear to develop AIDS. Called long-term nonprogressors, these individuals are believed to have genetic and immune response characteristics that slow, or may even halt, the course of disease progression. Much research interest centers on these people, because an understanding of their physiological characteristics that allow them to suppress the infection could be invaluable to the treatment of the disease in other patients.

After the HIV infection is established, the immune system regenerates cells only up to a certain point, which would explain a gradual progression to AIDS. The early regulatory functions of the immune system limit viral replication until a certain threshold is reached. When the number of different viral mutants becomes too large, the regulatory system is overwhelmed and shuts down, opening the door to opportunistic infections and eventual total decline.

When the total CD4+ T cell count falls from the normal 800 to 1,000 per cubic millimeter of blood to 200 per cubic millimeter, the rate of immune decline speeds up and the HIV-positive person becomes prone to the opportunistic infections and other illnesses that are characteristic of AIDS. In searching for an antiretroviral therapy, researchers find that rather than boosting the CD4+ T cell count, interruption of the viral replication may be the way to reverse immune deficiency in an HIV infection, though the nature of a reversing mechanism remains unknown.

SOME INCONSISTENCIES WITH CURRENT THEORIES. Most scientists agree that there are still gaps and inconsistencies in the knowledge of how HIV causes AIDS. One inconsistency concerns the infection and killing of the helper T cells. Initially, researchers thought that the main tactic of HIV was to infect and destroy the T cells. As these cells died, the numerical strength of the helper T cell force was depleted, thus causing the immune deficiency associated with AIDS patients.

Other scientists, however, consider this theory too simplistic, because so few T cells—no more than one infected cell in 500—are infected. Rather, two studies published in 2001 in the *Journal of Experimental Medicine*— Hiroshi Mohri et al.'s "Increased Turnover of T Lymphocytes in HIV-1 Infection and Its Reduction by Antiretroviral Therapy" (vol. 194, no. 9, November 5, 2001) and Joseph A. Kovacs et al.'s "Identification of Dynamically Distinct Subpopulations of T Lymphocytes That Are Differentially Affected by HIV" (vol. 194, no. 12, December 17, 2001)— support the idea that HIV does not block the production of T cells but instead accelerates the division of existing T cells. This causes the existing T cells to die off more quickly than normal.

Another inconsistency involves the observation that the rapid decline in the number of T cells comes relatively late in the infection, even though there are clear indications that the immune system has been impaired much earlier.

OPPORTUNISTIC INFECTIONS

Once HIV has destroyed the immune system, the body can no longer protect itself against bacterial, fungal, protozoal, and other viral agents that take advantage of the compromised condition and cause infections. These infections, which would not otherwise occur but for an impaired immune system, are known as opportunistic infections (OIs). In the non-AIDS community, OIs are problematic in hospitals, where ill, newborn, or elderly patients may also have less than adequately functioning immune systems. Because the patient is considered to have AIDS if at least one OI appears, OIs are also referred to as "AIDS-defining events," though OIs are not the only AIDS-defining events.

By 1997 the leading OI for Americans suffering from HIV/AIDS was *Pneumocystis carinii* pneumonia (PCP), a lung disease caused by a fungus. Before the discovery of HIV/AIDS, PCP was found almost exclusively in cancer and transplant patients with weakened immune systems. During the 1980s PCP was the AIDS-defining illness for two-thirds of people diagnosed with AIDS in the United States, and it was estimated that 75% of HIV-infected people would develop PCP during their lifetime. According to Laurence Huang et al., in "An Official ATS Workshop Summary: Recent Advances and Future Directions in Pneumocystis Pneumonia (PCP)" (*Proceedings of the American Thoracic Society*, vol. 3, no. 8, November 2006), the incidence of PCP decreased 3.4% per year from 1992 to 1995 and then declined 21.5% annually during 1996 to 1998, when powerful combinations of antiretroviral therapy were beginning to be used. Despite its decline, PCP remains the most frequently occurring serious OI among HIV-infected people.

Prescription drugs such as trimethoprim-sulfamethoxazole were found to be effective at preventing PCP during the late 1980s, and their widespread use along with the addition of antiretroviral therapy a decade later markedly reduced the cases of PCP. Nonetheless, James D. Heffelfinger et al. find in "Nonadherence to Primary Prophylaxis against *Pneumocystis jirovecii* Pneumonia" (*PLoS ONE*, vol. 4, no. 3, March 2009) that nearly one-fifth of HIV-infected people do not take the drugs prescribed to prevent PCP. The researchers identify illicit drug use and mental health issues including depression and low CD4 cell count as factors associated with nonadherence to treatment prescribed to prevent PCP.

Esophageal candidiasis, an infection of the esophagus, and extrapulmonary cryptococcosis, a systemic fungus that enters the body through the lungs and may invade any organ of the body, are also OIs frequently diagnosed in AIDS patients.

Other illnesses such as Burkitt's lymphoma, invasive cervical cancer, and primary brain lymphoma are also considered AIDS-defining events. Wasting syndrome (which is characterized by drastic weight loss and lethargy) is another illness that may be considered an AIDS-defining event. Other examples of AIDS-defining events include diagnosis of *Mycobacterium avium* complex, a serious bacterial infection that may occur in one part of the body such as the liver, bone marrow, and spleen or spread throughout the body; cytomegalovirus disease, a member of the herpesvirus group; Kaposi's sarcoma (see Figure 1.6), a once-rare cancer of the blood vessel walls that causes conspicuous purple lesions on the skin; and toxoplasmic encephalitis, an inflammation of the brain. Patients may experience more than one OI or AIDS-defining event.

In 2006 NIAID researchers identified a critical human cell surface molecule—protein xCT—as the receptor that can make cells vulnerable to infection with Kaposi's sarcoma herpesvirus (KSHV). Even though it is less common in the United States now than early in the AIDS pandemic, Kaposi's sarcoma remains the most common cancer associated with HIV infection. Figure 1.7 shows how KSHV fuses to and enters a human cell after binding to the protein xCT.

HIV and Tuberculosis

Tuberculosis (TB) is a communicable infection caused by the bacterium *Mycobacterium tuberculosis*. TB was a widespread pandemic in North America in the late 19th and early 20th centuries. Subsequently, it faded from prominence. However, TB regained a foothold in the 1990s, with the number of cases increasing in the United States. Part of this increase is the parallel increase in the occurrence of the infection in HIV-positive individuals. Indeed, HIV infection has become

FIGURE 1.6

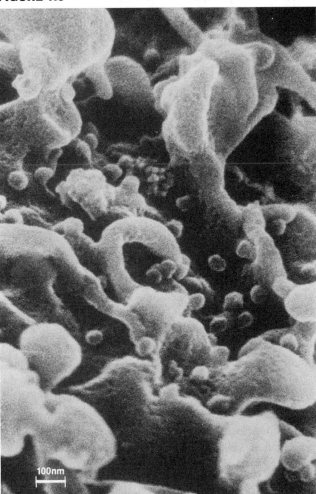

A skin biopsy of Kaposi's sarcoma. *(Centers for Disease Control and Prevention.)*

FIGURE 1.7

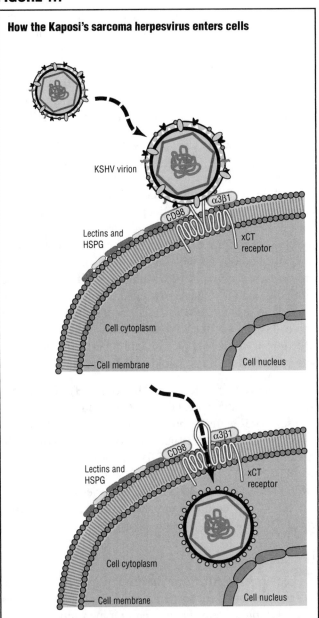

How the Kaposi's sarcoma herpesvirus enters cells

xCT = cystine/glutamic acid transporter.
HSPG = heparan sulfate proteoglycans.
KSVH = Kaposi's sarcoma-associated herpesvirus.

SOURCE: "This Illustration Shows How KSHV Fuses to and Enters a Human Cell after Binding to the Protein xCT," in *Landmark Discovery of a Kaposi's Sarcoma-Associated Herpesvirus Receptor Provides New Perspectives on Disease Associated with HIV/AIDS*, National Institute of Allergy and Infectious Disease, April 2006, http://www.nih.gov/ news/pr/apr2006/niaid-06.htm (accessed June 11, 2009)

one of the strongest known risk factors for the progression of TB from infection to disease.

A landmark report from the 1996 Conference on Retroviruses and Opportunistic Infections—Andrew D. Badley et al.'s "Enhanced Fas/Fas Ligand Dependent Activation Induced Apoptosis in CD4 Lymphocytes from HIV Seropositive Patients" (January 28–February 1, 1996)—first concluded that the decline in CD4+ T cells is greater in HIV-infected patients who develop TB than in those who remain free of TB. In some geographic areas up to 58% of those diagnosed with TB were also HIV positive. Of the many diseases associated with HIV infection, TB is one of the few that is transmissible (capable of being transmitted), treatable, and preventable.

TB is spread from person to person through the inhalation of airborne particles containing *M. tuberculosis*. The particles, called droplet nuclei, are produced when a person with infectious TB of the lung or larynx forcefully exhales, such as when coughing, sneezing,

speaking, or singing. These infectious particles remain suspended in the air and may be inhaled by someone sharing the same air. The risk of transmission is increased when ventilation is poor and when susceptible people share air for prolonged periods with a person who has untreated pulmonary TB.

Approximately 85% of TB infections occur in the lungs. This infection is called pulmonary TB. However,

TB may occur at any site of the body, such as the larynx, the lymph nodes, the brain, the kidneys, or the bones. These cases are called extrapulmonary TB. Except for laryngeal TB, people with extrapulmonary TB are usually not considered infectious to others. It is important to note that, as mentioned earlier, HIV is a bloodborne infection and cannot be spread through air. An HIV-positive person who has TB can spread TB nuclei through the air, but not HIV.

According to the CDC, in "Tuberculosis (TB)" (June 1, 2009, http://www.cdc.gov/tb/statistics/default.htm), the number of TB cases in the United States declined by 3.3% from 2006 to 2007; however, TB remains one of the leading causes of death of people who are HIV infected. This is because people who are not HIV infected can usually successfully defend themselves against TB infection. The risk that TB will develop in people infected only with *M. tuberculosis* is 10% within their lifetime. People with HIV, who may have weakened immune systems, are less able to resist infection and are more likely to develop active TB. HIV-infected people with either latent TB infection or active TB disease can be effectively treated with prescription drugs that kill the bacteria.

Extensively drug-resistant TB (XDR-TB), which does not respond to the conventional drugs used to combat the disease, poses a new threat to public health initiatives aimed at reducing the numbers of TB infections. In "Extensively Drug-Resistant Tuberculosis: New Strains, New Challenges" (*Expert Review of Anti-infective Therapy*, vol. 6, no. 5, October 2008), Ritu Banerjee et al. observe that high HIV coinfection rates in many parts of the world have contributed to the emergence of XDR-TB.

HIV and Cancer

People with AIDS are susceptible to cancer. Some malignant tumors, such as Kaposi's sarcoma and cancers of the lymph system, have been common among AIDS patients since the disease was first discovered in 1981. More recently, however, physicians and researchers have found that certain forms of cancer are more prevalent among HIV/AIDS patients who are living longer.

Most AIDS-related cancers are believed to be caused by viruses. These cancers are more common among HIV-infected people because HIV suppresses the immune system, enabling cancer-causing viruses to attack more successfully. These cancers include non-Hodgkin's lymphoma (found in lymph tissues) and primary lymphoma of the brain. People infected with HIV are also at greater risk of oral, lung, anal, liver, and skin cancers as well as myeloma (malignant tumors of the bone marrow), brain tumors, testicular cancers, and leukemia (cancer of the blood cells).

Because anti-HIV-combination drug therapies, such as highly active antiretroviral therapy (HAART), have become widely used, researchers report a decline in Kaposi's sarcoma and primary lymphoma of the brain. One possible explanation for the decline may be that the combination drug therapies enable the body to recover partial immunity, which in turn helps prevent the development of cancer.

Lung cancer is the third most commonly diagnosed cancer among people with HIV, after non-Hodgkin's lymphoma and Kaposi's sarcoma. Until recently it was assumed that the high rate of lung cancer in HIV-infected people was solely attributable to smoking, but recent research questions this assumption. In "HIV Infection Is Associated with an Increased Risk of Lung Cancer, Independent of Smoking" (*Clinical Infectious Diseases*, vol. 45, no. 1, July 1, 2007), Gregory D. Kirk et al. examine the relationship between HIV infection and lung cancer death, and smoking. They find strong evidence that HIV infection contributes to lung cancer, independent of smoking, and conclude that HIV infection alone increases the risk of developing lung cancer. They also find that HIV increased the lung cancer risk among smokers. Even though it is not known how HIV influences the development of lung cancer, Kirk et al. speculate that it might be directly involved in promoting the development of cancer or might increase susceptibility by compromising immune function. HIV might also increase susceptibility to the cancer-causing effects of tobacco.

Other researchers also report an association between HIV and lung cancer, independent of smoking. In "Smoke and Mirrors: HIV-Related Lung Cancer" (*Current Opinions in Oncology*, vol. 20, no. 5, September 2008), Alexandra Bazoes, Mark Bower, and Thomas Powles speculate that lung cancer in HIV-positive patients is a more aggressive and extensive disease.

TOWARD A VACCINE: THE HOPE AND THE REALITIES

The different routes of attack of HIV on the immune system and the ability of the virus to mutate has prompted the suggestion by some researchers that the development of an effective vaccine will be difficult to achieve. This admission is contrary to what Margaret M. Heckler (1931–), the secretary of the Department of Health and Human Services under President Ronald Reagan (1911–2004), announced in 1984, that the identification of HIV would lead to a vaccine within two years.

The intervening years have made many AIDS researchers believe that the chances of developing a vaccine that will prevent AIDS (confer immunity on the person receiving the vaccine) are remote. Testing the effectiveness of an AIDS vaccine is also difficult, because the deliberate contamination of people with HIV is both unethical and illegal. For example, recent studies, including one conducted in Thailand in 2009, overcome ethical concerns by offering vaccine trials in regions such as Thailand provinces that have some of the highest prevalence rates of HIV infection. Though some of the study's participants are given placebos rather than the vaccine being studied, those conducting the study advise all their subjects to practice safe sex and supply condoms to help prevent infection. As a result of ethical concerns, though, the focus of research has generally shifted to vaccines that do not prevent infections but lessen their effects and delay the progress of the disease.

According to Margaret I. Johnston and Anthony S. Fauci, in "An HIV Vaccine—Evolving Concepts" (*New England Journal of Medicine*, vol. 356, no. 20, May 17, 2007), such vaccine efforts continue. The huge genetic diversity and other unique features of the HIV envelope protein have frustrated attempts to identify an effective vaccine of the traditional type—one that imitates the effects of natural exposure and confers a high level of long-lasting protection against infection in the vast majority of recipients. As a result, much research focuses on harnessing T cells to stimulate cellular immunity to HIV. Research demonstrates the importance of cellular immunity in the early and later stages of HIV infection, and even though T cell vaccines have not completely eliminated the virus, they can produce cellular immune responses that may act to reduce virus levels or help people remain disease free for longer periods of time following infection. In animal studies, T cell vaccines decreased the amount of virus produced during early infection, prompted a reduction in virus levels after the acute stage of infection, delayed disease progression, or generated a combination of these beneficial effects. Figure 1.8 shows the steps involved in developing an HIV vaccine and the path to human clinical trials for vaccine candidates.

In "Challenges in the Development of an HIV-1 Vaccine" (*Nature*, vol. 455, no. 7213, October 2, 2008), Dan H. Barouch of the Harvard Medical School observes that despite advances in understanding HIV-1 and immunology, there are major scientific obstacles preventing the development of an effective vaccine. Vaccine candidates aimed at eliciting bloodborne and cellular immune responses have so far failed to protect against HIV infection or to reduce viral loads after infection in clinical studies.

In November 2008 the eagerly awaited results of the Step study—a landmark clinical trial of a Merck & Co. HIV vaccine candidate, known as a "test of concept" efficacy trial because it allows researchers to determine whether a vaccine can prevent HIV infection, lower HIV levels in people who become infected after vaccination, or both—were published in the *Lancet*: Susan P. Buchbinder et al.'s "Efficacy Assessment of a Cell-Mediated Immunity HIV-1 Vaccine (the Step Study): A Double-Blind, Randomised, Placebo-Controlled, Test-of-Concept Trial" and M. Juliana McElrath et al.'s "HIV-1 Vaccine-Induced Immunity in the Test-of-Concept Step Study: A Case-Cohort Analysis" (vol. 372, no. 9653, November 29, 2008). The study results were disappointing: they revealed that the vaccine did not prevent infection in those not previously infected with HIV, nor did the vaccine reduce the amount of virus in study participants who became infected with HIV through exposure from an infected person while in the trial.

Despite this setback, clinical trials of HIV vaccines continue. In "Clinical Trials" (September 16, 2009, http://www.aidsinfo.nih.gov/clinicaltrials), AIDSinfo, a service of the U.S. Department of Health and Human Services, notes that at least 15 trials were planned or under way in 2009.

FIGURE 1.8

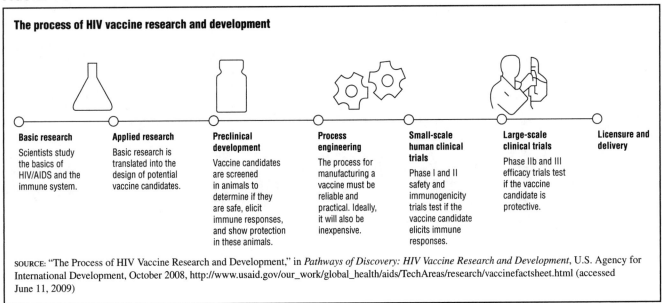

The process of HIV vaccine research and development

Basic research
Scientists study the basics of HIV/AIDS and the immune system.

Applied research
Basic research is translated into the design of potential vaccine candidates.

Preclinical development
Vaccine candidates are screened in animals to determine if they are safe, elicit immune responses, and show protection in these animals.

Process engineering
The process for manufacturing a vaccine must be reliable and practical. Ideally, it will also be inexpensive.

Small-scale human clinical trials
Phase I and II safety and immunogenicity trials test if the vaccine candidate elicits immune responses.

Large-scale clinical trials
Phase IIb and III efficacy trials test if the vaccine candidate is protective.

Licensure and delivery

SOURCE: "The Process of HIV Vaccine Research and Development," in *Pathways of Discovery: HIV Vaccine Research and Development*, U.S. Agency for International Development, October 2008, http://www.usaid.gov/our_work/global_health/aids/TechAreas/research/vaccinefactsheet.html (accessed June 11, 2009)

HAART Treatment Is Effective but Adherence May Be Difficult

In the mid-1990s a "hit-hard-early" strategy gained favor. In this strategy a cocktail of anti-HIV drugs was given to patients soon after diagnosis of the presence of the virus. The idea of HAART is to suppress the reproduction of the virus as much as possible. Some of the drugs target the virus's reverse transcriptase. By inhibiting the enzyme's activity, the ability of HIV to reproduce is thwarted. However, HAART has a downside. Even though it is able to suppress the viral load, it is unable to eradicate it, and once HAART is initiated, treatment must be continued over a lifetime. The therapy is expensive and hard to maintain, and its long-term use is associated with a number of serious side effects. If patients do not adhere to the treatment, then they may not adequately suppress the virus.

Historically, HAART treatment was initiated when CD4 cell counts fell below 350 cells per cubic millimeter and in many countries with limited resources, treatment was deferred until CD4 counts dropped below 200 cells per cubic millimeter. Emma Hitt reports in "Starting HAART at Higher T-Cell Counts Improves Survival in Early-Stage HIV" (*Medscape Medical News*, June 10, 2009) that early HAART treatment, when CD4 cell counts are between 200 and 350 cells per cubic millimeter, improves survival. Early treatment may also improve tolerability of antiviral drugs and reduce HIV transmission to other uninfected people.

CHAPTER 2
DEFINITION, SYMPTOMS, AND TRANSMITTAL

A DEFINITION OF AIDS

The Centers for Disease Control and Prevention (CDC) is the federal government's clearinghouse, research center, and monitoring agency for all infectious diseases, including HIV/AIDS. The CDC tracks the diseases in the United States and notifies health officials of their occurrence via *Morbidity and Mortality Weekly Report* notices and a Web site that is updated frequently.

The CDC defines AIDS as a specific group of diseases or conditions that are indicative of severe immunosuppression related to infection with HIV. The health agency first outlined a surveillance (a constant observation of a process) case definition in 1982, then revised it in 1983, 1985, 1987, 1993, and again in 2000 as knowledge about HIV infection increased and additional severe and common symptoms were included in the definitions. The 1993 definition emphasized the clinical importance of the CD4+ T cell count and included the addition of three clinical conditions.

THE 1993 CLASSIFICATION REVISION AND EXPANDED SURVEILLANCE CASE DEFINITION

In 1991 the CDC released a draft of the document that eventually became the "1993 Revised Classification System for HIV Infection and Expanded Surveillance Case Definition for AIDS among Adolescents and Adults" (*Morbidity and Mortality Weekly Report*, vol. 41, RR-17, December 18, 1992), by Kenneth G. Castro et al. of the CDC. This classification scheme was not revised in the intervening years and was the standard as of September 2009.

The revision addressed the concerns of many women, their attorneys, and physicians, who had strongly advocated the inclusion of diseases such as pelvic inflammatory disease (inflammation of the female reproductive organs by microorganisms) and vaginal candidiasis (a fungal infection, commonly termed a yeast infection

or thrush) as conditions that could precede the development of AIDS, so that women infected with HIV would be included in the revised definition. Advocates cautioned that if the CDC omitted such inclusive criteria, many women would be denied access to disability benefits, necessary treatment, and education.

Reasons for Expanding the Case Definition

The CDC reported three reasons for expanding the AIDS surveillance case definitions:

1. **To be consistent with standards of medical care for HIV-infected people**. The addition of a measurement for severe immunosuppression—a CD4+ T lymphocyte count of 200 per cubic millimeter or less than 14% of total lymphocytes—is consistent with the standard used to determine clinical and therapeutic treatment of HIV-infected people. (It is important to note that a person can be HIV infected and not have AIDS.) Some clinicians recommend a conservative approach, that all people with a count of 500 CD4+ T cells per cubic millimeter or less be given antiretroviral therapy. Others advocate more aggressive treatment and begin antiretroviral therapy as soon as the diagnosis of HIV infection is made. Prophylaxis (prevention treatment) against *Pneumocystis carinii* pneumonia (PCP), the most common serious opportunistic infection (OI), should be started on patients with a count of 200 CD4+ T cells per cubic millimeter or less.

2. **To include people with conditions of major public health importance in the HIV epidemic**. The inclusion of HIV-infected people with low CD4+ T cell counts allows the HIV/AIDS surveillance to reflect more accurately the number of people who have severe immunosuppression. These people are in the greatest need of close medical follow-up and are at the greatest risk for many or all the severe

HIV-related illnesses. The addition of three clinical conditions—pulmonary tuberculosis (TB), recurrent pneumonia, and invasive cervical cancer—to the 23 already accepted conditions of AIDS surveillance criteria indicates the documented or potential importance of these diseases in the HIV epidemic. The prognoses for both pulmonary TB and cervical cancer are improved with appropriate screening tests and proper follow-up. The third condition, recurrent pneumonia, was included to show the importance of pulmonary infections in the causes of HIV-related diseases and deaths.

3. **To simplify the AIDS case-reporting process**. The CDC tried to simplify the AIDS case-reporting process by allowing clinicians to report HIV-infected people on the basis of CD4+ T cell counts. Limited staff at outpatient clinics and the increasing proportion of AIDS cases necessitated the use of a simplified AIDS surveillance case definition.

New Definition and Classification—Tied to CD4+ Cells

One of the major obstacles in defining AIDS has been that it is not a single disease but several diseases making up a syndrome (a syndrome is a group or pattern of symptoms or abnormalities that are indicative of a certain disease). Newer preventive treatments delay the onset of many diseases such as PCP, which in the past helped define AIDS. To obtain a more realistic picture of the number of AIDS cases, the new classification system emphasized the importance of the CD4+ or helper T cell count.

Based on this, the 1993 definition included all HIV-infected people with a CD4+ T cell count of less than 200 per cubic millimeter or whose CD4+ T cell count was less than 14% of total lymphocytes. Essentially, most people with low T4 counts would be defined as having AIDS. As shown in Table 2.1, the 1993 classification system was based on three ranges of CD4+ T cell counts (1, 2, and 3) and three clinical categories (A, B, and C), with nine combinations being possible (A1, A2, A3, B1, B2, B3, C1, C2, and C3). People with AIDS-indicator conditions (category C) or those with CD4+ T cell counts of less than 200 per cubic millimeter meet the immunologic criteria for the AIDS surveillance case definition.

Table 2.2 gives a more detailed description of categories A and B, as well as the clinical conditions listed in category C. Note that for classification purposes, once a category C (AIDS indicator) condition occurs, the person remains in category C.

The Impact of the 1993 Definition on Case Reporting

CDC data indicate that expansion of the AIDS surveillance criteria changed both the process of AIDS surveillance and the number of reported cases. In "Current Trends

TABLE 2.1

Classification system for HIV infection and expanded surveillance case definition for AIDS among adolescents and adults

CD4+ T-cell categories	Clinical categories		
	(A) Asymptomatic, acute (primary) HIV or PGL*	(B) Symptomatic, not (A) or (C) conditions	(C) AIDS-indicator conditions
(1) ≥500/μL	A1	B1	C1
(2) 200–499/μL	A2	B2	C2
(3) <200/μL AIDS-indicator T-cell count2	A3	B3	C3

*PGL = persistent generalized lymphadenopathy. Clinical category A includes acute (primary) HIV infection.
Note: The shaded cells illustrate the expanded AIDS surveillance case definition. Persons with AIDS-indicator conditions (category C) as well as those with CD4+ T-lymphocyte counts <200/μL (categories A3 or B3) will be reportable as AIDS cases in the United States and territories, effective January 1, 1993.

SOURCE: Adapted from Kenneth G. Castro et al., "1993 Revised Classification System for HIV Infection and Expanded Surveillance Case Definition for AIDS among Adolescents and Adults," *Morbidity and Mortality Weekly Report*, vol. 41, no. RR-17, December 18, 1992, http://www.cdc.gov/mmwr/preview/mmwrhtml/00018871.htm (accessed June 18, 2009)

Update: Impact of the Expanded AIDS Surveillance Case Definition for Adolescents and Adults on Case Reporting—United States, 1993" (*Morbidity and Mortality Weekly Report*, vol. 43, no. 9, March 11, 1994), the CDC reports that in 1993, 103,500 AIDS cases were reported in the United States among adults and adolescents 13 years of age and older. This number was twice the 49,016 cases reported in 1992 and likely represented a one-time effect of the 1993 expansion of the AIDS definition. The steep increase probably represented the reporting of people who were diagnosed with the newly added conditions before 1993. New reported AIDS cases declined again beginning in 1996 in response to treatments, such as highly active antiretroviral therapy (HAART), that slowed the progression from HIV infection to AIDS. Between 1998 and 1999 the decline in the incidence of AIDS began to level. (See Figure 2.1.) From 1999 to 2003 essentially no change occurred. Between 2004 and 2005 the number of reported cases decreased slightly, and in 2006 it leveled off.

THE 2000 REVISED SURVEILLANCE CASE DEFINITION

In December 1999 the CDC released a revised surveillance case definition, updating the definition for HIV infection implemented in 1993. (See Table 2.3.) Effective January 1, 2000, the revision integrated the reporting for adult and pediatric HIV infection and AIDS into a single-case definition. The new definition was based on new data obtained using the more sensitive and specific HIV diagnostic tests that were not yet available at the time of the 1993 revision of the AIDS definition. These tests detect HIV deoxyribonucleic acid or ribonucleic acid (RNA); the earlier tests only detected anti-HIV antibod-

TABLE 2.2

Clinical categories of AIDS infection

Category A

Category A consists of one or more of the conditions listed below in an adolescent or adult (≥13 years) with documented HIV infection. Conditions listed in categories B and C must not have occurred.

- Asymptomatic HIV infection
- Persistent generalized lymphadenopathy
- Acute (primary) HIV infection with accompanying illness or history of acute HIV infection

Category B

Category B consists of symptomatic conditions in an HIV-infected adolescent or adult that are not included among conditions listed in clinical category C and that meet at least one of the following criteria: a) the conditions are attributed to HIV infection or are indicative of a defect in cell-mediated immunity; or b) the conditions are considered by physicians to have a clinical course or to require management that is complicated by HIV infection. Examples of conditions in clinical category B include, but are not limited to:

- Bacillary angiomatosis
- Candidiasis, oropharyngeal (thrush)
- Candidiasis, vulvovaginal; persistent, frequent, or poorly responsive to therapy
- Cervical dysplasia/moderate or severe cervical carcinoma in situ
- Constitutional symptoms, such as fever (38.5 C) or diarrhea lasting >1 month
- Hairy leukoplakia, oral
- Herpes zoster (shingles), involving at least two distinct episodes or more than one dermatome
- Idiopathic thrombocytopenic purpura
- Listeriosis
- Pelvic inflammatory disease, particularly if complicated by tubo-ovarian abscess
- Peripheral neuropathy

For classification purposes, category B conditions take precedence over those in category A. For example, someone previously treated for oral or persistent vaginal candidiasis (and who has not developed a category C disease) but who is now asymptomatic should be classified in clinical category B.

Category C

Category C includes the clinical conditions listed in the AIDS surveillance case definition. For classification purposes, once a category C condition has occurred, the person will remain in category C.

Conditions included in the 1993 AIDS surveillance case definition

- Candidiasis of bronchi, trachea, or lungs
- Candidiasis, esophageal
- Cervical cancer, invasive*
- Coccidioidomycosis, disseminated or extrapulmonary
- Cryptococcosis, extrapulmonary
- Cryptosporidiosis, chronic intestinal (>1 month's duration)
- Cytomegalovirus disease (other than liver, spleen, or nodes)
- Cytomegalovirus retinitis (with loss of vision)
- Encephalopathy, HIV-related
- Herpes simplex: chronic ulcer(s) (>1 month's duration); or bronchitis, pneumonitis, or esophagitis
- Histoplasmosis, disseminated or extrapulmonary
- Isosporiasis, chronic intestinal (>1 month's duration)
- Kaposi's sarcoma
- Lymphoma, Burkitt's (or equivalent term)
- Lymphoma, immunoblastic (or equivalent term)
- Lymphoma, primary, of brain
- *Mycobacterium avium* complex *or M. kansasii,* disseminated or extrapulmonary
- *Mycobacterium tuberculosis, any site* (pulmonary* or extrapulmonary)
- *Mycobacterium,* other species or unidentified species, disseminated or extrapulmonary
- *Pneumocystis carinii* pneumonia
- Pneumonia, recurrent*
- Progressive multifocal leukoencephalopathy
- *Salmonella* septicemia, recurrent
- Toxoplasmosis of brain
- Wasting syndrome due to HIV

*Added in the 1993 expansion of the AIDS surveillance case definition.

SOURCE: Kenneth G. Castro et al., "Clinical Categories," in "1993 Revised Classification System for HIV Infection and Expanded Surveillance Case Definition for AIDS among Adolescents and Adults," *Morbidity and Mortality Weekly Report*, vol. 41, no. RR-17, December 18, 1992, http://www.cdc.gov/mmwr/preview/mmwrhtml/00018871.htm (accessed June 18, 2009)

ies. The newer tests allow for HIV detection in nearly all infants aged one month and older. Because newborns might not have expressed anti-HIV antibodies—if their immune systems have even matured enough to be capable of antibody expression—they would be negative using an antibody-based test.

Even though reporting criteria include recommendations for diagnosing HIV infection, the primary purpose

of the original and updated case definitions for HIV and AIDS is public health surveillance as opposed to the diagnosis of individual patients.

DIAGNOSIS AND SYMPTOMS OF AIDS

Only a qualified health professional can diagnose AIDS. To evaluate a patient with a positive HIV test, the health care practitioner performs a complete physical

FIGURE 2.1

AIDS cases and deaths and persons living with AIDS, 1985–2006

[United States and dependent areas]

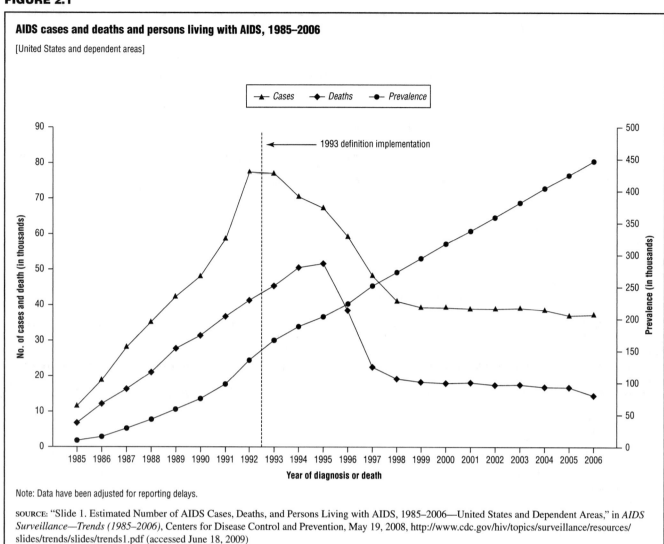

Note: Data have been adjusted for reporting delays.

SOURCE: "Slide 1. Estimated Number of AIDS Cases, Deaths, and Persons Living with AIDS, 1985–2006—United States and Dependent Areas," in *AIDS Surveillance—Trends (1985–2006)*, Centers for Disease Control and Prevention, May 19, 2008, http://www.cdc.gov/hiv/topics/surveillance/resources/ slides/trends/slides/trends1.pdf (accessed June 18, 2009)

examination and collects the patient's social and family history. Diagnostic laboratory tests are also performed. These tests typically include complete blood count and routine chemistry; CD4+ T cell count; assays (analyses) that measure the amount of HIV-1 RNA in plasma; tuberculin skin tests to detect the presence of the bacterium that causes tuberculosis; and assays for the microbial agents that cause syphilis, toxoplasmosis, and hepatitis B and C. Female patients are screened for cervical cancer using the *Papanicolaou* smear.

HIV infection progresses through a range of stages. Following the establishment of the infection (primary infection), there follows a typically prolonged asymptomatic (symptom free) period before the appearance of symptoms and the deterioration of the patient's health. Among the symptoms that develop are weight loss; profound, unexplained fatigue; nausea; fever; night sweats; swollen lymph glands; a heavy, persistent, dry cough; easy bruising or unexplained bleeding; watery diarrhea; loss of

memory; balance problems; mood changes; blurring or loss of vision; and oral lesions, such as thrush (a fungal infection caused by *Candida albicans*, which appears as a white coating on the tongue and throat). The infecting virus is basically the same in all infected people in terms of its structure and genetic makeup, but individual reactions to the virus vary greatly. Death is usually the result of the OIs and cancers that arise due to the impaired immune system—not HIV.

Dementia

Before the 1987 case definition many researchers were reluctant to include dementia as a symptom indicative of AIDS. Lawrence K. Altman notes in "New Study Is Easing Fears on AIDS and Mental Illness" (*New York Times*, June 3, 1989) that some observers cited early studies that showed as many as 40% to 70% of people infected with the virus developed neurological and psychological complications several years before other clinical symptoms, such as weight loss and fever, appeared.

TABLE 2.3

Revised surveillance case definition for HIV infection[a]

This revised definition of HIV infection, which applies to any HIV (e.g., HIV-1 or HIV-2), is intended for public health surveillance only. It incorporates the reporting criteria for HIV infection and AIDS into a single case definition. The revised criteria for HIV infection update the definition of HIV infection implemented in 1993; the revised HIV criteria apply to AIDS-defining conditions for adults and children, which require laboratory evidence of HIV. This definition is **not** presented as a guide to clinical diagnosis or for other uses.

I. In adults, adolescents, or children aged ≥18 months[b], a reportable case of HIV infection must meet at least one of the following criteria:
  Laboratory criteria

  Positive result on a screening test for HIV antibody (e.g., repeatedly reactive enzyme immunoassay), followed by a positive result on a confirmatory (sensitive and more specific) test for HIV antibody (e.g., Western blot or immunofluorescence antibody test)

  or

  Positive result or report of a detectable quantity on any of the following HIV virologic (nonantibody) tests:
  -HIV nucleic acid (DNA or RNA) detection (e.g., DNA polymerase chain reaction [PCR] or plasma HIV-1 RNA)[c]
  -HIV p24 antigen test, including neutralization assay
  -HIV isolation (viral culture)

  OR

  Clinical or other criteria (if the above laboratory criteria are not met)

  Diagnosis of HIV infection, based on the laboratory criteria above, that is documented in a medical record by a physician

  or

  Conditions that meet criteria included in the case definition for AIDS

II. In a child aged <18 months, a reportable case of HIV infection must meet at least one of the following criteria:
  Laboratory criteria

  Definitive
  Positive results on two separate specimens (excluding cord blood) using one or more of the following HIV virologic (nonantibody) tests:

  -HIV nucleic acid (DNA or RNA) detection
  -HIV p24 antigen test, including neutralization assay, in a child ≥1 month of age
  -HIV isolation (viral culture)

  or

  Presumptive
  A child who does not meet the criteria for definitive HIV infection but who has:
  Positive results on only one specimen (excluding cord blood) using the above HIV virologic tests and no subsequent negative HIV virologic or negative HIV antibody tests

  OR

  Clinical or other criteria (if the above definitive or presumptive laboratory criteria are not met)
  Diagnosis of HIV infection, based on the laboratory criteria above, that is documented in a medical record by a physician

  or

  Conditions that meet criteria included in the 1987 pediatric surveillance case definition for AIDS

This fear led the military and civilian authorities to bar infected people from certain jobs involving public safety, including commercial pilots and bus drivers.

Altman reports that officials at the World Health Organization (WHO) and the National Institutes of Health (NIH) jointly found these estimates to be false. They reported that even though neurological complications are common in the later stages of AIDS, dementia is rarely diagnosed in asymptomatic HIV-infected people, affecting fewer than 1% of those infected with HIV who have not yet developed AIDS.

A number of research studies were initiated in the 1990s to determine conclusively if there was any link between dementia and the subsequent diagnosis of AIDS. The data from studies conducted by the U.S. Air Force; a joint effort by the CDC and the San Francisco Health Department; and the Multicenter AIDS Cohort Study of men who have sex with other men in Baltimore, Maryland, Chicago, Illinois, Los Angeles, California, and Pittsburgh, Pennsylvania (sponsored by the National Institute of Allergy and Infectious Diseases and the National Cancer Institute)

confirmed that the 40% to 70% frequency rate of dementia for HIV-infected people was far higher than the actual rate. One explanation for the higher figures reported in the 1980s is that the data came from centers to which AIDS patients with dementia had been referred for treatment. Put another way, the sample population was skewed toward the increased prevalence of dementia.

HIV-associated dementia (also called AIDS dementia complex) is now recognized as a declining cognitive (thinking) function that generally occurs in the late stages of HIV infection. The dementia is caused directly by HIV infection of the central nervous system, which includes the brain, and is different from the forgetfulness and difficulty in concentrating that can be the by-products of depression and fatigue. Christopher Power et al. estimate in "NeuroAIDS: An Evolving Epidemic" (*Canadian Journal of Neurological Sciences*, vol. 36, no. 3, May 2009) that more than 50% of people infected with HIV will develop a neurological disorder, such as dementia, despite the availability of HAART.

III. A child aged <18 months born to an HIV-infected mother will be categorized for surveillance purposes as "not infected with HIV" if the child does not meet the criteria for HIV infection but meets the following criteria:

Laboratory criteria

Definitive

At least two negative HIV antibody tests from separate specimens obtained at ≥6 months of age

or

At least two negative HIV virologic tests[d] from separate specimens, both of which were performed at ≥1 month of age and one of which was performed at ≥4 months of age

AND

No other laboratory or clinical evidence of HIV infection (i.e., has not had any positive virologic tests, if performed, and has not had an AIDS-defining condition)

or

Presumptive

A child who does not meet the above criteria for definitive "not infected" status but who has:

One negative EIA HIV antibody test performed at ≥6 months of age and NO positive HIV virologic tests, if performed

or

One negative HIV virologic test[d] performed at ≥4 months of age and NO positive HIV virologic tests, if performed

or

One positive HIV virologic test with at least two subsequent negative virologic tests[d], at least one of which is at ≥4 months of age; or negative HIV antibody test results, at least one of which is at ≥6 months of age

AND

No other laboratory or clinical evidence of HIV infection (i.e., has not had any positive virologic tests, if performed, and has not had an AIDS-defining condition).

OR

Clinical or other criteria (if the above definitive or presumptive laboratory criteria are not met)

Determined by a physician to be "not infected" and a physician has noted the results of the preceding HIV diagnostic tests in the medical record

AND

NO other laboratory or clinical evidence of HIV infection (i.e., has not had any positive virologic tests, if performed, and has not had an AIDS-defining condition)

IV. A child aged <18 months born to an HIV-infected mother will be categorized as having perinatal exposure to HIV infection if the child does not meet the criteria for HIV infection (II) or the criteria for "not infected with HIV" (III).

[a]Draft revised surveillance criteria for HIV infection were approved and recommended by the membership of the Council of State and Territorial Epidemiologists (CSTE) at the 1998 annual meeting. Draft versions of these criteria were previously reviewed by state HIV/AIDS surveillance staffs, CDC, CSTE, and laboratory experts. In addition, the pediatric criteria were reviewed by an expert panel of consultants. [External Pediatric Consultants: C. Hanson, M. Kaiser, S. Paul, G. Scott, and P. Thomas. CDC staff: J. Bertolli, K. Dominguez, M. Kalish, M.L. Lindegren, M. Rogers, C. Schable, R.J. Simonds, and J. Ward]

[b]Children aged ≥18 months but <13 years are categorized as "not infected with HIV" if they meet the criteria in III.

[c]In adults, adolescents, and children infected by other than perinatal exposure, plasma viral RNA nucleic acid tests should **NOT** be used in lieu of licensed HIV screening tests (e.g., repeatedly reactive enzyme immunoassay). In addition, a negative (i.e., undetectable) plasma HIV-1 RNA test result does not rule out the diagnosis of HIV infection.

[d]HIV nucleic acid (DNA or RNA) detection tests are the virologic methods of choice to exclude infection in children aged <18 months. Although HIV culture can be used for this purpose, it is more complex and expensive to perform and is less well standardized than nucleic acid detection tests. The use of p24 antigen testing to exclude infection in children aged <18 months is not recommended because of its lack of sensitivity.

SOURCE: Patricia L. Fleming et al., "Appendix. Revised Surveillance Case Definition for HIV Infection," in "CDC Guidelines for National Human Immunodeficiency Virus Case Surveillance, Including Monitoring for Human Immunodeficiency Virus Infection and Acquired Immunodeficiency Syndrome," *Morbidity and Mortality Weekly Report*, vol. 48, no. RR-13, December 10, 1999, http://www.cdc.gov/mmwr/preview/mmwrhtml/rr4813a1.htm (accessed June 18, 2009)

Selected Cancers

Historically, the frequent diagnosis of specific AIDS-defining cancers—non-Hodgkin's lymphoma, Kaposi's sarcoma, and cervical cancer—have been attributed to compromised immune systems, and the occurrence of other cancers was thought to result from the fact that people with HIV/AIDS were living longer because of the widespread use of HAART.

In "Incidence of Non-AIDS-Defining Malignancies in HIV-Infected versus Noninfected Patients in the HAART Era: Impact of Immunosuppression" (*Journal of Acquired Immune Deficiency Syndromes*, vol. 52, no. 2, October 2009), Roger J. Bedimo et al. discuss the results of their study, which considered 33,420 HIV-infected and 66,840 HIV-uninfected patients. They find that other cancers, called non-AIDS-defining malignancies, appear to occur more frequently among people with HIV/AIDS. People with HIV/AIDS were found to be at 60% greater risk for anal, lung, and liver cancer as well as Hodgkin's lymphoma and melanoma than people who were not HIV infected.

Even though investigators do not yet know exactly why the rates of the cancers are higher among people with HIV infection, they hypothesize that:

- HIV or another as yet undetected virus may increase the risk of developing cancer.

- HAART may increase the risk of developing cancer.

- People with HIV may have lifestyle or other environmental exposures that increase their risk for cancer, such as smoking or excessive alcohol consumption.

From HIV to AIDS

Through 2009, among people who were not treated with antiretroviral therapy, the average amount of time from initial HIV infection to the development of AIDS was about 10 years. However, medical developments such as the use of HAART have significantly increased the life expectancy of AIDS patients.

In "The Lifetime Cost of Current Human Immunodeficiency Virus Care in the United States" (*Medical Care*, vol. 44, no. 11, November 2006), Bruce R. Schackman et al. note that a 1993 estimate of life expectancy for an asymptomatic person infected with HIV was less than seven years. During the 1990s life expectancy for HIV-infected people was about 10 years. A decade later, in 2006, life expectancy after HIV diagnosis averaged 24.2 years.

According to the Antiretroviral Therapy Cohort Collaboration, in "Life Expectancy of Individuals on Combination Antiretroviral Therapy in High-Income Countries: A Collaborative Analysis of 14 Cohort Studies" (*Lancet*, vol. 372, no. 9635, July 2008), a 20-year-old HIV-positive person starting antiretroviral therapy in 2008 could expect to live to age 69. The collaboration observes that this projection represents a 37% increase in life expectancy from the late 1990s, when a 20-year-old HIV-positive person starting antiretroviral could be expected to live an additional 36 years (to age 56).

THE EARLY STAGE. Even though the timing and progression of HIV infection vary among people, the disease follows a basic pattern. In the beginning of the early stage, shortly after the virus has entered the bloodstream, the T4 cell count is normal (around 1,000 per cubic millimeter). The virus is undetectable at this stage using assays that are geared to detect the presence of anti-HIV antibodies. The antibody assays can remain negative for up to six weeks. In unusual cases antibodies may remain undetectable for a year or more. Even after testing positive for the virus, or for the presence of the antiviral antibodies, many people remain asymptomatic for years. These people may develop a disorder similar to infectious mononucleosis with fatigue, fever, swollen glands, and possibly a rash. Often, these symptoms disappear within a few weeks, and a connection with an HIV infection is not made. Throughout this time, however, the virus is multiplying and destroying healthy cells. Most people continue to feel fine, though some may have chronically swollen lymph nodes. This stage usually lasts about five years.

THE MIDDLE STAGE. By the middle stage of infection, the CD4+ T cell count is reduced by half, to around 500 per cubic millimeter. Even with this physiological change, many people may still be asymptomatic. As the infection advances, skin tests will likely show that cell-mediated immunity, a form of immunological defense, is

disintegrating. The deterioration of the immune system has begun. This stage can also last up to five years.

In the 1980s a drug called azidothymidine (AZT; now called zidovudine), which had failed to fulfill its early potential as an anticancer compound, garnered a lot of publicity when it was shown to help slow the attachment of HIV to host cells. AZT delayed the onset of symptoms and extended this middle stage of the infection. However, AZT's benefits proved to be temporary, as HIV mutated to counteract the affect of the drug. The drug is still used today in conjunction with other medicines, and some studies suggest that people who receive AZT may develop AIDS later than those who do not take it.

Newer and more promising drugs have since been developed, in particular the protease inhibitors, which prevent the virus from destructively degrading cell protein. Protease inhibitors were licensed for use by the U.S. Food and Drug Administration (FDA) in December 1995.

Structured treatment interruptions (STIs), initially proposed in the late 1990s, in which the multiple drug therapy patients receive is stopped for short periods of time, have also shown promise. However, the disastrous consequences that have resulted from patients taking self-initiated "drug holidays" underscore the importance of receiving a physician's approval before embarking on an STI program.

Considerable research indicates that STI may be associated with worse health outcomes in terms of immune function and viral load than continuous antiretroviral therapy. Nonetheless, some investigators believe there is a role for STI, especially as a short-term strategy to help patients experiencing severe side effects of treatment such as drug toxicity. Calvin J. Cohen et al. report in "Pilot Study of a Novel Short-Cycle Antiretroviral Treatment Interruption Strategy: 48-Week Results of the Five-Days-On, Two-Days-Off (FOTO) Study" (*HIV Clinical Trials*, vol. 8, no. 1, January–February 2007), a study of STI that treated 30 patients on a five-day-on antiretroviral therapy and two-day-off cycle, that after eight weeks on this schedule 90% of the patients maintained adequate suppression of the virus. In "Virologic Determinants of Success after Structured Treatment Interruptions of Antiretrovirals in Acute HIV-1 Infection" (*Journal of Acquired Immune Deficiency Syndromes*, vol. 47, no. 2, February 1, 2008), Sharon R. Lewin et al. hypothesize that the total pool of infected cells and the degree of persistent viral replication would determine the likelihood of successful control of the virus after STIs. The researchers also posit that starting antiretroviral therapy early—during primary HIV infection—might help limit viral replication during STIs.

THE LATE STAGE. The third and final stage of HIV infection is reached when the CD4+ T cell count per cubic millimeter drops to 200 or below. Though many patients are still asymptomatic at this point, the functioning of the immune system has by now been markedly weakened. The body is far less able to defend itself from invasion. As a consequence, the risk of infection due to opportunistic bacteria, viruses, fungi, and parasites and the possibility of cancer increase dramatically. To prevent PCP, one of the most common OIs, patients are usually treated with antibiotics during this stage.

At the onset of the late stage, patients may experience weight loss, diarrhea, lethargy, and recurring fever. Skin and mucous membrane infections increase. Oral fungal infections such as thrush and chronic infection caused by the herpes simplex virus are common.

As the late stage progresses, the immune system collapses. OIs move deeper into the body. It is not uncommon for a parasitic infection called toxoplasmosis to attack the brain, while the cryptococcosis fungus attacks the nervous system, liver, bones, and skin. Cytomegalovirus can cause pneumonia, encephalitis, and retinitis. The latter, an inflammation of the retina, can cause blindness. Many other infections can occur. The consequences and complications of compromised immune function are many, and death becomes a matter of time. The average survival rate, once the late stage has been reached, is two years.

THE TRANSMISSION OF HIV

When AIDS was first identified, it was often compared with the Black Death of the 14th century, in terms of the public panic surrounding the disease and its possible spread. The comparison has not proved to be valid. The bacterium that caused the Black Death (and that still causes bubonic plague) is highly contagious, largely because it is readily transmitted via food, water, and air. HIV is not nearly as contagious. Moreover, by observing precautions that prevent the sharing of bodily fluids, the transmission of HIV can be almost entirely prevented.

The accumulated knowledge of more than 25 years of research and observations have definitively established that the HIV infection can only be transmitted by the following routes:

- Oral, anal, or vaginal sex with an infected person. Sexual intercourse—particularly heterosexual sex— is the most common mode of HIV transmission worldwide.

- Sharing drug needles or syringes with an infected person.

- Maternal transmission to a baby at the time of birth and possibly through breast milk. Even though breast-feeding is a known source of HIV transmission, there is also some evidence that in some instances it may confer protection against HIV infection. Furthermore, in many developing countries where alternative

sources of nutrition are unavailable, the benefits of breastfeeding outweigh the risks. For this reason, the WHO recommends in *HIV Transmission through Breastfeeding: A Review of Available Evidence* (2008, http://whqlibdoc.who.int/publications/2008/9789241596596_eng.pdf) that HIV-infected women "breastfeed their infants exclusively for the first six months of life, unless replacement feeding is acceptable, feasible, affordable, sustainable and safe for them and their infants before that time. When those conditions are met, WHO recommends avoidance of all breastfeeding by HIV-infected women."

- Transplantation of HIV-infected organs or transfusion of infected bodily fluids, such as blood or blood products. In the mid-1980s the transfusion of HIV-infected blood caused thousands of cases of AIDS and led to many deaths in separate incidents in Europe, the United States, and Canada. The blood agencies of the affected countries have revamped their blood-testing policies so that molecular assay techniques, which detect HIV genetic material, are used to screen every donated blood sample.

Confirming the involvement of bodily fluids in HIV transmission, high concentrations of HIV have been found in blood, semen, and cerebrospinal fluid. Not all body fluids seem to be involved, because HIV concentrations 1,000 times less have been found in saliva, tears, vaginal secretions, breast milk, and feces. However, there have been no reports of HIV transmission from saliva, tears, or human bites. In fact, Altman reports in "Protein in Saliva Found to Block AIDS Virus in Test Tube Study" (*New York Times*, February 7, 1995) that a small protein found in human saliva actually blocks the virus from entering the system. Table 2.4 shows the estimated distribution of HIV/AIDS diagnoses in adolescents and adults by gender and transmission category in the United States in 2007 and the cumulative totals from the beginning of the epidemic through 2007.

Casual Contact

Even though HIV is an infectious, contagious disease, it is not spread in the same manner as a common cold or chicken pox. It is not spread by sneezing or coughing, as are airborne illnesses. HIV is not spread by sharing a bathroom, swimming in a pool, or by hugging or shaking hands. Studies of family members who lived with and cared for AIDS patients have not found definitive evidence that anyone has become infected through casual contact. Still, myths abound. To combat misinformation, the U.S. Surgeon General's office and public health education initiatives continue to stress that HIV is not spread by:

- Bites from mosquitoes or other insects.

- Bites from animals.

TABLE 2.4

AIDS cases by transmission category, 2007 and cumulative through 2007

Transmission category	Estimated # of AIDS cases, in 2007		
	Adult and adolescent male	Adult and adolescent female	Total
Male-to-male sexual contact	16,749	—	16,749
Injection drug use	3,750	2,260	6,010
Male-to-male sexual contact and injection drug use	1,664	—	1,664
High-risk heterosexual contact[a]	4,011	7,100	11,111
Other[b]	181	220	401

[a]Heterosexual contact with a person known to have, or to be at high risk for, HIV infection.
[b]Includes hemophilia, blood transfusion, perinatal exposure, and risk not reported or not identified.

Transmission category	Estimated # of AIDS cases, through 2007[a]		
	Adult and adolescent male	Adult and adolescent female	Total
Male-to-male sexual contact	487,695	—	487,695
Injection drug use	175,704	80,155	255,859
Male-to-male sexual contact and injection drug use	71,242	—	71,242
High-risk heterosexual contact[b]	63,927	112,230	176,157
Other[c]	12,108	6,158	18,266

[a]Includes persons with a diagnosis of AIDS from the beginning of the epidemic through 2007.
[b]Heterosexual contact with a person known to have, or to be at high risk for, HIV infection.
[c]Includes hemophilia, blood transfusion, perinatal exposure, and risk not reported or not identified.

SOURCE: "AIDS Cases by Transmission Category," in *Basic Statistics*, Centers for Disease Control and Prevention, Divisions of HIV/AIDS Prevention, February 26, 2009, http://www.cdc.gov/hiv/topics/surveillance/basic.htm#exposure (accessed June 20, 2009)

- Food handled, prepared, or served by HIV-infected people.

- Forks, spoons, knives, or drinking glasses used by HIV-infected people.

- Chairs previously occupied by people with HIV.

- Casual contact such as touching, hugging, or kissing a person who is HIV positive (open-mouth kissing with a person who is HIV positive is not recommended because of potential exposure to blood).

Donating Blood

Health officials agree that donating blood poses no danger of HIV infection for the donors. The needles used to draw blood from donors are new and are thrown away after one use. Therefore, contact with HIV from donating blood is impossible.

SAFETY OF BLOOD AND TRANSPLANT PROCEDURES

To safeguard the nation's transplant recipients, the CDC suggests that all donors of blood products, tissue, and organs be screened and tested. The recommendations include screening for behaviors—risk factors—associated with the acquisition of HIV infection, a physical examination for signs and symptoms related to HIV infection, and laboratory screening for antibodies to HIV. It is important to remember that the CDC does not regulate medical protocol; its main function is to offer health care guidelines and information to the nation and its health care providers.

The U.S. Blood Supply

Before HIV-antibody testing began in 1985, it is estimated that 70% of hemophiliacs (people with inherited bleeding disorders) who received blood products were given tainted blood-clotting factor (a concentrate of blood used to stem bleeding) and were therefore infected with HIV. According to Steve Sternberg, in "A Legacy of Tainted Blood" (*USA Today*, July 11, 2006), approximately 10,000 of these patients developed AIDS and 5,000 have died.

The widespread use of two blood-screening tests, both of which are also used on plasma and other blood products, has strengthened the safety of the U.S. blood and plasma supply. Since 1992 the Public Health Service, an arm of the U.S. Department of Health and Human Services, has required that all blood and plasma donations be screened for the rare HIV-2 antibody, as well as the more common HIV-1 antibody.

In 2001 the FDA approved the first nucleic acid test (NAT) system to screen plasma donors for HIV. Rather than relying on the identification of antigens or antibodies, the new test provides extremely sensitive detection of RNA from HIV-1. Even with the new test, however, there is still some risk due to the "window period," during which a person who has acquired the HIV-1 infection may still test negative. For HIV-1 antigen and antibody detection, the window period is 16 and 21 days, respectively, following infection. NAT systems reduce the window period to 12 days. Put another way, anyone who is infected with HIV and who donates blood more than 12 days after exposure to the virus will register HIV positive.

Barbee I. Whitaker et al. indicate in *The 2007 National Blood Collection and Utilization Survey Report* (October 2008, http://www.hhs.gov/ophs/bloodsafety/2007nbcus_survey.pdf) that in 2006, 16.2 million units of blood were donated in the United States. There are many measures in place to ensure the safety of the U.S. blood supply; however, the FDA admits that it is impossible to ensure zero risk of transmitting infectious disease. So even though the U.S. blood supply is considered safe, blood banks across the country nonetheless encourage individuals concerned about tainted blood to bank their own blood for possible future use.

Foreign Blood Supplies

HIV infection from contaminated blood has been much more common in other countries. In "Top French Officials Cleared over Blood with AIDS Virus" (*New York Times*, March 10, 1999), Craig R. Whitney reports that a French court ruled in 1998 that a former prime minister and two former cabinet members would be tried on charges that they allowed HIV-contaminated blood to be used for transfusions during 1984 and 1985. Relatives of the patients argued that the French government had refused U.S. technology that would have detected antibodies in the tainted blood in favor of a French procedure that was in development. Approximately 4,400 people acquired HIV as a result of this action. Many of the victims were hemophiliacs, and about 40% of the total number infected had died of AIDS. The former French officials, Prime Minister Laurent Fabius (1946–), Minister of Social Affairs Georgina Dufoix (1943–), and Minister of Health Edmond Herve (1942–), faced charges of involuntary homicide and went to trial in 1999. Herve was convicted without a penalty and Dufoix and Fabius were acquitted. The tragedy resulted in the overhaul of the blood supply and donation networks in France.

Jane Perlez notes in "Parents Sue Romania over Child's H.I.V. Infection" (*New York Times*, August 31, 1995) that the WHO reported in 1995 that 3,000 children in Romania—home to thousands of abandoned babies left in squalid institutions after the fall of the Romanian dictator Nicolae Ceausescu (1918–1989)—were infected by contaminated blood and syringes in the late 1980s. The WHO estimated that 1,000 of those children had died. According to Perlez, "Romania has more than half of the juvenile AIDS cases in Europe. More than 90 percent of the country's reported AIDS cases are among children, most of whom were infected by contaminated needles and syringes." The Romanian Health Ministry faced litigation for causing the spread of HIV.

According to the article "Another German Trial for H.I.V.-Tainted Blood" (*New York Times*, November 30, 1995), Gunter Kurt Eckert, the owner of a German drug laboratory, was charged in 1995 with nearly 6,000 counts of murder or attempted murder for selling HIV-tainted blood products to German hospitals in 1987. Nearly 90% of the 6,000 batches had not been tested for HIV. Testing has been mandatory in Germany since 1986.

The article "Canada's Tainted Blood Scandal: A Timeline" (CBC News, October 1, 2007) notes that the Canadian blood collection, testing, and distribution system was completely overhauled in the wake of the distribution of blood that was contaminated with HIV and the hepatitis C virus. It was discovered that 95% of hemophiliacs who received blood products prior to 1990 had been infected with hepatitis C. In 2001 the Canadian supreme court ruled that the negligence of the blood

agency during the early years of the AIDS crisis entitled several thousand affected Canadians to a $1.2 billion federal-provincial government compensation offer. Legal wrangling in the intervening years delayed the implementation of the court's ruling.

Canada was not the only country to endure charges that tainted blood had been distributed. The article "AIDS Scandals around the World" (BBC News, August 9, 2001) explains that China, Iran, Italy, Japan, and Portugal also acknowledged that tainted blood supplies infected people from the mid-1980s to 1990.

UNSCREENED BLOOD JEOPARDIZED U.S. SERVICEMEN According to Travis J. Tritten, in "Report: Unscreened Blood Posed Danger" (*Stars & Stripes*, April 11, 2009), "battlefield attacks that resulted in mass casualties or severe injuries often overtaxed the military's blood supply system until 2007, meaning medics collected fresh blood from those on site for emergency treatment of the wounded," which resulted in many service members receiving unscreened blood that "did not meet federal safety standards required of all other military blood supplies." Tritten notes that there have been no known cases of HIV transmission from unscreened transfusions and that even though the practice is still used when screened blood is unavailable, rapid testing for HIV and other bloodborne pathogens helps ensure the safety of transfusions conducted in the field.

Organ and Tissue Transplants

In several instances HIV has been transmitted through organ (kidney, liver, heart, lung, and pancreas) and other tissue transplants. The risk of such transmission is low simply because there are far fewer transplant cases than blood transfusions.

In 1994 the FDA began regulating the sale of bone, skin, corneas, cartilage, tendons, and similar nonblood vessel-bearing tissues used for transplants. The FDA requires that all procurement agencies conduct behavioral screening and infectious-disease (HIV-1, HIV-2, hepatitis B virus, and hepatitis C virus) testing of donors.

TESTING PEOPLE FOR HIV

A person infected with HIV produces antibodies specific to the virus as part of the body's immune response to the invader. Even though the antibodies are not enough to successfully fight HIV, they are of diagnostic value, as they can indicate the presence of the virus.

Antibody-based HIV testing is done, rather than a direct test for the virus itself, because it is too difficult to isolate the virus from the blood. Testing serves to determine if there is a viral infection in donated blood, tissues, or organs. This protects the recipients of the donated material and can be used to identify HIV-infected donors.

An antibody-based test cannot detect all HIV-positive blood. It can typically take between four and 12 weeks following HIV infection for antibodies to appear, although in rare cases this period can be up to one year. The introduction of tests that detect the viral nucleic acid rather than the HIV antibodies has markedly increased the detection sensitivity of blood screening. Still, even nucleic acid detection has a window period, albeit a shorter one, of about 12 days.

The fact that detection is not absolute from the moment of HIV infection means that the possibility exists that some HIV-infected donors may not be diagnosed and their blood may enter the nation's blood supply. However, the number of predicted contaminated blood samples is extremely small. To try to further reduce the chances of contaminated blood entering the blood supply, blood banks routinely question potential donors about high-risk behaviors. Any donor whose behavior might indicate an increased risk of HIV infection (such as injection drug use or unsafe sex) is automatically excluded from donating blood.

Diagnostic Tools for HIV Antibodies

Two tests commonly used to detect HIV antibodies are believed to be about 99% reliable. These tests are the enzyme-linked immunosorbent assay (ELISA) and the Western blot.

Introduced in 1985, ELISA is a test designed for screening rather than diagnosing. The assay uses purified HIV antigens to probe for the presence of complimentary antibodies in a sample such as blood. If anti-HIV antibodies are present in the sample, they attach themselves to the viral proteins that have been immobilized on a plastic surface. A second antibody that has been raised against the anti-HIV antibody (antibodies are proteins, too, so they can function as antigens, stimulating the formation of antibodies) is bound to the anti-HIV antibodies. The second antibody contains a chemical that can be made to change color. The color change reveals the presence of the anti-HIV antibody. If no color change appears, no anti-HIV antibody is present in the blood sample. This test is reliable, simple to conduct, and inexpensive.

The Western blot, introduced in 1987, is a confirmatory test. This means the test is commonly used to verify the results of the less-specific assays. The Western blot technique separates the various HIV proteins from one another, based on their speed of movement through a gel under the influence of electricity. The separated proteins are transferred from the gel to a membrane made of a material such as nitrocellulose. When the nitrocellulose is exposed to a blood sample, antibodies that recognize one of the proteins on the nitrocellulose will bind to the particular protein. As with ELISA, a color reaction can be induced to indicate the site of the bound antibodies.

The Western blot provides a positive, negative, or intermediate result. The presence of three or more of the color bands confirms an HIV infection. If fewer—one or two—bands appear, the test is considered intermediate and retesting is performed six months later. If no color bands appear, the test is considered negative with no HIV present, though many people who test negative also repeat the test six months later.

Urine Tests

In June 1998 the FDA approved a urine-based diagnostic kit for HIV marketed by Calypte Biomedical Corporation that does not require confirmation by a blood test. Urine tests are easier to use and cost less than blood tests for health care providers. According to the NIH, there is no evidence that HIV is spread through urine. Therefore, the chances of accidental infection through needle sticks or handling of samples are lessened. The urine test and its urine-based confirmation test, like most blood tests, recognize the existence of antibodies, not the actual virus.

The test is marketed to life insurance companies, clinical laboratories, public health agencies, the military, immigration authorities, and the criminal justice system. In the press release "Calypte Appoints Distributor for Its HIV-1 Urine Test in People's Republic of China" (Business Wire, June 12, 2000), Calypte announced its partnership with the Chinese National Center for AIDS Prevention and Control (NCAIDS) to distribute the first HIV-1 antibody urine test in the People's Republic of China. NCAIDS estimated in 2000 that the total number of HIV infections in China could rise to as high as 10 million before 2010 if proper countermeasures are not taken.

In July 2005 Calypte began marketing its products in developing countries; however, as of September 2009, Calypte rapid test products, which detect HIV-1 and HIV-2 antibodies in the blood, oral fluids, and urine, were not yet available in the United States. In 2009 Calypte (2009, http://www.calypte.com/products.asp) was developing a rapid test for professional use at its Portland, Oregon, facility. An over-the-counter version for consumers was slated to follow. In September 2007 the U.S. Agency for International Development (USAID) placed the Calypte oral test on its rapid HIV test waiver list, which, under the U.S. Acquisition and Assistance Policy Directive, permits the test to be used in USAID-funded projects. The USAID decision allows countries whose governments have approved the test to purchase it with funds from the President's Emergency Plan for AIDS Relief (this program was launched in 2003 to combat global HIV/AIDS).

Home Testing

As of 2009, the FDA had approved only one method of home testing for HIV-1, the Home Access Express

HIV-1 Test System, which is produced by the Home Access Health Corporation. The FDA warned that the more than one dozen nonapproved home HIV tests advertised could produce inaccurate results. Proponents of home testing state that it offers the advantages of privacy and ease of use. Users mail an anonymous blood sample to a laboratory and receive results seven days after the sample arrives at the laboratory, or if they choose the "express" option, results are available the same day the sample arrives at the laboratory. Critics of home testing point out that it is expensive; a kit costs as much as $65 and may be prohibitively expensive for poorer populations—for whom such a test is most needed. Critics also question the impersonal practice of relaying HIV-positive results and follow-up counseling by telephone.

A. David Paltiel and Harold A Pollack maintain in "Price, Performance, and the FDA Approval Process: The Example of Home HIV Testing" (*Medical Decision Making*, May 8, 2009) that in addition to evidence of the test's performance and its sensitivity (the ability of the test to accurately detect disease in people who have the disease) and specificity (the ability of the test to accurately identify people who do not have the disease) when administered by untrained users, the FDA should consider the population of end-users. Paltiel and Pollack assert that the performance of the home HIV test, which is measured in terms of its ability to correctly detect the presence and absence of HIV infection among the people who purchase it, depends on market factors such as its retail price. For example, their analysis suggests that a cheaper test may work better when marketed at a lower price because there is a greater chance that it will be used by people likely to be infected, rather than by the uninfected "worried well" who can afford to purchase it.

Rapid-Response Tests

According to Bernard M. Branson, in "Point-of-Care Rapid Tests for HIV Antibody" (September 12, 2006, http://www.cdc.gov/hiv/topics/testing/resources/journal _article/J_Lab_Med_20031.htm), during the mid-to late 1990s the CDC recommended the development of a new HIV test that would give results instantly. The CDC hoped that this would encourage people to learn the results of their tests. Currently, about half of the people who are tested at voluntary counseling and testing clinics and at perinatal screening do not return to collect their results, so the benefit of testing is lost. The CDC stresses the importance of obtaining results quickly. It contends that people are not only more likely to take a test that gives results instantly but also will benefit from the opportunity to learn they are infected before their immune systems have been seriously damaged. Furthermore, rapid results may lead to earlier, more effective treatment and might reduce transmission of the virus.

The FDA has approved a number of rapid-response tests designed for use in clinics in the United States. The first test to be approved is manufactured by Murex Diagnostics Inc. This test detects the presence of HIV antibody in about 10 minutes. The test is as accurate as the standard Western blot test. However, because the Western blot test also looks for protein bands, this test remains the absolute antibody-based indicator of HIV.

In late 2002 the FDA announced approval of another blood-based antibody test (OraQuick Rapid HIV-1 by OraSure Technologies Inc.) for use. As of 2007 the test, which produces results within about 10 minutes, was not licensed for home use and could only be performed in a clinical setting. However, the fact that the test does not require any specialized equipment or refrigeration offers the possibility of home use in the future.

Another similar rapid-response test kit, developed and manufactured by the Canadian-based MedMira Inc., was granted FDA approval in April 2003 for sale in the United States. The kit is also approved in China, where HIV infection rates dramatically increased during the first decade of the 21st century.

Table 2.5 shows the body fluids used by the rapid HIV tests that have been approved by the FDA. It also shows the sensitivity and specificity of each of the rapid HIV tests. Sensitivity is the ability or extent to which a diagnostic test detects a disease when it is truly present. Specificity is the ability or extent to which a diagnostic test excludes the presence of a disease when it is truly not present. In other words, a sensitive test will produce a positive test result when in fact the patient has the disease, whereas a specific test will give a negative result when the patient does not have the disease.

Rapid HIV tests are used more frequently in other countries, such as China. In developing countries, quick-response tests are used to screen blood before transfusions and to screen pregnant women so medical interventions can be given to prevent mother-to-child transmission of the virus. They are also used in rural clinics.

Revised Recommendations for HIV Testing

In 2006 Bernard M. Branson et al. of the CDC published "Revised Recommendations for HIV Testing of Adults, Adolescents, and Pregnant Women in Health-Care Settings" (*Morbidity and Mortality Weekly Report*, vol. 55, RR-14, September 22, 2006). The new recommendations updated and replaced guidelines issued in 1993. The major revisions from the 1993 guidelines are to advise routine HIV screening of adults, adolescents, and pregnant women in health care settings in the United States; to screen people at high risk for HIV infection at least annually; to eliminate the requirement for separate written consent for HIV testing, making general consent sufficient to permit HIV testing; and to remove the

TABLE 2.5

FDA-approved rapid HIV tests, 2008

	FDA approval received	Specimen type	CLIA category[a]	Sensitivity[b]	Specificity[b]	Manufacturer	Approved for HIV-2 detection?	List price per device[c]	External controls
OraQuick Advance Rapid HIV-1/2 Antibody Test	Nov 2002	Oral fluid Whole blood (finger stick or venipuncture) Plasma	Waived Waived Moderate complexity	99.3% 99.6% 99.6%	99.8% 100% 99.9%	OraSure Technologies, Inc. www.orasure.com	Yes	$17.50	Sold separately ($25 each)
Uni-Gold Recombigen HIV	Dec 2003	Whole blood (finger stick or venipuncture) Serum & plasma	Waived Moderate complexity	100% 100%	99.7% 99.8%	Trinity Biotech www.unigoldhiv.com	No	$15.75 *$8.00[d]*	Sold separately ($26.25 each)
Reveal G-3 Rapid HIV-1	Apr 2003	Serum Plasma	Moderate complexity Moderate complexity	99.8% 99.8%	99.1% 98.6%	MedMira, Inc. www.medmira.com	No	$14.00	Included
MultiSpot HIV-1/HIV-2 Rapid Test	Nov 2004	Serum Plasma	Moderate complexity Moderate complexity	100% 100%	99.93% 99.91%	BioRad Laboratories www.biorad.com	Yes -differentiates HIV-1 from HIV-2	$25.00	Included
Clearview HIV 1/2 STAT-PAK	May 2006	Whole blood (finger stick or venipuncture) Serum & plasma	Waived Non-waived	99.7% 99.7%	99.9% 99.9%	Inverness Medical Professional Diagnostics www.invernessmedicalpd.com	Yes	$17.50 *$8.00[d]*	Sold separately ($50/set)
Clearview COMPLETE HIV 1/2	May 2006	Whole blood (finger stick or venipuncture) Serum & plasma	Waived Non-waived	99.7% 99.7%	99.90% 99.9%	Inverness Medical Professional Diagnostics www.invernessmedicalpd.com	Yes	$18.50 *$9.00[d]*	Sold separately ($50/set)

[a]Clinical Laboratory Improvement Amendments: CLIA regulations identify three categories of tests: waived, moderate complexity, or high complexity.

[b]Sensitivity is the probability that the test result will be reactive if the specimen is a true positive; specificity is the probability that the test result will be nonreactive if the specimen is a true negative. Data are from the FDA summary basis of approval, for HIV-1 only.

[c]Actual price may vary by purchasing agreements with manufacturers.

[d]"Public health" price for public health programs that are recipients of CDC funds for expanded HIV testing.

Note: Trade names are for identification purposes only and do not imply endorsement. This information was compiled from package inserts and direct calls to manufacturers.

SOURCE: "FDA-Approved Rapid HIV Antibody Screening Tests, February 4, 2008," in *Rapid HIV Testing*, Centers for Disease Control and Prevention, February 15, 2008, http://www.cdc.gov/hiv/topics/testing/rapid/pdf/RT_Comparison-Chart_2-4-08.pdf (accessed July 6, 2009) requirement to provide prevention counseling as part of HIV screening and testing programs in health care settings. The 2006 guidelines also advise that HIV screening be part of routine prenatal screening for all pregnant women and that repeat screening during the third trimester of pregnancy be performed in areas where there are high levels of HIV infection among pregnant women.

Test Tracks HIV/AIDS Progression

In June 1996 the FDA approved a test to help determine how fast an HIV infection progressed to full-blown AIDS. Developed by Roche Diagnostic Systems Inc., the Amplicor HIV-1 monitor test is not intended to screen for HIV or to confirm an HIV diagnosis. Instead, the test detects the amount of HIV in the blood (the viral load) by measuring HIV genetic material. An increased viral load indicates the advancement of the infection toward AIDS and an increasing predisposition to the development of OIs. The test is based on a technique developed in 1984 called the polymerase chain reaction (PCR). PCR uses a heat-resistant bacterial enzyme to amplify the copies of target stretches of genetic material to detectable amounts. The process can be completed in less than one hour. This test was the first PCR-based test to be approved.

FDA approval was granted in 1997 to expand the use of the test as an aid in managing HIV in patients undergoing antiretroviral therapy. In 1999 a more sensitive version of the test became available, and this test has been widely used since then—to help evaluate and track the progression of HIV infection and disease and to predict the risk of complications and debilitating infections.

David March reports in "Viral Load Testing: Way to Predict Anti-HIV Failures in Africa" (*JHU Gazette*, March 23, 2009) that in February 2009 a research team led by Steven Reynolds presented its findings about how to track the progress of HIV and predict treatment failures at the 2009 Conference on Retroviruses and Opportunistic Infections in Montreal, Canada. According to March, Reynolds and his colleagues asserted that "counting the number of HIV viruses in the blood rather than relying solely on counting the number of circulating HIV-fighting CD4 immune system cells" is a more effective way to detect early signs that antiretroviral drugs are no longer working. Reynolds observed that "detecting antiretroviral drug failures accurately and early is essential to avoiding HIV drug resistance, which could result in HIV disease progressing to AIDS and leading to illness and death."

CHAPTER 3

PATTERNS AND TRENDS IN HIV/AIDS SURVEILLANCE

DETERMINING THE NUMBER OF PEOPLE INFECTED WITH HIV

The Centers for Disease Control and Prevention (CDC) keeps track of the number of people in the United States who are infected with HIV, the virus that causes AIDS.

These CDC figures, which have always been acknowledged as estimates, have been criticized as being inaccurate—either too high or too low. Nonetheless, the historical continuity of CDC data permits trend analyses. Therefore, when viewed over a number of years, the figures provide a reasonable indication of the progress of the disease in the United States.

Estimates of HIV infection are important, as they directly influence public health and medical resource allocation as well as political and economic decisions. Definitive figures are difficult to obtain because laws prevent testing for HIV without consent and permission. Furthermore, many people are understandably reluctant to participate in community or household surveys because of confidentiality concerns and fear of losing or failing to obtain insurance coverage.

Health officials contend that knowing the prevalence of HIV infections (prevalence is a measure of all cases of illness existing at a given point in time) is not as crucial as knowing whether the number of HIV infections is rising or falling. The rate at which people develop HIV/AIDS during a specified period is known as the incidence rate. Because there are no national studies to collect these data (not all states require reporting of new HIV cases), estimates are based on reports from states that mandate confidential reporting of HIV cases, along with other small studies and surveys. CDC officials explain that a major problem has been the lack of knowledge about how many people had become infected before the beginning of the agency's regular collection of data. This would help determine how the current incidence of HIV compares to previous years. The comparison of incidence rates is important because they are a direct measure of the rate at which individuals become ill and provide data to help estimate the risk or probability of illness.

CDC data through 2007 from the states and U.S.-dependent areas with confidential HIV reporting indicate that 263,936 people were living with HIV that had not yet progressed to AIDS. (See Table 3.1.) Of the 2007 total, 2,195 were children younger than 13 and 261,741 were adults and adolescents.

In the 39 areas—34 states and five U.S. dependent areas—with confidential name-based HIV infection reporting since at least 2003, the prevalence rate of HIV infection among adults and adolescents was estimated at 154.2 per 100,000 at the end of 2007. Figure 3.1 shows that the rates of HIV infection vary widely from state to state, from a low of 16.2 per 100,000 in North Dakota to 282 per 100,000 in New York.

The CDC also compiles figures on the numbers of people living with AIDS. Table 3.1 shows the numbers of adults, adolescents, and children living with AIDS in 2007. Through 2007, 467,664 adults and adolescents were estimated to be living with AIDS. The number of children younger than 13 living with AIDS through 2007 was 914.

AIDS CASE NUMBERS

The first cases of what came to be recognized as AIDS were reported in the United States in June 1981. Five young, homosexual males in Los Angeles, California, were diagnosed with *Pneumocystis carinii* pneumonia and other opportunistic infections. The CDC notes in *HIV/AIDS Surveillance Report, 1997* (December 1997, http://www.cdc.gov/hiv/topics/surveillance/resources/reports/pdf/hivsur92.pdf) that by August 1989 approximately 100,000 cases of AIDS had been reported to the agency. By December 1997 that number had risen to 641,086; of these, 390,692 people had died. Cumulatively, through 2007 there were 1,030,832 reported cases of AIDS in the United States—1,021,242

TABLE 3.1

Estimated numbers of persons living with HIV infection or AIDS at the end of 2007

[By area of residence—United States and dependent areas]

Area of residence	Living with HIV infection (not AIDS)			Living with AIDS		
	Adults or adolescents	Children (<13 years)	Total	Adults or adolescents	Children (<13 years)	Total
Alabama	5,721	18	5,740	4,036	10	4,046
Alaska	288	1	289	342	1	343
Arizona	6,168	58	6,226	5,104	6	5,110
Arkansas	2,419	6	2,425	2,280	6	2,286
California	—	—	—	65,498	84	65,582
Colorado	6,052	14	6,067	4,284	2	4,286
Connecticut	—	—	—	6,922	9	6,930
Delaware	—	—	—	1,836	8	1,844
District of Columbia	—	—	—	8,871	24	8,895
Florida[a]	39,385	301	39,686	47,907	152	48,059
Georgia	13,721	152	13,873	17,968	43	18,011
Hawaii	—	—	—	1,313	3	1,316
Idaho	406	3	409	318	0	318
Illinois	—	—	—	17,037	38	17,075
Indiana	3,921	18	3,939	4,009	10	4,019
Iowa	643	1	644	915	2	917
Kansas	1,365	5	1,370	1,388	2	1,390
Kentucky	—	—	—	2,813	13	2,826
Louisiana	7,646	92	7,738	8,476	14	8,491
Maine	—	—	—	537	0	537
Maryland	—	—	—	15,652	30	15,682
Massachusetts	—	—	—	9,162	19	9,181
Michigan	6,455	46	6,501	7,077	11	7,088
Minnesota	3,361	19	3,380	2,434	5	2,439
Mississippi	4,348	28	4,376	3,333	8	3,341
Missouri	5,106	33	5,139	5,719	6	5,725
Montana	—	—	—	205	0	205
Nebraska	699	8	708	833	2	835
Nevada	3,554	10	3,564	2,994	3	2,997
New Hampshire	—	—	—	585	3	588
New Jersey	17,493	119	17,612	17,628	43	17,671
New Mexico	962	0	962	1,335	4	1,339
New York	45,712	677	46,390	75,146	106	75,253
North Carolina	13,056	67	13,122	9,116	13	9,129
North Dakota	87	0	87	78	2	80
Ohio	8,499	57	8,557	7,398	28	7,426
Oklahoma	2,221	16	2,237	2,272	2	2,274
Oregon	—	—	—	2,948	3	2,951
Pennsylvania	—	—	—	19,180	57	19,236
Rhode Island	—	—	—	1,343	7	1,350
South Carolina	6,591	35	6,626	7,489	21	7,510
South Dakota	203	4	207	146	1	147
Tennessee	7,105	49	7,154	6,826	8	6,834
Texas	26,361	244	26,605	34,899	41	34,940
Utah	944	10	954	1,207	0	1,207
Vermont	—	—	—	237	2	239
Virginia	10,542	34	10,577	8,855	16	8,872
Washington	—	—	—	5,625	4	5,629
West Virginia	665	5	670	781	4	785
Wisconsin	2,415	17	2,432	2,286	10	2,296
Wyoming	96	2	98	105	1	106
Subtotal	**254,212**	**2,151**	**256,363**	**454,746**	**889**	**455,636**

among adults and adolescents and 9,590 in children under the age of 13. (See Table 3.2.) According to the CDC, in *HIV/AIDS Surveillance Report, 2007* (2009, http://www.cdc .gov/hiv/topics/surveillance/resources/reports/2007report/pdf/ 2007SurveillanceReport.pdf), as of 2007, 583,298 people had died of the disease.

During the mid-1990s the number of AIDS cases rose dramatically. This surge was not an actual numerical increase, but was due to the expanded 1993 AIDS surveillance definition, which added diseases and conditions that had not been part of the previous definition of AIDS. By the

late 1990s the number of AIDS cases leveled off and began to decline, probably as a result of the increasing use of effective antiretroviral drugs that delay the progression of AIDS. Except for a slight decline from 2004 to 2005, the total number of cases of HIV/AIDS diagnosed each year had increased, rising from 38,398 in 2004 to 44,084 in 2007. (See Table 3.3.) However, it is important to bear in mind that this increasing number does not mean that more people are becoming infected with HIV each year; it includes people who may have been HIV positive for years and have been recently diagnosed as well as new cases of AIDS. In fact, the

TABLE 3.1

Estimated numbers of persons living with HIV infection or AIDS at the end of 2007 [CONTINUED]

[By area of residence—United States and dependent areas]

Area of residence	Living with HIV infection (not AIDS)			Living with AIDS		
	Adults or adolescents	Children (<13 years)	Total	Adults or adolescents	Children (<13 years)	Total
U.S. dependent areas						
American Samoa	1	0	1	1	0	1
Guam	61	0	61	35	0	35
Northern Mariana Islands	7	0	7	3	0	3
Puerto Rico	7,221	41	7,261	11,484	19	11,503
U.S. Virgin Islands	240	3	243	330	1	331
Total[b]	**261,741**	**2,195**	**263,936**	**467,664**	**914**	**468,578**

Note: These numbers do not represent reported case counts. Rather, these numbers are point estimates, which result from adjustments of reported case counts. The reported case counts have been adjusted for reporting delays, but not for incomplete reporting. Dashes indicate data not shown because the state has not had laws or regulations requiring confidential name-based HIV infection reporting since at least 2003.
[a]Florida has confidential name-based HIV infection reporting for only the diagnoses made during July 1997 or later.
[b]Total number of persons living with HIV infection (not AIDS) includes persons reported from areas with confidential name-based HIV infection reporting who were residents of other states or whose area of residence is unknown. Total number of persons living with AIDS includes persons whose area of residence is unknown. Because column totals were calculated independently of the values for the subpopulations, the values in each column may not sum to the column total.

SOURCE: "Table 14. Estimated Numbers of Persons Living with HIV Infection (not AIDS) or with AIDS at the End of 2007, by Area of Residence—United States and Dependent Areas," in *HIV/AIDS Surveillance Report, 2007*, vol. 19, Centers for Disease Control and Prevention, 2009, http://www.cdc.gov/hiv/topics/surveillance/resources/reports/2007report/pdf/table14.pdf (accessed June 20, 2009)

article "Ban Urges End to Prejudice against People Living with HIV/AIDS" (UN News Centre, August 4, 2008) explains that in the United States and in many other countries fewer people are becoming infected with HIV.

THE NATURE OF THE EPIDEMIC

Changes in the distribution of HIV infection illustrate the increasing diversity of those affected by the epidemic in the more than 25 years since AIDS was first diagnosed. The CDC notes in "Current Trends Update: Acquired Immunodeficiency Syndrome—United States, 1981–1990" (*Morbidity and Mortality Weekly Report*, vol. 40, no. 22, June 7, 1991) that all the 189 AIDS cases reported in 1981 in the United States were males. Three-fourths (76%) of them were men who had sex with men (MSM) living in New York and California. In 1990, of the 43,339 AIDS cases reported by all states, approximately 30% were from New York and California, 11.5% were women, and about 2% were children. In 1999 the proportions of reported cases among women, African-Americans, Hispanics, and people exposed through heterosexual contact all increased. By contrast, the percentage of reported cases among whites and MSM declined somewhat.

Table 3.3 shows that between 2004 and 2007 MSM sexual contact continued to account for the largest proportion of diagnosed cases; however, the numbers of cases attributable to intravenous drug use and high-risk heterosexual contact also grew among males and females. By contrast, the number of cases diagnosed in children under the age of 13 declined during this period.

Regional Differences

AIDS cases have been reported in all 50 states, the District of Columbia, and dependent areas. However, the distribution of cases is far from even. (See Figure 3.2.) In 2006 the highest rate by far was in the District of Columbia, where the rate was 2016.5 per 100,000. There was a concentration in the states on the East Coast (particularly in New York, Connecticut, Maryland, New Jersey, and Delaware, with respective rates of 438.1, 252.1, 311.8, 236.8, and 247.2, and in Florida, with a rate of 304.8). Also prominent were Puerto Rico (341.8) and the U.S. Virgin Islands (355). Figure 3.3 shows the corresponding AIDS rates for children younger than 13 in 2006. The estimated rates for children living with AIDS ranged from 0 per 100,000 in Idaho, Montana, Utah, American Samoa, Guam, and the Northern Mariana Islands to 36.5 per 100,000 in the District of Columbia.

RATES IN MAJOR METROPOLITAN AREAS. Most AIDS cases are concentrated in larger metropolitan regions (the city and surrounding suburbs). The cumulative total for metropolitan areas with populations of 500,000 or more was 871,192 (or 85%) of all reported cases (the cumulative total includes both those who have died and those still living). (See Table 3.4.) In 2006 and 2007 the annual metropolitan AIDS incidence rates per 100,000 people were highest on the coasts, such as in the New York division (40.3 and 36.6, respectively); Miami, Florida, division (48.9 and 35.4); Baltimore–Towson, Maryland (37.5 and 29.6); Fort Lauderdale, Florida, division (43.4 and 36.5); the Washington division (35.8 and 34.5); Baton Rouge, Louisiana (30.1 and 31.4); Columbia, South Carolina (28.4 and 25.3); and the San Francisco division

FIGURE 3.1

Estimated rates for adults and adolescents living with HIV infection or with AIDS, 2007

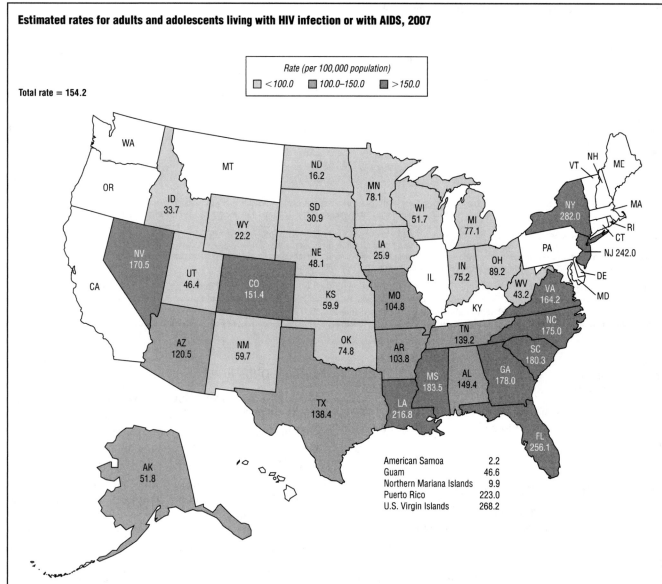

Note: Data from 34 states and 5 U.S. dependent areas with confidential name-based HIV infection reporting since at least 2003. Data have been adjusted for reporting delays.

SOURCE: "Slide 14. Estimated Prevalence Rates for Adults and Adolescents Living with HIV Infection (not AIDS), 2007—34 States and 5 U.S. Dependent Areas," in *HIV/AIDS Surveillance—General Epidemiology (through 2007)*, Centers for Disease Control and Prevention, April 3, 2009, http://www.cdc.gov/ hiv/topics/surveillance/resources/slides/general/slides/general_14.pdf (accessed June 20, 2009)

(26.7 and 41.7). By contrast, Midwest metropolitan areas displayed some of the lowest rates: Akron, Ohio (4.6 and 3.3), Grand Rapids, Michigan (6.5 and 5), and Youngstown–Warren–Boardman, Ohio (4.9 and 9.5). Ogden–Clearfield, Utah, had the lowest overall rate (1.4 and 1.5), followed by Boise City–Nampa, Idaho (2.5 and 2), Colorado Springs, Colorado (3.5 and 3.8), and Des Moines, Iowa (4.3 and 4.8).

There are several reasons for the higher rates in urban areas. First, metropolitan areas are more cosmopolitan and, by definition, more tolerant of alternative lifestyles such as those of MSM, a group with high-risk sexual behaviors. Second, large metropolitan areas also have greater numbers of intravenous drug users, another major risk factor for HIV infection. Third, even though HIV infection and transmission are not restricted to more populated areas, those who need and seek treatment may migrate to these areas for access to medical care and social services. In many smaller communities medical care may be unavailable and financial and/or social barriers may limit access to health care services.

Rates among MSM: A Decline?

Table 3.5 displays CDC data on reported AIDS cases among adults, adolescents, and children younger than age

TABLE 3.2

Reported AIDS cases and annual rates, by area of residence, 2006, 2007, and cumulative

[United States and dependent areas]

Area of residence	2006 No.	2006 Rate	2007 No.	2007 Rate	Cumulative[a] Adults or adolescents	Cumulative[a] Children (<13 yrs)	Total
Alabama	462	10.1	391	8.4	9,015	76	9,091
Alaska	39	5.8	32	4.7	682	7	689
Arizona	511	8.3	585	9.2	10,929	46	10,975
Arkansas	253	9.0	196	6.9	4,083	36	4,119
California	3,990	11.0	4,952	13.5	148,274	675	148,949
Colorado	320	6.7	355	7.3	9,098	31	9,129
Connecticut	410	11.7	528	15.1	15,216	183	15,399
Delaware	117	13.7	171	19.8	3,715	26	3,741
District of Columbia	820	140.1	871	148.1	18,008	188	18,196
Florida	4,922	27.3	3,961	21.7	107,980	1,544	109,524
Georgia	1,589	17.0	1,877	19.7	33,607	240	33,847
Hawaii	89	7.0	78	6.1	3,002	17	3,019
Idaho	25	1.7	23	1.5	626	2	628
Illinois	1,341	10.5	1,348	10.5	34,783	283	35,066
Indiana	344	5.5	329	5.2	8,572	56	8,628
Iowa	84	2.8	76	2.5	1,802	13	1,815
Kansas	121	4.4	132	4.8	2,919	14	2,933
Kentucky	203	4.8	292	6.9	4,869	35	4,904
Louisiana	819	19.3	879	20.5	18,480	132	18,612
Maine	68	5.2	46	3.5	1,156		,163
Maryland	1,615	28.8	1,394	24.8	31,611	320	31,931
Massachusetts	530	8.2	612	9.5	19,819	218	20,037
Michigan	661	6.5	628	6.2	15,558	114	15,672
Minnesota	211	4.1	197	3.8	5,016	28	5,044
Mississippi	358	12.3	352	12.1	6,976	56	7,032
Missouri	464	7.9	542	9.2	11,585	61	11,646
Montana	7	0.7	25	2.6	401	3	404
Nebraska	119	6.7	80	4.5	1,561	11	1,572
Nevada	292	11.7	335	13.1	6,095	29	6,124
New Hampshire	54	4.1	51	3.9	1,124	10	1,134
New Jersey	1,063	12.3	1,164	13.4	49,907	787	50,694
New Mexico	93	4.8	113	5.7	2,712	9	2,721
New York	5,473	28.4	4,810	24.9	179,116	2,345	181,461
North Carolina	1,243	14.0	1,024	11.3	17,007	120	17,127
North Dakota	6	0.9	8	1.3	151	2	153
Ohio	760	6.6	703	6.1	15,698	140	15,838
Oklahoma	203	5.7	264	7.3	5,079	26	5,105
Oregon	278	7.5	239	6.4	6,229	19	6,248
Pennsylvania	1,887	15.2	1,750	14.1	35,120	369	35,489
Rhode Island	112	10.5	66	6.2	2,648	28	2,676
South Carolina	704	16.3	742	16.8	14,055	108	14,163
South Dakota	18	2.3	15	1.9	270	5	275
Tennessee	679	11.2	658	10.7	13,114	59	13,173
Texas	2,958	12.6	2,964	12.4	72,434	394	72,828
Utah	57	2.2	68	2.6	2,363	20	2,383
Vermont	19	3.1	6	1.0	468	6	474
Virginia	599	7.8	634	8.2	17,431	177	17,608
Washington	377	5.9	427	6.6	12,202	35	12,237
West Virginia	65	3.6	76	4.2	1,575	11	1,586
Wisconsin	216	3.9	199	3.6	4,716	33	4,749
Wyoming	8	1.6	13	2.5	242	2	244
Subtotal	**37,656**	**12.6**	**37,281**	**12.4**	**989,099**	**9,156**	**998,255**

13 at the time of diagnosis by transmission category and gender. There were 38,297 newly reported adult and adolescent AIDS cases in 2007. Of the 2007 total, 28,320 were adult and adolescent males. Of these males, the portion attributable to transmission among MSM who did not also inject drugs was 14,383 cases (51% of total). An additional 1,514 (5%) of MSM in 2007 also used intravenous drugs, and in this group it is unclear whether AIDS was acquired from sexual behavior or intravenous drug use. An examination of data from 1981 (when record keeping began) until 2007 reveals that men in the MSM exposure category who did not use intravenous drugs accounted for 54% of the cumulative reported AIDS cases in men and 44% of the total cumulative reported AIDS cases.

Between 2004 and 2007 the greatest proportion of transmission occurred as a result of MSM. (See Table 3.3.) The numbers of AIDS cases attributable to MSM rose throughout this period, rising sharply from 17,898 in 2004 to 22,472 in 2007. AIDS cases in women attributable to high-risk heterosexual contact also rose, increasing from 7,967 in 2004 to 9,076 in 2007.

TABLE 3.2

Reported AIDS cases and annual rates, by area of residence, 2006, 2007, and cumulative [CONTINUED]

[United States and dependent areas]

Area of residence	2006 No.	2006 Rate	2007 No.	2007 Rate	Cumulative[a] Adults or adolescents	Cumulative[a] Children (<13 yrs)	Total
U.S. dependent areas							
American Samoa	0	0.0	0	0.0	1	0	1
Guam	0	0.0	0	0.0	68	1	69
Northern Mariana Islands	0	0.0	0	0.0	3	0	3
Puerto Rico	844	21.5	847	21.5	30,333	403	30,736
U.S. Virgin Islands	32	29.5	34	31.4	663	18	681
Other[b]	0	0.0	0	0.0	3	0	3
Total[c]	**38,751**	**12.8**	**38,384**	**12.5**	**1,021,242**	**9,590**	**1,030,832[d]**

[a]From the beginning of the epidemic through 2007.
[b]Persons reported from areas with confidential name-based AIDS reporting but who are residents of other areas.
[c]Includes persons whose state or area of residence is unknown.
[d]Includes 1,084 persons whose state or area of residence is unknown.

SOURCE: "Table 16. Reported AIDS Cases and Annual Rates (per 100,000 Population), by Area of Residence, 2006, 2007, and Cumulative—United States and Dependent Areas," in *HIV/AIDS Surveillance Report, 2007*, vol. 19, Centers for Disease Control and Prevention, 2009, http://www.cdc.gov/hiv/topics/surveillance/resources/reports/2007report/pdf/table16.pdf (accessed June 21, 2009)

TABLE 3.3

Estimated numbers of HIV/AIDS cases, by year of diagnosis and selected characteristics, 2004–07

[34 states and 5 U.S. dependent areas with confidential name-based HIV infection reporting]

	Year of diagnosis 2004	2005	2006	2007
Data for 34 states				
Age at diagnosis (year)				
<13	212	189	169	159
13–14	41	40	45	40
15–19	1,081	1,216	1,409	1,703
20–24	3,714	3,875	4,184	4,907
25–29	4,524	4,547	4,884	5,771
30–34	5,353	5,024	4,686	5,089
35–39	6,359	5,907	5,678	6,088
40–44	6,011	5,889	6,003	6,554
45–49	4,286	4,338	4,377	5,172
50–54	2,645	2,698	2,862	3,489
55–59	1,473	1,531	1,512	1,938
60–64	771	729	741	942
≥65	696	657	643	803
Race/ethnicity				
American Indian/Alaska Native	177	180	163	228
Asian[a]	308	329	332	455
Black/African American	19,309	18,479	18,975	21,549
Hispanic/Latino[b]	6,183	6,383	6,590	7,484
Native Hawaiian/other Pacific Islander	39	43	49	46
White	10,836	10,818	10,815	12,556
Transmission category				
Male adult or adolescent				
Male-to-male sexual contact	17,898	18,333	18,894	22,472
Injection drug use	3,198	2,990	2,931	3,133
Male-to-male sexual contact and injection drug use	1,413	1,308	1,195	1,260
High-risk heterosexual contact[c]	4,167	3,923	4,029	4,551
Other[d]	140	120	132	102
Subtotal	26,814	26,673	27,182	31,518
Female adult or adolescent				
Injection drug use	2,065	1,834	1,729	1,806
High-risk heterosexual contact[c]	7,967	7,852	8,033	9,076
Other[d]	103	90	80	96
Subtotal	10,135	9,775	9,842	10,977

TABLE 3.3

Estimated numbers of HIV/AIDS cases, by year of diagnosis and selected characteristics, 2004–07 [CONTINUED]

[34 states and 5 U.S. dependent areas with confidential name-based HIV infection reporting]

	Year of diagnosis 2004	2005	2006	2007
Child (<13 years at diagnosis)				
Perinatal	177	162	134	139
Other[e]	37	30	36	20
Subtotal	214	192	170	159
Subtotal for 34 states	**37,164**	**36,640**	**37,193**	**42,655**
Data for U.S. dependent areas	1,234	1,391	1,338	1,429
Total[f]	**38,398**	**38,032**	**38,531**	**44,084**

Notes: These numbers do not represent reported case counts. Rather, these numbers are point estimates, which result from adjustments of reported case counts. The reported case counts have been adjusted for reporting delays and missing risk-factor information, but not for incomplete reporting.
Data include persons with a diagnosis of HIV infection (not AIDS), a diagnosis of HIV infection and a later diagnosis of AIDS, or concurrent diagnoses of HIV infection and AIDS.
[a]Includes Asian/Pacific Islander legacy cases.
[b]Hispanics/Latinos can be of any race.
[c]Heterosexual contact with a person known to have, or to be at high risk for, HIV infection.
[d]Includes hemophilia, blood transfusion, perinatal exposure, and risk factor not reported or not identified.
[e]Includes hemophilia, blood transfusion, and risk factor not reported or not identified.
[f]Includes persons of unknown race or multiple races and persons of unknown sex. Because column totals were calculated independently of the values for the subpopulations, the values in each column may not sum to the column total.

SOURCE: "Table 1. Estimated Numbers of Cases of HIV/AIDS, by Year of Diagnosis and Selected Characteristics, 2004–2007—34 States and 5 U.S. Dependent Areas with Confidential Name-Based HIV Infection Reporting," in *HIV/AIDS Surveillance Report, 2007*, vol. 19, Centers for Disease Control and Prevention, 2009, http://www.cdc.gov/hiv/topics/surveillance/resources/reports/2007report/pdf/table1.pdf (accessed June 21, 2009)

FIGURE 3.2

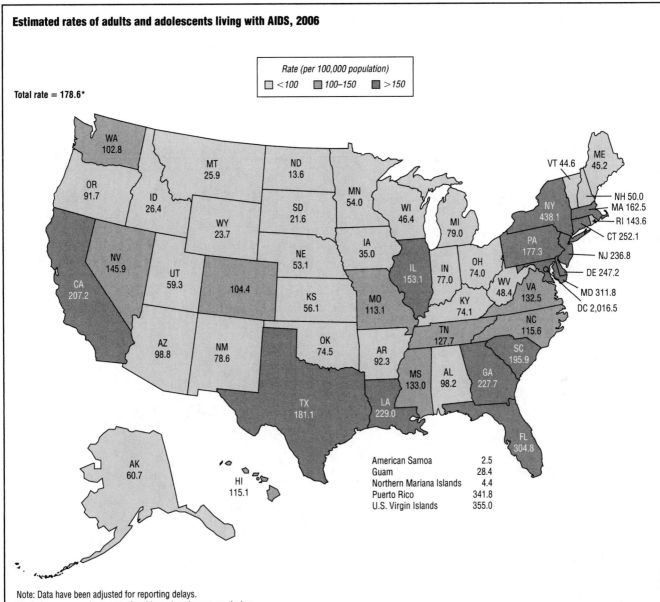

Estimated rates of adults and adolescents living with AIDS, 2006

Rate (per 100,000 population)
☐ <100   ▨ 100–150   ■ >150

Total rate = 178.6*

	Rate
American Samoa	2.5
Guam	28.4
Northern Mariana Islands	4.4
Puerto Rico	341.8
U.S. Virgin Islands	355.0

Note: Data have been adjusted for reporting delays.
*Includes persons whose area of residence is unknown or missing.

SOURCE: "Slide 22. Estimated Prevalence Rates for Adults and Adolescents Living with AIDS (per 100,000 Population), 2006, United States and Dependent Areas," in *AIDS Surveillance—General Epidemiology (through 2006)*, Centers for Disease Control and Prevention, May 20, 2008, http://www.cdc.gov/hiv/topics/surveillance/resources/slides/epidemiology/slides/EPI-AIDS_22.pdf (accessed June 21, 2009)

Rates among Women

In 2007 reported AIDS cases among women that were attributable to intravenous drug use (1,633) accounted for 16% of the total number of cases. (See Table 3.5.) The number of AIDS cases attributable to intravenous drug use varied very little between 2005 and 2007, hovering around 1,800 cases per year. (See Table 3.3.)

When considering the role of heterosexual contact in the acquisition of AIDS, the proportion was far higher for women in 2007 (9,076 cases, representing 83% of the total of 10,944) than for men (4,551, representing 14% of the total of 31,518). (See Table 3.3.)

Decline in AIDS Due to Blood Transfusions

As a result of screening procedures for blood and blood products that began in 1985, the CDC indicates that the number of AIDS cases among adult and adolescent transfusion recipients decreased between 1995 (664 cases) and 1997 (409 cases). A pronounced decrease in 1999 (256 cases) was followed by a steady decline after an initial slight increase to 282 cases in 2000: 218 cases in 2001, 219 in 2003, 160 in 2005, and 109 in 2007. (See Table 3.5.)

The number of AIDS cases among adults and adolescents with hemophilia has also decreased. In 1996, 318

FIGURE 3.3

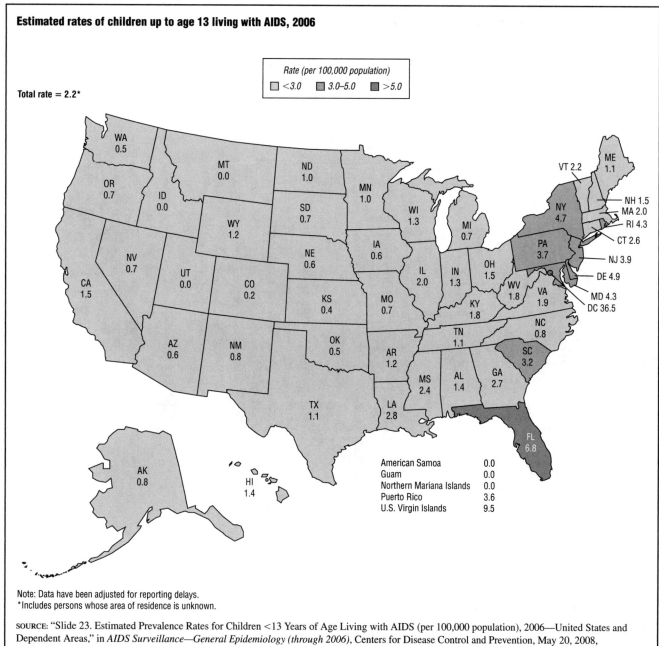

Estimated rates of children up to age 13 living with AIDS, 2006

Total rate = 2.2*

Rate (per 100,000 population)
☐ <3.0   ▨ 3.0–5.0   ◼ >5.0

WA 0.5
MT 0.0
ND 1.0
MN 1.0
OR 0.7
ID 0.0
WY 1.2
SD 0.7
WI 1.3
MI 0.7
VT 2.2
ME 1.1
NY 4.7
NH 1.5
MA 2.0
RI 4.3
CT 2.6
NV 0.7
UT 0.0
CO 0.2
NE 0.6
IA 0.6
IL 2.0
IN 1.3
OH 1.5
PA 3.7
NJ 3.9
DE 4.9
MD 4.3
DC 36.5
CA 1.5
KS 0.4
MO 0.7
KY 1.8
WV 1.8
VA 1.9
AZ 0.6
NM 0.8
OK 0.5
AR 1.2
TN 1.1
NC 0.8
SC 3.2
MS 2.4
AL 1.4
GA 2.7
TX 1.1
LA 2.8
FL 6.8
AK 0.8
HI 1.4

American Samoa 0.0
Guam 0.0
Northern Mariana Islands ... 0.0
Puerto Rico 3.6
U.S. Virgin Islands 9.5

Note: Data have been adjusted for reporting delays.
*Includes persons whose area of residence is unknown.

SOURCE: "Slide 23. Estimated Prevalence Rates for Children <13 Years of Age Living with AIDS (per 100,000 population), 2006—United States and Dependent Areas," in *AIDS Surveillance—General Epidemiology (through 2006)*, Centers for Disease Control and Prevention, May 20, 2008, http://www.cdc.gov/hiv/topics/surveillance/resources/slides/epidemiology/slides/EPI-AIDS_23.pdf (accessed June 21, 2009)

cases were reported. The number of new cases among hemophiliacs declined to 151 in 1999, to 106 in 2001, to 85 in 2003, to 79 cases in 2005, and to 46 in 2007. (See Table 3.5.)

Current Age and Gender Distribution

Of the 1,030,832 cumulative total reported cases of AIDS in 2007, 1,021,242 (99% of the cumulative total) were among adults and adolescents. (See Table 3.5.) The remaining 9,590 cases (1%) were children under the age of 13. According to the CDC, in 2007 more people between the ages of 40 to 44 (107,923) and 45 to 49 (103,625) were living with AIDS (211,548,

37% of all cases) than in any other age category. (See Table 3.6.)

Cumulatively, the total number of AIDS cases that were reported in adults and adolescents up to 2007 occurred predominantly in males (824,921 cases, or 80% of the cumulative total). (See Table 3.5.) Adult and adolescent females accounted for 205,911 cumulative cases (20% of the cumulative total).

Race or Ethnicity and AIDS

The changing racial and ethnic profile and characteristics of Americans with HIV/AIDS from 1993 through 2005 reflect a shift in the population at risk for HIV/AIDS. In

TABLE 3.4

Reported AIDS cases and annual rates, by metropolitan area of residence and age category, 2006, 2007, and cumulative

	2006		2007		Cumulative		
Area of residence	No.	Rate	No.	Rate	Adults or adolescents	Children (<13 yrs)	Total
MSA (population ≥500,000)							
Akron, OH	32	4.6	23	3.3	786	1	787
Albany—Schenectady—Troy, NY	106	12.5	67	7.9	2,325	24	2,349
Albuquerque, NM	51	6.2	65	7.8	1,470	3	1,473
Allentown—Bethlehem—Easton, PA—NJ	118	14.8	91	11.3	1,441	17	1,458
Atlanta—Sandy Springs—Marietta, GA	991	19.3	1,216	23.0	23,106	135	23,241
Augusta—Richmond County, GA—SC	35	6.7	77	14.6	1,937	24	1,961
Austin—Round Rock, TX	193	12.6	210	13.1	5,042	26	5,068
Bakersfield, CA	141	18.2	164	20.7	1,739	9	1,748
Baltimore—Towson, MD	998	37.5	791	29.6	21,153	218	21,371
Baton Rouge, LA	230	30.1	242	31.4	3,971	20	3,991
Birmingham—Hoover, AL	111	10.1	89	8.0	2,701	25	2,726
Boise City—Nampa, ID	14	2.5	12	2.0	293	0	293
Boston, MA—NH[a]	353	7.9	371	8.3	13,864	149	14,013
Boston division	183	9.9	229	12.3	8,697	91	8,788
Cambridge division	103	7.0	93	6.3	3,220	36	3,256
Essex division	51	7.0	39	5.3	1,617	21	1,638
Bridgeport—Stamford—Norwalk, CT	136	15.2	140	15.6	3,865	57	3,922
Buffalo—Niagara Falls, NY	98	8.6	102	9.0	2,578	20	2,598
Cape Coral—Fort Myers, FL	88	15.4	84	14.2	1,773	24	1,797
Charleston—North Charleston, SC	89	14.4	99	15.7	2,135	18	2,153
Charlotte—Gastonia—Concord, NC—SC	285	18.0	259	15.7	3,502	22	3,524
Chattanooga, TN—GA	49	9.6	47	9.1	1,034	3	1,037
Chicago, IL—IN—WI	1,127	11.9	1,254	13.2	31,226	262	31,488
Chicago division	1,043	13.2	1,152	14.5	29,314	249	29,563
Gary division	49	7.1	71	10.2	1,109	8	1,117
Lake division	35	4.0	31	3.6	803	5	808
Cincinnati—Middletown, OH—KY—IN	196	9.2	132	6.2	2,868	18	2,886
Cleveland—Elyria—Mentor, OH	168	8.0	135	6.4	4,368	48	4,416
Colorado Springs, CO	21	3.5	23	3.8	599	5	604
Columbia, SC	200	28.4	181	25.3	3,457	24	3,481
Columbus, OH	163	9.4	146	8.3	3,268	16	3,284
Dallas, TX	920	15.4	806	13.1	20,960	63	21,023
Dallas division	709	17.7	618	15.0	16,597	37	16,634
Fort Worth division	211	10.7	188	9.2	4,363	26	4,389
Dayton, OH	55	6.6	65	7.8	1,286	15	1,301
Deltona—Daytona Beach—Ormond Beach, FL	88	17.7	63	12.6	1,519	16	1,535
Denver—Aurora, CO	237	9.8	271	11.0	7,174	22	7,196
Des Moines, IA	23	4.3	26	4.8	556	4	560
Detroit, MI	438	9.7	413	9.2	10,778	74	10,852
Detroit division	323	16.1	294	14.8	8,554	58	8,612
Warren division	115	4.6	119	4.8	2,224	16	2,240
El Paso, TX	40	5.5	135	18.4	1,609	10	1,619
Fresno, CA	66	7.5	98	10.9	1,544	11	1,555
Grand Rapids—Wyoming, MI	50	6.5	39	5.0	854	6	860
Greensboro—High Point, NC	66	9.6	64	9.2	1,328	14	1,342
Greenville, SC	67	11.2	50	8.1	1,343	4	1,347
Harrisburg—Carlisle, PA	69	13.2	78	14.7	1,330	8	1,338
Hartford—West Hartford—East Hartford, CT	127	10.7	202	17.0	5,317	46	5,363
Honolulu, HI	66	7.3	55	6.1	2,175	14	2,189
Houston—Baytown—Sugar Land, TX	1,097	19.9	1,001	17.8	26,782	172	26,954
Indianapolis, IN	147	8.8	121	7.1	3,944	25	3,969
Jackson, MS	115	21.6	139	26.0	2,555	30	2,585
Jacksonville, FL	310	24.2	301	23.1	6,316	76	6,392
Kansas City, MO—KS	161	8.2	297	15.0	4,984	15	4,999
Knoxville, TN	35	5.2	45	6.6	927	5	932
Lakeland, FL	113	20.3	77	13.4	1,890	21	1,911
Las Vegas—Paradise, NV	256	14.4	278	15.1	4,923	28	4,951
Little Rock—North Little Rock, AR	76	11.6	74	11.1	1,460	14	1,474

HIV/AIDS Surveillance Report, 2001 (December 2001, http://www.cdc.gov/hiv/topics/surveillance/resources/reports/2001report/pdf/2001surveillance-report_year-end.pdf), the CDC indicates that in 1993 there were 60,587 cases reported among African-Americans. By 2007 the number of cases had reached 426,003. (See Table 3.7.) As Table 3.6 shows, the number of African-Americans living with HIV/AIDS

continued to outpace the number of whites living with HIV/AIDS from 2004 to 2007.

In 1999 African-Americans accounted for 40.6% (127,169) of people estimated to be living with HIV/AIDS. By 2007 this figure had risen to 47% (267,116). (See Table 3.6.) In contrast, the proportion of non-Hispanic

TABLE 3.4

Reported AIDS cases and annual rates, by metropolitan area of residence and age category, 2006, 2007, and cumulative [CONTINUED]

	2006		2007		Cumulative		
Area of residence	No.	Rate	No.	Rate	Adults or adolescents	Children (<13 yrs)	Total
Los Angeles, CA	1,667	13.0	1,927	15.0	60,289	294	60,583
Los Angeles division	1,472	14.9	1,638	16.6	53,183	250	53,433
Santa Ana division	195	6.5	289	9.6	7,106	44	7,150
Louisville, KY—IN	96	7.9	177	14.3	2,451	25	2,476
Madison, WI	29	5.3	30	5.4	550	4	554
McAllen—Edinburg—Pharr, TX	44	6.4	55	7.7	688	12	700
Memphis, TN—MS—AR	345	27.1	255	19.9	5,382	19	5,401
Miami, FL	2,284	42.2	1,792	33.1	57,554	1,000	58,554
Fort Lauderdale division	769	43.4	642	36.5	17,045	263	17,308
Miami division	1,162	48.9	846	35.4	30,522	514	31,036
West Palm Beach division	353	27.9	304	24.0	9,987	223	10,210
Milwaukee—Waukesha—West Allis, WI	109	7.1	110	7.1	2,621	18	2,639
Minneapolis—St Paul—Bloomington, MN—WI	184	5.8	168	5.2	4,431	22	4,453
Modesto, CA	22	4.3	36	7.0	711	6	717
Nashville—Davidson—Murfreesboro, TN	172	11.6	223	14.7	4,071	20	4,091
New Haven—Milford, CT	106	12.6	142	16.8	4,707	73	4,780
New Orleans—Metairie—Kenner, LA	271	27.4	325	31.5	9,158	69	9,227
New York, NY—NJ—PA	5,469	29.1	5,095	27.1	199,402	2,903	202,305
Edison division	131	5.7	166	7.2	6,871	140	7,011
Nassau division	253	9.1	213	7.7	8,404	111	8,515
New York division	4,672	40.3	4,249	36.6	163,738	2,313	166,051
Newark division	413	19.4	467	21.9	20,389	339	20,728
Ogden—Clearfield, UT	7	1.4	8	1.5	273	4	277
Oklahoma City, OK	89	7.6	112	9.4	2,365	5	2,370
Omaha—Council Bluffs, NE—IA	82	10.0	60	7.2	1,097	3	1,100
Orlando, FL	517	25.9	461	22.7	9,108	94	9,202
Oxnard—Thousand Oaks—Ventura, CA	19	2.4	34	4.3	1,046	3	1,049
Palm Bay—Melbourne—Titusville, FL	61	11.5	45	8.4	1,556	11	1,567
Philadelphia, PA—NJ—DE—MD	1,364	23.5	1,275	21.9	29,476	315	29,791
Camden division	112	9.0	96	7.7	3,217	42	3,259
Philadelphia division	1,157	29.8	1,053	27.1	23,144	252	23,396
Wilmington division	95	13.8	126	18.2	3,115	21	3,136
Phoenix—Mesa—Scottsdale, AZ	355	8.8	452	10.8	7,883	31	7,914
Pittsburgh, PA	134	5.7	145	6.2	3,322	20	3,342
Portland—South Portland, ME	34	6.6	24	4.7	586	0	586
Portland—Vancouver—Beaverton, OR—WA	212	9.9	186	8.6	5,006	10	5,016
Poughkeepsie—Newburgh—Middletown, NY	109	16.4	67	10.0	3,231	24	3,255
Providence—New Bedford—Fall River, RI—MA	155	9.7	104	6.5	4,007	44	4,051
Raleigh—Cary, NC	205	20.5	153	14.6	2,153	13	2,166
Richmond, VA	121	10.1	97	8.0	3,465	35	3,500
Riverside—San Bernardino—Ontario, CA	319	8.0	427	10.5	9,078	61	9,139
Rochester, NY	132	12.8	122	11.8	3,267	13	3,280
Sacramento—Arden—Arcade—Roseville, CA	166	8.0	131	6.3	4,155	26	4,181
St. Louis, MO—IL	364	12.9	233	8.2	6,220	40	6,260
Salt Lake City, UT	40	3.7	48	4.4	1,792	10	1,802
San Antonio, TX	246	12.7	239	12.0	5,223	30	5,253
San Diego—Carlsbad—San Marcos, CA	380	12.9	478	16.1	13,489	65	13,554
San Francisco, CA	705	16.9	1,091	26.0	41,498	98	41,596
Oakland division	250	10.2	373	15.0	9,987	50	10,037
San Francisco division	455	26.7	718	41.7	31,511	48	31,559
San Jose—Sunnyvale—Santa Clara, CA	145	8.2	152	8.4	3,924	15	3,939
San Juan—Caguas—Guaynabo, PR	571	22.0	590	22.7	21,993	279	22,272
Sarasota—Bradenton—Venice, FL	105	15.4	61	8.9	2,040	28	2,068
Scranton—Wilkes-Barre, PA	46	8.4	47	8.6	587	5	592
Seattle, WA	271	8.3	312	9.4	9,468	28	9,496
Seattle division	248	9.9	277	10.9	8,423	19	8,442
Tacoma division	23	3.0	35	4.5	1,045	9	1,054
Springfield, MA	46	6.7	106	15.5	2,189	27	2,216
Stockton, CA	54	8.1	60	8.9	1,142	16	1,158
Syracuse, NY	51	7.9	44	6.8	1,369	9	1,378
Tampa—St Petersburg—Clearwater, FL	603	22.4	469	17.2	11,639	115	11,754

whites living with HIV/AIDS in 1999 was 38% (120,731), and by 2007 it was 32% (181,380).

In 2007 Hispanics accounted for 6,921 new reported AIDS cases. (See Table 3.7.) The corresponding figures for whites and African-Americans were 10,407 and 17,507, respectively. The total number of male and female adult and adolescent reported AIDS cases in native Hawaiians/

Other Pacific Islanders (76) and Native Americans/Alaskan natives (158) were the lowest of all racial and ethnic groups in the United States.

In 2007 the total (male and female) reported AIDS incidence rate per 100,000 adults and adolescents among African-Americans (96.2) was nearly nine times higher than that among non-Hispanic white Americans (10.8), about six

TABLE 3.4

Reported AIDS cases and annual rates, by metropolitan area of residence and age category, 2006, 2007, and cumulative [CONTINUED]

Area of residence	2006		2007		Cumulative		
	No.	Rate	No.	Rate	Adults or adolescents	Children (<13 yrs)	Total
Toledo, OH	66	10.1	40	6.1	855	14	869
Tucson, AZ	95	10.0	84	8.7	2,075	10	2,085
Tulsa, OK	62	6.9	103	11.4	1,594	10	1,604
Virginia Beach—Norfolk—Newport News, VA—NC	131	7.9	211	12.7	4,923	63	4,986
Washington, DC—VA—MD—WV	1,643	31.2	1,618	30.5	32,494	315	32,809
Bethesda division	172	15.0	185	16.0	2,956	24	2,980
Washington division	1,471	35.8	1,433	34.5	29,538	291	29,829
Wichita, KS	38	6.4	30	5.0	880	2	882
Worcester, MA	77	9.9	62	7.9	1,840	21	1,861
Youngstown—Warren—Boardman, OH—PA	28	4.9	54	9.5	576	0	576
Subtotal for MSAs (population ≥500,000)	**31,261**	**15.8**	**31,088**	**15.6**	**862,954**	**8,238**	**871,192**
Metropolitan areas (population of 50,000 to 499,999)	**4,331**	**7.8**	**4,295**	**7.7**	**96,828**	**830**	**97,658**
Nonmetropolitan areas	**2,753**	**5.5**	**2,555**	**5.1**	**57,151**	**454**	**57,605**
Total[b]	**38,500**	**12.7**	**38,128**	**12.5**	**1,019,432**	**9,559**	**1,028,991**

Note: Because of the lack of U.S. census information for all U.S. dependent areas, includes data for only the 50 states, the District of Columbia, and Puerto Rico.

MSA = metropolitan statistical area.

[a]Reported case counts for the metropolitan divisions do not sum to the MSA total. MSA total includes data from 1 metropolitan division with population of <500,000.

[b]Includes persons whose county of residence is unknown.

SOURCE: "Table 17. Reported AIDS Cases and Annual Rates (per 100,000 Population), by Metropolitan Statistical Area of Residence, 2006, 2007, and Cumulative—United States and Puerto Rico," in *HIV/AIDS Surveillance Report, 2007*, vol. 19, Centers for Disease Control and Prevention, 2009, http://www .cdc.gov/hiv/topics/surveillance/resources/reports/2007report/pdf/table17.pdf (accessed June 21, 2009)

times than that of Native Americans/Alaskan natives (16.1), and more than twice that of Hispanics (36.9). (See Table 3.8.) The rates were lowest among Asian-Americans (9.3).

The racial and ethnic difference is particularly alarming among children under the age of 13. As shown in Table 3.8, in 2007 the rate of HIV/AIDS per 100,000 population for African-American children (1.9) was nearly five times the rate for Hispanic and Asian-American children (both at 0.4). The other racial and ethnic categories were negligible.

The racial disparity is also reflected in the acquisition of HIV/AIDS by infants born to HIV-infected mothers. From 1994 through 2007 the number of reported cases of HIV/AIDS among African-American infants has been significantly greater than the reported cases for non-Hispanic whites and Hispanic infants born to HIV-infected mothers. In 2007 more than six times as many infants were born to African-American HIV-infected mothers (57) as to white HIV-infected mothers (9). (See Table 3.9.)

HOW HIV IS TRANSMITTED

HIV can be transmitted by sexual contact with an infected person; by needle sharing among infected intravenous drug users; through the receipt of infected blood, blood products, or tissue; and directly from an infected mother to her infant during pregnancy, delivery, or breastfeeding.

In the United States MSM remain the majority of HIV carriers, although prevalence among heterosexuals is on the rise. The CDC reports in *HIV/AIDS Surveillance Report, 1988* (January 1989, http://www.cdc.gov/hiv/ topics/surveillance/resources/reports/pdf/surveillance88 .pdf) that 70% of adult and adolescent males with AIDS had a single risk factor of a history of high-risk sexual activity in 1987. Even though more than half (51%) of reported cases of AIDS among male adults and adolescents were attributable to MSM in 2007, cumulatively the percentage of affected MSM was 54%. (See Table 3.10.) Adult and adolescent males with a history of intravenous drug use as their only risk factor made up 14% of all cases in 1987. This proportion has remained relatively constant in the intervening years; and even though a cumulative of 20% of AIDS cases in adult and adolescent males were attributable to intravenous drug use, it accounted for only 11% of cases in 2007.

The proportion of adult and adolescent females with AIDS whose only risk factor was intravenous drug use had dropped from 49% in 1987 to 16% in 2007. (See Table 3.11.) Adult and adolescent females with a history of heterosexual contact as their only risk factor made up 31% of all female cases in 1987. By 2007 it had increased to 47%. Researchers suggest that one reason for steadily increasing HIV infection and AIDS among heterosexuals is that an increased proportion report multiple sex partners, which is a risk factor for HIV infection.

Undetermined Risk

In 2007 there were 10,005 adult and adolescent (both male and female) cases of AIDS with an undetermined risk. (See Table 3.10 and Table 3.11.) That is, there was no reported history of exposure to HIV through any of the routes listed in the exposure categories. These include

TABLE 3.5

Reported AIDS cases, by age category, transmission category, and sex, 2007 and cumulative

[United States and dependent areas]

	Males				Females				Total			
	2007		Cumulative[a]		2007		Cumulative[a]		2007		Cumulative[a]	
Transmission category	No.	%	No.	%	No.	%	No.	%	No.	%	No.	%
Adult or adolescent												
Male-to-male sexual contact	14,383	51	445,645	54	—	—	—	—	14,383	38	445,645	44
Injection drug use	3,103	11	166,251	20	1,633	16	69,591	35	4,736	12	235,842	23
Male-to-male sexual contact and injection drug use	1,514	5	67,797	8	—	—	—	—	1,514	4	67,797	7
Hemophilia/coagulation disorder	37	0	5,212	1	9	0	355	0	46	0	5,567	1
High-risk heterosexual contact[b]	2,791	10	52,623	6	4,713	47	90,229	45	7,504	20	142,852	14
Sex with injection drug user	281	1	11,941	1	704	7	26,825	13	985	3	38,766	4
Sex with bisexual male	—	—	—	—	233	2	5,415	3	233	1	5,415	1
Sex with person with hemophilia	4	0	90	0	10	0	513	0	14	0	603	0
Sex with HIV-infected transfusion recipient	31	0	584	0	25	0	819	0	56	0	1,403	0
Sex with HIV-infected person, risk factor not specified	2,475	9	40,008	5	3,741	37	56,657	28	6,216	16	96,665	9
Receipt of blood transfusion, blood components, or tissue[c]	50	0	5,181	1	59	1	4,134	2	109	0	9,315	1
Other/risk factor not reported or identified[d]	6,442	23	77,328	9	3,563	36	36,896	18	10,005	26	114,224	11
Subtotal	28,320	100	820,037	100	9,977	100	201,205	100	38,297	100	1,021,242	100
Child (<13 yrs at diagnosis)												
Hemophilia/coagulation disorder	0	0	222	5	0	0	7	0	0	0	229	2
Mother with documented HIV infection or 1 of the following risk factors	30	77	4,333	89	43	90	4,464	95	73	84	8,797	92
Injection drug use	8	21	1,675	34	10	21	1,673	36	18	21	3,348	35
Sex with injection drug user	2	5	783	16	3	6	752	16	5	6	1,535	16
Sex with bisexual male	1	3	103	2	1	2	111	2	2	2	214	2
Sex with person with hemophilia	0	0	20	0	0	0	16	0	0	0	36	0
Sex with HIV-infected transfusion recipient	0	0	11	0	0	0	15	0	0	0	26	0
Sex with HIV-infected person, risk factor not specified	8	21	746	15	8	17	804	17	16	18	1,550	16
Receipt of blood transfusion, blood components, or tissue	0	0	70	1	0	0	82	2	0	0	152	2
Has HIV infection, risk factor not specified	11	28	925	19	21	44	1,011	21	32	37	1,936	20
Receipt of blood transfusion, blood components, or tissue[e]	1	3	242	5	0	0	141	3	1	1	383	4
Other/risk factor not reported or identified[f]	8	21	87	2	5	10	94	2	13	15	181	2
Subtotal	39	100	4,884	100	48	100	4,706	100	87	100	9,590	100
Total	**28,359**	**100**	**824,921**	**100**	**10,025**	**100**	**205,911**	**100**	**38,384**	**100**	**1,030,832[g]**	**100**

[a]From the beginning of the epidemic through 2007.
[b]Heterosexual contact with a person known to have, or to be at high risk for, HIV infection.
[c]AIDS developed in 43 adults/adolescents after they received transfusion of HIV-infected blood that had tested negative for HIV antibodies. AIDS developed in 13 additional adults after they received tissue, organs, or artificial insemination from HIV-infected donors.
[d]Includes 37 adults/adolescents who were exposed to HIV-infected blood, body fluids, or concentrated virus in health care, laboratory, or household settings, as supported by seroconversion, epidemiologic, or laboratory evidence. One person was infected after intentional inoculation with HIV-infected blood. Includes an additional 908 persons who acquired HIV infection perinatally but who were more than 12 years of age when AIDS was diagnosed. These 908 persons are not counted in the values for the pediatric transmission category.
[e]AIDS developed in 3 children after they received transfusion of HIV-infected blood that had tested negative for HIV antibodies.
[f]Includes 25 children who had sexual contact with an HIV-infected man and an additional 4 children who were exposed to HIV-infected blood in household, health care, or other settings, as supported by seroconversion, epidemiologic, or laboratory evidence.
[g]Includes 2 persons of unknown sex.

SOURCE: "Table 19. Reported AIDS Cases, by Transmission Category and Sex, 2007 and Cumulative—United States and Dependent Areas," in *HIV/AIDS Surveillance Report, 2007*, vol. 19, Centers for Disease Control and Prevention, 2009, http://www.cdc.gov/hiv/topics/ surveillance/resources/reports/2007report/ pdf/table19.pdf (accessed June 21, 2009)

people currently being investigated by local health departments, people whose exposure history was incomplete at the time of their death, those who refused to be interviewed or whose cases were not followed up, and those who were interviewed but for whom no follow-up occurred. When an exposure mode is identified during follow-up, patients are subsequently reclassified into the appropriate exposure category.

MORTALITY FROM AIDS

In "Deaths: Final Data for 2006" (*National Vital Statistics Reports*, vol. 57, no. 14, April 17, 2009), Melonie

TABLE 3.6

Estimated numbers of persons living with HIV/AIDS, by year and selected characteristics, 2004–07

[34 states and 5 U.S. dependent areas with confidential name-based HIV infection reporting]

	2004	2005	2006	2007
Data for 34 states				
Age at end of year				
<13	3,996	3,568	3,119	2,736
13–14	1,316	1,297	1,242	1,159
15–19	3,864	4,286	4,828	5,400
20–24	13,699	14,367	15,347	16,965
25–29	28,681	30,081	31,659	33,857
30–34	50,564	48,057	46,931	47,390
35–39	82,730	80,663	78,206	76,365
40–44	102,941	106,420	108,069	107,923
45–49	82,043	89,050	95,752	103,625
50–54	53,903	60,030	67,082	74,582
55–59	28,077	33,023	38,186	43,985
60–64	13,363	15,309	17,705	20,962
≥65	10,512	12,361	14,363	16,982
Race/ethnicity				
American Indian/Alaska Native	1,895	2,010	2,111	2,281
Asian[a]	2,171	2,468	2,752	3,160
Black/African American	230,138	241,029	252,612	267,116
Hispanic/Latino[b]	78,480	82,810	87,469	92,943
Native Hawaiian/other Pacific Islander	124	161	207	248
White	158,258	165,178	172,509	181,380
Transmission category				
Male adult or adolescent				
Male-to-male sexual contact	208,401	221,945	236,309	253,804
Injection drug use	62,422	62,743	63,281	64,335
Male-to-male sexual contact and injection drug use	26,984	27,346	27,649	28,081
High-risk heterosexual contact[c]	40,546	43,010	45,474	48,515
Other[d]	3,071	3,129	3,231	3,322
Subtotal	341,425	358,173	375,944	398,057
Female adult or adolescent				
Injection drug use	36,977	37,313	37,725	38,266
High-risk heterosexual contact[c]	88,092	93,706	99,440	106,139
Other[d]	1,993	2,082	2,155	2,287
Subtotal	127,061	133,101	139,319	146,692

TABLE 3.6

Estimated numbers of persons living with HIV/AIDS, by year and selected characteristics, 2004–07 [CONTINUED]

[34 states and 5 U.S. dependent areas with confidential name-based HIV infection reporting]

	2004	2005	2006	2007
Child (<13 yrs at diagnosis)				
Perinatal	6,524	6,557	6,541	6,505
Other[e]	676	679	684	676
Subtotal	7,200	7,236	7,225	7,181
Subtotal for 34 states	475,688	498,512	522,490	551,932
Data for U.S. dependent areas	16,985	17,767	18,483	19,445
Total[f]	492,673	516,279	540,972	571,378

Notes: These numbers do not represent reported case counts. Rather, these numbers are point estimates, which result from adjustments of reported case counts. The reported case counts have been adjusted for reporting delays and missing risk-factor information, but not for incomplete reporting.
Data include persons with a diagnosis of HIV infection (not AIDS), a diagnosis of HIV infection and a later diagnosis of AIDS, or concurrent diagnoses of HIV infection and AIDS.
[a]Includes Asian/Pacific Islander legacy cases.
[b]Hispanics/Latinos can be of any race.
[c]Heterosexual contact with a person known to have, or to be at high risk for, HIV infection.
[d]Includes hemophilia, blood transfusion, perinatal exposure, and risk factor not reported or not identified.
[e]Includes hemophilia, blood transfusion, and risk factor not reported or not identified.
[f]Includes persons of unknown race or multiple races and persons of unknown sex. Because column totals were calculated independently of the values for the subpopulations, the values in each column may not sum to the column total.

SOURCE: "Table 9. Estimated Numbers of Persons Living with HIV/AIDS, by Year and Selected Characteristics, 2004–2007—34 States and 5 U.S. Dependent Areas with Confidential Name-Based HIV Infection Reporting," in *HIV/AIDS Surveillance Report, 2007*, vol. 19, Centers for Disease Control and Prevention, 2009, http://www.cdc.gov/hiv/topics/surveillance/resources/reports/2007report/pdf/table9.pdf (accessed June 21, 2009)

P. Heron et al. of the CDC note that in 2006 the average life expectancy for Americans was 77.7 years, an all-time high. This figure would have been higher were it not for heart diseases (the leading cause of death for all age categories), malignant neoplasms (cancers, which were the leading cause of death for those aged 45 to 64), and accidents (the leading cause of death for those aged 15 to 44). (See Table 1.1 in Chapter 1.) AIDS is also among the top 10 leading causes of death among those aged 15 to 44. Cumulatively, through 2007 there were 376,924 reported AIDS deaths among Americans aged 15 to 44, representing nearly two-thirds (64%) of the 583,298 people who had died from AIDS. (See Table 3.12.)

Nearly 100% of AIDS patients die within seven years of the initial diagnosis of the late stage of HIV infection.

Figure 3.4 shows the duration of survival in months, following diagnosis, from 1998 through 2005. Some deaths are not reported to the CDC or are reported as deaths from other causes. As such, the reported case-fatality rate (the number of deaths from a disease divided by the number of cases of that disease) is probably an underestimate. The case-fatality rate is frequently used as a measure of the severity of a disease and to estimate the probability of death among diagnosed cases.

According to the CDC, in *HIV/AIDS Surveillance Report, 2001*, the number of deaths due to AIDS peaked at 51,670 in 1995. Since then the number of deaths each year has been dropping. In 2007 the disease killed 14,561 Americans. (See Table 3.12.) As a result of more effective treatment, fewer people are dying from AIDS. However, the statistics for children under the age of 13 at the time of diagnosis remain grim: half die before their first birthday, whereas the other half do not live to adolescence.

TABLE 3.7

Estimated number of AIDS cases by year of diagnosis and selected characteristics, 2003–07 and cumulative

[United States and dependent areas]

	Year of diagnosis					
	2003	2004	2005	2006	2007	Cumulative[a]
Data for 50 states and the District of Columbia						
Age at diagnosis (yr)						
<13	73	55	54	38	28	9,209
13–14	72	71	70	71	80	1,169
15–19	302	333	409	392	455	6,089
20–24	1,577	1,635	1,669	1,603	1,927	38,175
25–29	3,073	3,191	3,071	3,283	3,380	120,464
30–34	5,578	5,126	4,637	4,200	4,187	201,906
35–39	8,096	7,050	6,417	6,185	5,888	219,601
40–44	7,708	7,687	7,261	7,106	6,813	177,250
45–49	5,676	5,506	5,662	5,456	5,749	112,896
50–54	3,393	3,466	3,472	3,578	3,636	63,408
55–59	1,711	1,830	1,839	2,005	2,040	34,160
60–64	865	898	856	949	980	18,249
≥65	770	786	711	829	800	15,853
Race/ethnicity						
American Indian/Alaska Native	181	184	164	148	158	3,492
Asian[b]	394	389	378	425	475	7,511
Black/African American	19,580	18,719	17,690	17,257	17,507	426,003
Hispanic/Latino[c]	7,214	6,817	6,804	6,875	6,921	169,138
Native Hawaiian/other Pacific Islander	52	51	58	61	76	721
White	11,061	11,064	10,580	10,521	10,407	404,465
Transmission category						
Male adult or adolescent						
Male-to-male sexual contact	16,782	16,627	16,172	16,235	16,749	487,695
Injection drug use	5,098	4,527	4,243	3,940	3,750	175,704
Male-to-male sexual contact and injection drug use	2,129	1,964	1,972	1,748	1,664	71,242
High-risk heterosexual contact[d]	4,140	4,204	3,909	4,054	4,011	63,927
Other[e]	220	222	230	209	181	12,108
Subtotal	28,370	27,545	26,525	26,185	26,355	810,676
Female adult or adolescent						
Injection drug use	3,002	2,884	2,604	2,331	2,260	80,155
High-risk heterosexual contact[d]	7,247	6,956	6,768	6,955	7,100	112,230
Other[e]	202	193	176	186	220	6,158
Subtotal	10,450	10,033	9,548	9,471	9,579	198,544
Child (<13 yrs at diagnosis)						
Perinatal	66	53	48	33	24	8,434
Other[f]	7	2	5	6	4	775
Subtotal	73	55	54	38	28	9,209
Region of residence						
Northeast	10,432	9,349	9,115	9,143	8,973	314,277
Midwest	4,264	4,074	4,328	4,082	4,074	105,573
South	17,643	18,089	16,641	16,271	16,683	390,479
West	6,555	6,122	6,043	6,199	6,232	208,099
Subtotal for 50 states and the District of Columbia	38,893	37,633	36,127	35,695	35,962	1,018,428
Data for U.S. dependent areas	1,085	917	955	832	812	32,051
Total[g]	**40,054**	**38,695**	**37,256**	**36,791**	**37,041**	**1,051,875[h]**

Note: These numbers do not represent reported case counts. Rather, these numbers are point estimates, which result from adjustments of reported case counts. The reported case counts have been adjusted for reporting delays and missing risk-factor information, but not for incomplete reporting.
[a]From the beginning of the epidemic through 2007.
[b]Includes Asian/Pacific Islander legacy cases.
[c]Hispanics/Latinos can be of any race.
[d]Heterosexual contact with a person known to have, or to be at high risk for, HIV infection.
[e]Includes hemophilia, blood transfusion, perinatal exposure, and risk factor not reported or not identified.
[f]Includes hemophilia, blood transfusion, and risk factor not reported or not identified.
[g]Includes persons of unknown race or multiple races and persons of unknown sex. Because column totals were calculated independently of the values for the subpopulations, the values in each column may not sum to the column total.
[h]Includes 7,099 persons of unknown race or multiple races, 1,393 persons of unknown state of residence, and 3 persons who were residents of other areas.

SOURCE: "Table 4. Estimated Numbers of AIDS Cases, by Year of Diagnosis and Selected Characteristics, 2003–2007 and Cumulative—United States and Dependent Areas," in *HIV/AIDS Surveillance Report, 2007*, vol. 19, Centers for Disease Control and Prevention, 2009, http://www.cdc.gov/hiv/topics/surveillance/resources/reports/2007report/pdf/table4.pdf (accessed June 21, 2009)

TABLE 3.8

Estimated numbers of cases and rates of AIDS, by race/ethnicity, age, and gender, 2007

[34 states with confidential name-based HIV infection reporting]

	Adults or adolescents						Children (<13 yrs)		Total, all[a]	
	Males		Females		Total[a]					
Race/ethnicity	No.	Rate	No.	Rate	No.	Rate	No.	Rate	No.	Rate
American Indian/Alaska Native	160	23.1	68	9.4	228	16.1	0	0.0	228	12.8
Asian[b]	363	15.5	88	3.5	451	9.3	4	0.4	455	7.7
Black/African American	14,247	136.8	7,196	60.6	21,442	96.2	107	1.9	21,549	76.7
Hispanic/Latino[c]	5,906	56.2	1,555	16.0	7,460	36.9	24	0.4	7,484	27.7
Native Hawaiian/other Pacific Islander	42	76.7	5	9.0	46	43.4	0	0.0	46	34.6
White	10,563	18.7	1,971	3.3	12,534	10.8	21	0.1	12,556	9.2
Total[d]	**31,518**	**38.8**	**10,977**	**12.9**	**42,496**	**25.6**	**159**	**0.4**	**42,655[e]**	**21.1**

Notes: These numbers do not represent reported case counts. Rather, these numbers are point estimates, which result from adjustments of reported case counts. The reported case counts have been adjusted for reporting delays, but not for incomplete reporting.
Data include persons with a diagnosis of HIV infection (not AIDS), a diagnosis of HIV infection and a later diagnosis of AIDS, or concurrent diagnoses of HIV infection and AIDS.
[a]Because row totals were calculated independently of the values for the subpopulations, the values in each row may not sum to the row total.
[b]Includes Asian/Pacific Islander legacy cases.
[c]Hispanics/Latinos can be of any race.
[d]Includes persons of unknown race or multiple races. Because column totals were calculated independently of the values for the subpopulations, the values in each column may not sum to the column total.
[e]Includes 336 persons of unknown race or multiple races.

SOURCE: "Table 6a. Estimated Numbers of Cases and Rates (per 100,000 Population) of HIV/AIDS, by Race/Ethnicity, 2007—34 States with Confidential Name-Based HIV Infection Reporting," in *HIV/AIDS Surveillance Report, 2007*, vol. 19, Centers for Disease Control and Prevention, 2009, http://www.cdc .gov/hiv/topics/surveillance/resources/reports/2007report/pdf/table6ab.pdf (accessed June 21, 2009)

TABLE 3.9

Reported cases of HIV/AIDS in infants born to HIV-infected mothers, by year of report and selected characteristics, 1994–2007

[25 states with confidential name-based HIV infection reporting]

	Year of report													
	1994	1995	1996	1997	1998	1999	2000	2001	2002	2003	2004	2005	2006	2007
Child's race/ethnicity														
American Indian/Alaska Native	5	1	0	1	0	1	0	0	1	1	0	1	2	0
Asian[a]	1	0	0	1	1	0	1	0	0	1	0	2	2	2
Black/African American	215	200	158	120	94	77	77	84	66	62	61	70	47	57
Hispanic/Latino[b]	31	20	19	14	10	11	15	13	18	10	15	18	8	9
Native Hawaiian/other Pacific Islander	0	0	0	0	0	0	0	0	0	0	0	0	0	0
White	76	73	45	25	27	18	10	17	20	15	10	15	11	9
Perinatal transmission category														
Mother with documented HIV infection or 1 of the following risk factors Injection drug use	120	90	77	49	23	23	24	21	13	9	6	18	7	11
Sex with injection drug user	65	43	40	27	19	21	8	9	11	7	5	8	6	5
Sex with bisexual male	8	11	5	5	2	5	3	5	2	5	4	6	2	0
Sex with person with hemophilia	2	2	0	0	1	1	1	1	0	1	0	0	0	0
Sex with HIV-infected transfusion recipient	1	0	0	0	0	0	0	0	0	0	0	0	0	1
Sex with HIV-infected person, risk factor not specified	82	86	49	53	46	29	42	47	40	40	33	35	24	15
Receipt of blood transfusion, blood components, or tissue	6	4	3	2	2	1	0	2	1	0	0	0	0	0
Has HIV infection, risk factor not specified	46	59	50	30	39	29	25	30	40	32	38	40	35	47
Child's diagnosis[c]														
HIV infection	123	130	114	89	90	68	73	74	71	76	68	88	58	64
AIDS	207	165	110	77	42	41	30	41	36	18	18	19	16	15
Total[d]	**330**	**295**	**224**	**166**	**132**	**109**	**103**	**115**	**107**	**94**	**86**	**107**	**74**	**79**

Notes: Since 1994, the following 25 states have had laws and regulations requiring confidential name-based HIV infection reporting: Alabama, Arizona, Arkansas, Colorado, Idaho, Indiana, Louisiana, Michigan, Minnesota, Mississippi, Missouri, Nevada, New Jersey, North Carolina, North Dakota, Ohio, Oklahoma, South Carolina, South Dakota, Tennessee, Utah, Virginia, West Virginia, Wisconsin, and Wyoming.
Data include children with a diagnosis of HIV infection (not AIDS), a diagnosis of HIV infection and a later diagnosis of AIDS, or concurrent diagnoses of HIV infection and AIDS.
[a]Includes Asian/Pacific Islander legacy cases.
[b]Hispanics/Latinos can be of any race.
[c]In the surveillance system as of June 2008.
[d]Includes children of unknown race or multiple races.

SOURCE: "Table 25. Reported Cases of HIV/AIDS in Infants Born to HIV-Infected Mothers, by Year of Report and Selected Characteristics, 1994–2007—25 States with Confidential Name-Based HIV Infection Reporting," in *HIV/AIDS Surveillance Report, 2007*, vol. 19, Centers for Disease Control and Prevention, 2009, http://www.cdc.gov/hiv/topics/surveillance/resources/reports/2007report/pdf/table25.pdf (accessed June 21, 2009)

TABLE 3.10

Reported AIDS cases for male adults and adolescents, by transmission category and race/ethnicity, 2007 and cumulative

[United States and dependent areas]

Transmission category	2007 No.	2007 %	Cumulative[a] No.	Cumulative[a] %
American Indian/Alaska Native				
Male-to-male sexual contact	71	54	1,473	55
Injection drug use	18	14	410	15
Male-to-male sexual contact and injection drug use	15	11	477	18
Hemophilia/coagulation disorder	0	0	25	1
High-risk heterosexual contact[b]	6	5	119	4
Sex with injection drug user	1	1	31	1
Sex with person with hemophilia	0	0	0	0
Sex with HIV-infected transfusion recipient	0	0	3	0
Sex with HIV-infected person, risk factor not specified	5	4	85	3
Receipt of blood transfusion, blood components, or tissue	1	1	8	0
Other/risk factor not reported or identified	20	15	171	6
Total	**131**	**100**	**2,683**	**100**
Asian[c]				
Male-to-male sexual contact	216	57	4,154	67
Injection drug use	16	4	299	5
Male-to-male sexual contact and injection drug use	10	3	260	4
Hemophilia/coagulation disorder	1	0	63	1
High-risk heterosexual contact[b]	34	9	378	6
Sex with injection drug user	4	1	49	1
Sex with person with hemophilia	0	0	1	0
Sex with HIV-infected transfusion recipient	2	1	12	0
Sex with HIV-infected person, risk factor not specified	28	7	316	5
Receipt of blood transfusion, blood components, or tissue	4	1	104	2
Other/risk factor not reported or identified	96	25	973	16
Total	**377**	**100**	**6,231**	**100**
Black/African American				
Male-to-male sexual contact	4,497	39	108,134	37
Injection drug use	1,391	12	84,645	29
Male-to-male sexual contact and injection drug use	460	4	22,917	8
Hemophilia/coagulation disorder	9	0	614	0
High-risk heterosexual contact[b]	1,677	15	31,669	11
Sex with injection drug user	149	1	6,949	2
Sex with person with hemophilia	2	0	41	0
Sex with HIV-infected transfusion recipient	11	0	249	0
Sex with HIV-infected person, risk factor not specified	1,515	13	24,430	8
Receipt of blood transfusion, blood components, or tissue	20	0	1,195	0
Other/risk factor not reported or identified	3,497	30	42,527	15
Total	**11,551**	**100**	**291,701**	**100**
Hispanic/Latino[d]				
Male-to-male sexual contact	2,926	48	68,278	44
Injection drug use	903	15	47,344	30
Male-to-male sexual contact and injection drug use	297	5	11,366	7
Hemophilia/coagulation disorder	4	0	468	0
High-risk heterosexual contact[b]	626	10	11,698	8
Sex with injection drug user	67	1	2,489	2
Sex with person with hemophilia	1	0	12	0
Sex with HIV-infected transfusion recipient	8	0	133	0
Sex with HIV-infected person, risk factor not specified	550	9	9,064	6
Receipt of blood transfusion, blood components, or tissue	8	0	663	0
Other/risk factor not reported or identified	1,350	22	15,743	10
Total	**6,114**	**100**	**155,560**	**100**

TABLE 3.10

Reported AIDS cases for male adults and adolescents, by transmission category and race/ethnicity, 2007 and cumulative

[CONTINUED]

[United States and dependent areas]

Transmission category	2007 No.	2007 %	Cumulative[a] No.	Cumulative[a] %
Native Hawaiian/other Pacific Islander				
Male-to-male sexual contact	39	70	430	76
Injection drug use	2	4	26	5
Male-to-male sexual contact and injection drug use	3	5	29	5
Hemophilia/coagulation disorder	0	0	5	1
High-risk heterosexual contact[b]	1	2	28	5
Sex with injection drug user	0	0	5	1
Sex with person with hemophilia	0	0	0	0
Sex with HIV-infected transfusion recipient	0	0	0	0
Sex with HIV-infected person, risk factor not specified	1	2	23	4
Receipt of blood transfusion, blood components, or tissue	0	0	3	1
Other/risk factor not reported or identified	11	20	42	7
Total	**56**	**100**	**563**	**100**
White				
Male-to-male sexual contact	6,490	66	260,797	73
Injection drug use	737	8	32,425	9
Male-to-male sexual contact and injection drug use	711	7	32,325	9
Hemophilia/coagulation disorder	23	0	4,013	1
High-risk heterosexual contact[b]	417	4	8,260	2
Sex with injection drug user	56	1	2,348	1
Sex with person with hemophilia	1	0	36	0
Sex with HIV-infected transfusion recipient	10	0	183	0
Sex with HIV-infected person, risk factor not specified	350	4	5,693	2
Receipt of blood transfusion, blood components, or tissue	17	0	3,176	1
Other/risk factor not reported or identified	1,410	14	17,302	5
Total	**9,805**	**100**	**358,298**	**100**
Total				
Male-to-male sexual contact	14,383	51	445,645	54
Injection drug use	3,103	11	166,251	20
Male-to-male sexual contact and injection drug use	1,514	5	67,797	8
Hemophilia/coagulation disorder	37	0	5,212	1
High-risk heterosexual contact[b]	2,791	10	52,623	6
Sex with injection drug user	281	1	11,941	1
Sex with person with hemophilia	4	0	90	0
Sex with HIV-infected transfusion recipient	31	0	584	0
Sex with HIV-infected person, risk factor not specified	2,475	9	40,008	5
Receipt of blood transfusion, blood components, or tissue	50	0	5,181	1
Other/risk factor not reported or identified	6,442	23	77,328	9
Total	**28,320[e]**	**100**	**820,037[f]**	**100**

[a]From the beginning of the epidemic through 2007.
[b]Heterosexual contact with a person known to have, or to be at high risk for, HIV infection.
[c]Includes Asian/Pacific Islander legacy cases.
[d]Hispanics/Latinos can be of any race.
[e]Includes 286 males of unknown race or multiple races.
[f]Includes 5,001 males of unknown race or multiple races.

SOURCE: "Table 21. Reported AIDS Cases for Male Adults and Adolescents, by Transmission Category and Race/Ethnicity, 2007 and Cumulative—United States and Dependent Areas," in *HIV/AIDS Surveillance Report, 2007*, vol. 19, Centers for Disease Control and Prevention, 2009, http://www.cdc.gov/hiv/topics/surveillance/resources/reports/2007report/pdf/table21.pdf (accessed June 21, 2009).

TABLE 3.11

Reported AIDS cases for female adults and adolescents, by transmission category and race/ethnicity, 2007 and cumulative

[United States and dependent areas]

Transmission category	2007 No.	2007 %	Cumulative[a] No.	Cumulative[a] %
American Indian/Alaska Native				
Injection drug use	8	18	286	40
Hemophilia/coagulation disorder	0	0	3	0
High-risk heterosexual contact[b]	22	50	299	42
Sex with injection drug user	7	16	115	16
Sex with bisexual male	1	2	28	4
Sex with person with hemophilia	0	0	2	0
Sex with HIV-infected transfusion recipient	0	0	6	1
Sex with HIV-infected person, risk factor not specified	14	32	148	21
Receipt of blood transfusion, blood components, or tissue	1	2	18	3
Other/risk factor not reported or identified	13	30	105	15
Total	**44**	**100**	**711**	**100**
Asian[c]				
Injection drug use	2	2	95	9
Hemophilia/coagulation disorder	0	0	7	1
High-risk heterosexual contact[b]	47	53	540	54
Sex with injection drug user	5	6	92	9
Sex with bisexual male	2	2	74	7
Sex with person with hemophilia	0	0	3	0
Sex with HIV-infected transfusion recipient	0	0	18	2
Sex with HIV-infected person, risk factor not specified	40	45	353	35
Receipt of blood transfusion, blood components, or tissue	3	3	87	9
Other/risk factor not reported or identified	36	41	274	27
Total	**88**	**100**	**1,003**	**100**
Black/African American				
Injection drug use	817	13	39,793	33
Hemophilia/coagulation disorder	7	0	149	0
High-risk heterosexual contact[b]	2,928	46	52,928	44
Sex with injection drug user	345	5	13,871	12
Sex with bisexual male	139	2	2,498	2
Sex with person with hemophilia	3	0	122	0
Sex with HIV-infected transfusion recipient	17	0	297	0
Sex with HIV-infected person, risk factor not specified	2,424	38	36,140	30
Receipt of blood transfusion, blood components, or tissue	33	1	1,517	1
Other/risk factor not reported or identified	2,516	40	25,761	21
Total	**6,301**	**100**	**120,148**	**100**
Hispanic/Latino[d]				
Injection drug use	313	18	13,298	35
Hemophilia/coagulation disorder	0	0	68	0
High-risk heterosexual contact[b]	894	52	18,991	50
Sex with injection drug user	152	9	6,705	17
Sex with bisexual male	33	2	857	2
Sex with person with hemophilia	1	0	46	0
Sex with HIV-infected transfusion recipient	3	0	142	0
Sex with HIV-infected person, risk factor not specified	705	41	11,241	29
Receipt of blood transfusion, blood components, or tissue	8	0	613	2
Other/risk factor not reported or identified	490	29	5,370	14
Total	**1,705**	**100**	**38,340**	**100**

TABLE 3.11

Reported AIDS cases for female adults and adolescents, by transmission category and race/ethnicity, 2007 and cumulative
[CONTINUED]

[United States and dependent areas]

Transmission category	2007 No.	2007 %	Cumulative[a] No.	Cumulative[a] %
Native Hawaiian/other Pacific Islander				
Injection drug use	2	14	22	19
Hemophilia/coagulation disorder	0	0	0	0
High-risk heterosexual contact[b]	8	57	63	54
Sex with injection drug user	1	7	23	20
Sex with bisexual male	1	7	7	6
Sex with person with hemophilia	0	0	1	1
Sex with HIV-infected transfusion recipient	0	0	2	2
Sex with HIV-infected person, risk factor not specified	6	43	30	26
Receipt of blood transfusion, blood components, or tissue	1	7	6	5
Other/risk factor not reported or identified	3	21	25	22
Total	**14**	**100**	**116**	**100**
White				
Injection drug use	471	28	15,473	40
Hemophilia/coagulation disorder	2	0	125	0
High-risk heterosexual contact[b]	756	45	16,541	42
Sex with injection drug user	188	11	5,839	15
Sex with bisexual male	55	3	1,915	5
Sex with person with hemophilia	6	0	336	1
Sex with HIV-infected transfusion recipient	5	0	344	1
Sex with HIV-infected person, risk factor not specified	502	30	8,107	21
Receipt of blood transfusion, blood components, or tissue	12	1	1,858	5
Other/risk factor not reported or identified	452	27	5,046	13
Total	**1,693**	**100**	**39,043**	**100**
Total				
Injection drug use	1,633	16	69,591	35
Hemophilia/coagulation disorder	9	0	355	0
High-risk heterosexual contact[b]	4,713	47	90,229	45
Sex with injection drug user	704	7	26,825	13
Sex with bisexual male	233	2	5,415	3
Sex with person with hemophilia	10	0	513	0
Sex with HIV-infected transfusion recipient	25	0	819	0
Sex with HIV-infected person, risk factor not specified	3,741	37	56,657	28
Receipt of blood transfusion, blood components, or tissue	59	1	4,134	2
Other/risk factor not reported or identified	3,563	36	36,896	18
Total	**9,977[e]**	**100**	**201,205[f]**	**100**

[a]From the beginning of the epidemic through 2007.
[b]Heterosexual contact with a person known to have, or to be at high risk for, HIV infection.
[c]Includes Asian/Pacific Islander legacy cases.
[d]Hispanics/Latinos can be of any race.
[e]Includes 132 females of unknown race or multiple races.
[f]Includes 1,844 females of unknown race or multiple races.

SOURCE: "Table 23. Reported AIDS Cases for Female Adults and Adolescents, by Transmission Category and Race/Ethnicity, 2007 and Cumulative—United States and Dependent Areas," in *HIV/AIDS Surveillance Report, 2007*, vol. 19, Centers for Disease Control and Prevention, 2009, http://www.cdc.gov/hiv/topics/surveillance/resources/reports/2007report/pdf/table23.pdf (accessed June 21, 2009)

TABLE 3.12

Estimated numbers of deaths of persons with AIDS by year of death and selected characteristics, 2003–07 and cumulative

[United States and dependent areas]

	Year of death					
	2003	2004	2005	2006	2007	Cumulative[a]
Data for 50 states and the District of Columbia						
Age at death (yr)						
<13	24	14	6	16	5	4,891
13–14	7	15	10	4	17	292
15–19	36	34	38	44	41	1,143
20–24	162	173	143	164	155	8,880
25–29	522	489	452	437	440	44,219
30–34	1,298	1,147	1,062	841	766	96,379
35–39	2,821	2,443	2,078	1,815	1,600	118,886
40–44	3,582	3,434	3,316	2,857	2,660	107,417
45–49	3,307	3,283	3,287	3,103	2,865	76,249
50–54	2,442	2,543	2,622	2,494	2,411	47,022
55–59	1,368	1,425	1,558	1,532	1,476	26,767
60–64	721	738	798	813	817	15,244
≥65	792	830	879	868	858	15,404
Race/ethnicity						
American Indian/Alaska Native	75	85	70	79	70	1,792
Asian[b]	73	92	71	99	84	3,114
Black/African American	8,926	8,656	8,546	7,886	7,124	226,879
Hispanic/Latino[c]	2,627	2,601	2,450	2,256	2,312	82,894
Native Hawaiian/other Pacific Islander	5	17	14	4	11	291
White	5,231	4,963	4,933	4,398	4,187	245,127
Transmission category						
Male adult or adolescent						
Male-to-male sexual contact	6,131	5,896	5,888	5,329	5,373	274,184
Injection drug use	3,655	3,356	3,245	2,820	2,397	112,068
Male-to-male sexual contact and injection drug use	1,343	1,262	1,318	1,154	1,054	42,551
High-risk heterosexual contact[d]	1,436	1,514	1,467	1,543	1,433	25,860
Other[e]	163	137	126	98	83	8,728
Subtotal	12,728	12,166	12,044	10,945	10,339	463,392
Female adult or adolescent						
Injection drug use	1,955	1,966	1,816	1,594	1,446	46,624
High-risk heterosexual contact[d]	2,257	2,312	2,283	2,321	2,211	43,432
Other[e]	86	71	70	75	57	3,928
Subtotal	4,298	4,350	4,169	3,991	3,714	93,984
Child (<13 yrs at diagnosis)						
Perinatal	50	52	33	46	50	4,842
Other[f]	7	2	3	7	7	575
Subtotal	57	54	37	53	57	5,417
Region of residence						
Northeast	4,992	4,708	4,435	4,076	3,463	183,292
Midwest	1,700	1,491	1,387	1,478	1,368	56,137
South	7,735	7,678	7,812	7,282	7,080	206,654
West	2,655	2,693	2,615	2,152	2,200	116,710
Subtotal for 50 states and the District of Columbia	17,082	16,570	16,249	14,989	14,110	562,793
Data for U.S. dependent areas	574	568	535	541	403	20,178
Total[g]	**17,679**	**17,154**	**16,823**	**15,564**	**14,561**	**583,298[h]**

Notes: These numbers do not represent reported death counts. Rather, these numbers are point estimates, which result from adjustments of reported death counts. The reported death counts have been adjusted for reporting delays and missing risk-factor information, but not for incomplete reporting.
[a]From the beginning of the epidemic through 2007.
[b]Includes Asian/Pacific Islander legacy cases.
[c]Hispanics/Latinos can be of any race.
[d]Heterosexual contact with a person known to have, or to be at high risk for, HIV infection.
[e]Includes hemophilia, blood transfusion, perinatal exposure, and risk factor not reported or not identified.
[f]Includes hemophilia, blood transfusion, and risk factor not reported or not identified.
[g]Includes persons of unknown race or multiple races and persons of unknown sex. Because column totals were calculated independently of the values for the subpopulations, the values in each column may not sum to the column total.
[h]Includes 2,704 persons of unknown race or multiple races, 325 persons of unknown state of residence, and 2 persons who were residents of other areas.

SOURCE: "Table 8. Estimated Numbers of Deaths of Persons with AIDS, by Year of Death and Selected Characteristics, 2003–2007 and Cumulative—United States and Dependent Areas," in *HIV/AIDS Surveillance Report, 2007*, vol. 19, Centers for Disease Control and Prevention, 2009, http://www.cdc.gov/hiv/topics/surveillance/resources/reports/2007report/pdf/table8.pdf (accessed June 21, 2009).

FIGURE 3.4

Proportion of persons surviving, by number of months after AIDS diagnosis, 1998–2005

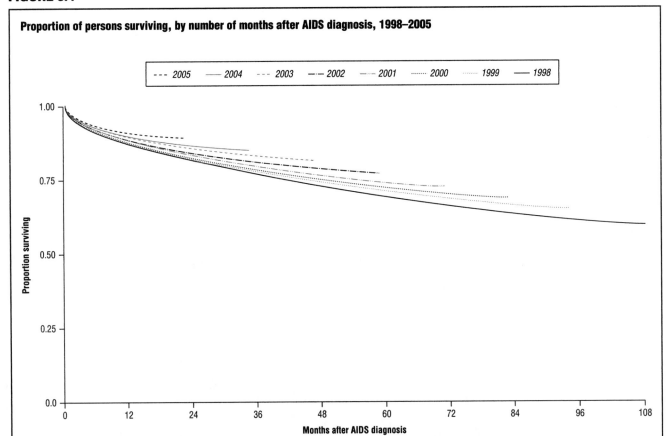

SOURCE: "Slide 24. Proportion of Persons Surviving, by Months after AIDS Diagnosis during 1998–2005 and by Year of Diagnosis—United States and Dependent Areas," in *AIDS Surveillance—General Epidemiology (through 2006)*, Centers for Disease Control and Prevention, May 20, 2008 http://www .cdc.gov/hiv/topics/surveillance/resources/slides/epidemiology/slides/EPI-AIDS_24.pdf (accessed June 21, 2009)

CHAPTER 4
POPULATIONS AT RISK

This chapter examines the prevalence rates of HIV infection—that is, the number of people who have the disease in a specified time period as opposed to (often at the end of a given year) the total number of people in the population being examined. Prevalence rates are based on surveys of selected segments of the general population and the prevalence rates of people in high-risk groups. These are not absolute numbers. The actual number of cases of HIV infection is likely to be higher than those reported in this chapter, because reporting is not universal and, as of September 2009, only 34 U.S. states and five U.S. dependent areas subscribed to confidential reporting practices. However, information on prevalence rates serves as a road map that reveals trends such as the geographic distribution of disease or changes in how the disease is transmitted.

INCREASE IN AIDS
AMONG HETEROSEXUALS

The increase in the number and proportion of HIV/AIDS cases among heterosexuals signals a major shift in the patterns of the epidemic. In 1997 the Centers for Disease Control and Prevention (CDC) reported that people diagnosed with AIDS who acquired HIV through heterosexual transmission accounted for the largest proportional increase of all cases in the previous year. During 2007, 38,384 new cases of AIDS among adults and adolescents were reported to the CDC. (See Table 3.5 in Chapter 3.) Twenty percent (7,504) of these new cases were people who reported that their only exposure was through heterosexual contact. In comparison, the CDC reports in *Weekly Surveillance Report, 1985* (December 30, 1985, http://www.cdc.gov/hiv/topics/surveillance/resources/reports/pdf/surveillance85.pdf) that 1% of all AIDS cases were attributable to heterosexual transmission in 1985.

The CDC notes that between 1997 and 2000 the number of new AIDS cases dropped significantly, and that the proportions of those infected in each exposure category

also changed. Cases attributed to male-to-male sexual contact (MSM) represented 35% of all cases in 1997 and 1998, dropping to 34% in 1999, 32% in 2000, and 31% in 2001. In 2003 the MSM rate rebounded to 35% and by 2007 it accounted for 51% of new cases. (See Table 3.5 in Chapter 3.) Despite the decline from the late 1990s, MSM continued to represent the largest proportion (46% in both 2000 and 2001, 45% in 2003, and 44% in 2007) of cumulative AIDS cases since 1981.

In 2007 the majority of HIV/AIDS cases in women were attributed to high-risk heterosexual contact, which accounted for 83% of cases in female adults and adolescents (though this figure includes those who acquired HIV/AIDS through blood transfusion, perinatal exposure, and other risk factors not reported or not identified). (See Figure 4.1.) Among women, 16% of HIV/AIDS cases were attributed to injection drug use (IDU) in 2007.

The proportion of women who contracted AIDS through heterosexual contact remained relatively constant at 37% in 2001 and 38% in 2002. However, in 2003 the proportion increased to 45%, and in 2007 it had risen to 47%. (See Table 3.5 in Chapter 3.)

Risks of Heterosexual Contact

Figure 4.2 shows how African-American females continue to be disproportionately affected—in 2007 two-thirds (66%) of HIV/AIDS cases among female adults and adolescents were among African-American females, even though African-Americans accounted for just 14% of the female population in the United States. Although not as dramatically, Hispanic females are also disproportionately affected. In 2007 Hispanic females made up 11% of the female population but accounted for 14% of HIV/AIDS cases among females. In contrast, white females made up 70% of the female adult and adolescent population but accounted for 18% of HIV/AIDS cases among females.

FIGURE 4.1

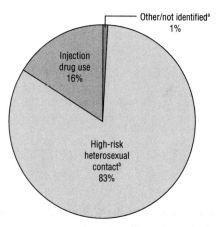

Percentages of HIV/AIDS cases among female adults and adolescents, by transmission category, 2007

[34 states]

Notes: Data include persons with a diagnosis of HIV infection regardless of their AIDS status at diagnosis. Data from 34 states with confidential name-based HIV infection reporting since at least 2003. Data have been adjusted for reporting delays and missing risk-factor information.
^aHeterosexual contact with a person known to have, or to be at high risk for, HIV infection.
^bIncludes blood transfusion, perinatal exposure, and risk factor not reported or not identified.

SOURCE: "Slide 9. Percentages of HIV/AIDS Cases among Female Adults and Adolescents, by Transmission Category 2007—34 States," in *HIV/AIDS Surveillance in Women*, Centers for Disease Control and Prevention, May 5, 2009, http://www.cdc.gov/hiv/topics/surveillance/resources/slides/women/slides/Women9.pdf (accessed June 21, 2009)

High-risk heterosexual contact accounted for 3,333 cases of HIV infection among male adults and adolescents in 2007. (See Table 4.1.) Of those 3,333 cases, 60% were African-American (2,009 cases), 20% were Hispanic (677 cases), and 17% were white males (571 cases).

INJECTION DRUG USERS

In *Preventing HIV Transmission: The Role of Sterile Needles and Bleach* (1995), Jacques Normand, David Vlahov, and Lincoln E. Moses of the National Academy of Sciences concluded that "the HIV epidemic in this country is now clearly driven by infections occurring in the population of injection drug users, their sexual partners, and their offspring." During the 1990s the proportions of both HIV infection and AIDS deaths attributable to IDU among adults and adolescents increased. According to the CDC, in 1995 IDU was the exposure category for 25% of male and 47% of female AIDS deaths. To prevent a rise in IDU-associated HIV infection and AIDS, Normand, Vlahov, and Moses urged policymakers to adequately fund needle exchange programs. Since 1995 the percentage of HIV/AIDS cases attributable to IDU has been steadily decreasing. By 2007 IDU accounted for 8% of cases of HIV infection in male adults and adolescents and 16% of

FIGURE 4.2

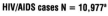

Percentages of HIV/AIDS cases among female adults and adolescents, by race/ethnicity, 2007

[34 states]

HIV/AIDS cases N = 10,977^a

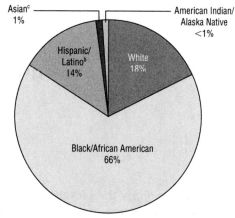

Female population, 34 States N = 85,031,796

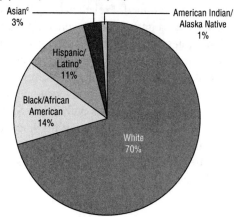

Notes: Data include persons with a diagnosis of HIV infection regardless of their AIDS status at diagnosis.
Data from 34 states with confidential name-based HIV infection reporting since at least 2003. Data have been adjusted for reporting delays.
^aIncludes 95 female adults and adolescents of unknown race or multiple races.
^bHispanics/Latinos can be of any race.
^cIncludes Asian and Pacific Islander legacy cases.

SOURCE: "Slide 10. Percentages of HIV/AIDS Cases and Population among Female Adults and Adolescents, by Race/Ethnicity 2007—34 States," in *HIV/AIDS Surveillance in Women*, Centers for Disease Control and Prevention, May 5, 2009, http://www.cdc.gov/hiv/topics/surveillance/resources/slides/women/slides/Women10.pdf (accessed June 21, 2009)

cases in female adults and adolescents. (See Table 4.1 and Figure 4.1.)

How HIV Is Transmitted through Injection Drug Use

HIV can be transmitted through IDU when the blood of an HIV-infected drug user is transferred to a drug user who is not yet infected with HIV. This transfer occurs almost

TABLE 4.1

Reported cases of HIV infection for male adults and adolescents, by transmission category and race/ethnicity, 2007 and cumulative

[47 states, the District of Columbia, and 5 U.S. dependent areas with confidential name-based HIV infection reporting]

Transmission category	2007 No.	2007 %	Cumulative[a] No.	Cumulative[a] %
American Indian/Alaska Native				
Male-to-male sexual contact	123	61	614	58
Injection drug use	13	6	106	10
Male-to-male sexual contact and injection drug use	21	10	130	12
Hemophilia/coagulation disorder	1	0	1	0
High-risk heterosexual contact[b]	10	5	63	6
Sex with injection drug user	1	0	16	2
Sex with person with hemophilia	0	0	0	0
Sex with HIV-infected transfusion recipient	0	0	0	0
Sex with HIV-infected person, risk factor not specified	9	4	47	4
Receipt of blood transfusion, blood components, or tissue	0	0	1	0
Other/risk factor not reported or identified	33	16	143	14
Total	**201**	**100**	**1,058**	**100**
Asian[c]				
Male-to-male sexual contact	596	77	1,362	68
Injection drug use	11	1	56	3
Male-to-male sexual contact and injection drug use	22	3	46	2
Hemophilia/coagulation disorder	0	0	1	0
High-risk heterosexual contact[b]	41	5	120	6
Sex with injection drug user	0	0	6	0
Sex with person with hemophilia	0	0	0	0
Sex with HIV-infected transfusion recipient	3	0	5	0
Sex with HIV-infected person, risk factor not specified	38	5	109	5
Receipt of blood transfusion, blood components, or tissue	4	1	9	0
Other/risk factor not reported or identified	102	13	400	20
Total	**776**	**100**	**1,994**	**100**
Black/African American				
Male-to-male sexual contact	7,320	45	36,389	39
Injection drug use	1,510	9	13,189	14
Male-to-male sexual contact and injection drug use	526	3	3,958	4
Hemophilia/coagulation disorder	13	0	120	0
High-risk heterosexual contact[b]	2,009	12	12,470	13
Sex with injection drug user	180	1	1,662	2
Sex with person with hemophilia	1	0	16	0
Sex with HIV-infected transfusion recipient	10	0	83	0
Sex with HIV-infected person, risk factor not specified	1,818	11	10,709	11
Receipt of blood transfusion, blood components, or tissue	24	0	228	0
Other/risk factor not reported or identified	4,877	30	27,421	29
Total	**16,279**	**100**	**93,775**	**100**

TABLE 4.1

Reported cases of HIV infection for male adults and adolescents, by transmission category and race/ethnicity, 2007 and cumulative
[CONTINUED]

[47 states, the District of Columbia, and 5 U.S. dependent areas with confidential name-based HIV infection reporting]

Transmission category	2007 No.	2007 %	Cumulative[a] No.	Cumulative[a] %
Hispanic/Latino[d]				
Male-to-male sexual contact	6,077	60	21,173	51
Injection drug use	1,115	11	7,327	17
Male-to-male sexual contact and injection drug use	401	4	1,825	4
Hemophilia/coagulation disorder	3	0	32	0
High-risk heterosexual contact[b]	677	7	3,557	8
Sex with injection drug user	98	1	534	1
Sex with person with hemophilia	2	0	8	0
Sex with HIV-infected transfusion recipient	5	0	23	0
Sex with HIV-infected person, risk factor not specified	572	6	2,992	7
Receipt of blood transfusion, blood components, or tissue	16	0	67	0
Other/risk factor not reported or identified	1,768	18	7,931	19
Total	**10,057**	**100**	**41,912**	**100**
Native Hawaiian/other Pacific Islander				
Male-to-male sexual contact	69	76	161	74
Injection drug use	4	4	7	3
Male-to-male sexual contact and injection drug use	4	4	10	5
Hemophilia/coagulation disorder	0	0	0	0
High-risk heterosexual contact[b]	5	5	13	6
Sex with injection drug user	1	1	3	1
Sex with person with hemophilia	0	0	0	0
Sex with HIV-infected transfusion recipient	0	0	0	0
Sex with HIV-infected person, risk factor not specified	4	4	10	5
Receipt of blood transfusion, blood components, or tissue	0	0	1	0
Other/risk factor not reported or identified	9	10	27	12
Total	**91**	**100**	**219**	**100**
White				
Male-to-male sexual contact	15,345	74	69,234	70
Injection drug use	978	5	6,247	6
Male-to-male sexual contact and injection drug use	1,307	6	6,827	7
Hemophilia/coagulation disorder	48	0	403	0
High-risk heterosexual contact[b]	571	3	3,075	3
Sex with injection drug user	62	0	577	1
Sex with person with hemophilia	1	0	8	0
Sex with HIV-infected transfusion recipient	10	0	44	0
Sex with HIV-infected person, risk factor not specified	498	2	2,446	2
Receipt of blood transfusion, blood components, or tissue	19	0	197	0
Other/risk factor not reported or identified	2,393	12	12,541	13
Total	**20,661**	**100**	**98,524**	**100**

exclusively through the sharing of injecting equipment, primarily needles and syringes.

Blood enters and makes contact with the needle and syringe in two ways. The first occurs when blood is drawn into the syringe to verify that the needle is inside a vein, before the injection of the drug. The second occurs follow-

ing the injection, when the syringe is refilled several times with blood from the vein to "wash out" any heroin, cocaine, or other drug left in the syringe after the first injection. Even the smallest amount of HIV-infected blood left in the syringe can cause the virus to be transmitted to the next user of the contaminated syringe and needle.

TABLE 4.1

Reported cases of HIV infection for male adults and adolescents, by transmission category and race/ethnicity, 2007 and cumulative

[CONTINUED]

[47 states, the District of Columbia, and 5 U.S. dependent areas with confidential name-based HIV infection reporting]

Transmission category	2007 No.	2007 %	Cumulative[a] No.	Cumulative[a] %
Total				
Male-to-male sexual contact	29,713	61	129,915	54
Injection drug use	3,653	8	27,158	11
Male-to-male sexual contact and injection drug use	2,298	5	12,920	5
Hemophilia/coagulation disorder	65	0	560	0
High-risk heterosexual contact[b]	3,333	7	19,490	8
Sex with injection drug user	345	1	2,825	1
Sex with person with hemophilia	4	0	32	0
Sex with HIV-infected transfusion recipient	28	0	155	0
Sex with HIV-infected person, risk factor not specified	2,956	6	16,478	7
Receipt of blood transfusion, blood components, or tissue	64	0	510	0
Other/risk factor not reported or identified	9,221	19	49,207	21
Total	**48,347[e]**	**100**	**239,760[f]**	**100**

[a]From the beginning of the epidemic through 2007.
[b]Heterosexual contact with a person known to have, or to be at high risk for, HIV infection.
[c]Includes Asian/Pacific Islander legacy cases.
[d]Hispanics/Latinos can be of any race.
[e]Includes 282 males of unknown race or multiple races.
[f]Includes 2,278 males of unknown race or multiple races.

SOURCE: "Table 22. Reported Cases of HIV Infection (not AIDS) for Male Adults and Adolescents, by Transmission Category and Race/Ethnicity, 2007 and Cumulative—47 States, the District of Columbia, and 5 U.S. Dependent Areas with Confidential Name-Based HIV Infection Reporting," in *HIV/AIDS Surveillance Report, 2007*, vol. 19, Centers for Disease Control and Prevention, 2009, http://www.cdc.gov/hiv/topics/surveillance/resources/reports/2007report/pdf/table22.pdf (accessed June 21, 2009)

Among IDUs the risk of HIV infection increases in proportion to the duration of IDU. Put another way, the longer the drug use, the greater the risk of infection. Diseases such as hepatitis show this same pattern. Risk also increases with the frequency of needle sharing and IDU in a geographic area, such as a large city, where there is a high prevalence of HIV infection.

General Trends

Table 3.5 in Chapter 3 shows that, of the cumulative AIDS cases among adults and adolescents reported from 1981 through 2007 (1,021,242), 235,842 (or 23% of the cumulative total) were attributable to IDU. Cumulatively, 67,797 cases (7%) were attributable to MSM in conjunction with IDU, and an additional 38,766 cases (4%) were the result of heterosexual contact with an IDU.

HIV is also spread among non-IDUs who trade sex for drugs, especially crack cocaine, as well as the partners of these users. Those who trade sex for drugs often engage in unprotected sex and have multiple sex partners.

People who exchange sex for drugs and have a sexually transmitted disease (STD) that causes ulcers or sores on the genitals, such as syphilis or herpes simplex, are at a higher risk for HIV infection. Drug and/or alcohol users may also be at greater risk for infection because these substances often lessen inhibitions and reduce the reluctance to have unsafe, unprotected sex.

Gender and Racial/Ethnic Differences

Annual adult and adolescent rates for HIV/AIDS reported in 2007 were far higher for African-Americans (96.2 per 100,000 people) and Hispanics (36.9 per 100,000) than for whites (10.8 per 100,000) and Native Americans/Alaskan natives (16.1 per 100,000). (See Table 3.8 in Chapter 3.) The lowest rate was for Asian-Americans (9.3 per 100,000).

The CDC reports that 7,506 cases (7,473 adults and adolescents and 33 children under the age of 13) of AIDS reported in 2001 were transmitted by IDUs. By 2007 this number had dropped to 4,754 (4,736 adults and adolescents and 18 children under the age of 13). (See Table 3.5 in Chapter 3.) The number of women acquiring AIDS through IDU in 2000 (2,609), in 2001 (2,212), in 2003 (2,262), in 2005 (2,047), and in 2007 (1,633) was less than the number of women who were infected through heterosexual contact (3,981 in 2000, 4,142 in 2001, 5,234 in 2003, 4,918 in 2005, and 4,713 in 2007). In 2000, 2001, 2003, 2005, and 2007 about 19%, 16%, 15%, 13%, and 11%, respectively, of AIDS cases reported in males was attributable to IDUs, and approximately another 5% to 6% (in 2000, 2001, 2003, 2005, and 2007) were MSM who also injected drugs. (See Table 3.5 in Chapter 3.)

Of the 855 women who became infected with HIV through IDU during 2000, 53% were African-American, 38% were white, and 7% were Hispanic. By 2007 the number of cases of HIV transmission to women via IDU had increased to 2,041. (See Table 4.2.) Of women infected with HIV via IDU in 2007, whites accounted for 36% (733), Hispanics for 18% (375), and African-Americans for 44% (894) of cases. Of the women who were infected with HIV in 2007, 25% of white women acquired the virus from IDU (733 of 2,971 cases in white women); 13% of Hispanic women acquired the virus through IDU (375 of 2,795 cases in Hispanic women); and 11% of African-American women acquired the virus through IDU (894 of 8,119 cases in African-American women).

In men with HIV infection, IDU was second only to MSM as a risk factor from 2000 through 2007. Of the 3,653 men infected with HIV via IDU in 2007, 1,510 (41%) were African-American, 1,115 (31%) were Hispanic, and 978 (27%) were white. (See Table 4.1.) Of men infected with HIV in 2007, 11% of Hispanic men, 9% of African-American men, 6% of Native American and Alaskan Natives, 5% of white men, 4% of Native Hawaiian

TABLE 4.2

Reported cases of HIV infection for female adults and adolescents, by transmission category and race/ethnicity, 2007 and cumulative

[47 states, the District of Columbia, and 5 U.S. dependent areas with confidential name-based HIV infection reporting]

Transmission category	2007		Cumulative[a]	
	No.	%	No.	%
American Indian/Alaska Native				
Injection drug use	18	26	121	28
Hemophilia/coagulation disorder	0	0	0	0
High-risk heterosexual contact[b]	27	39	204	47
Sex with injection drug user	5	7	56	13
Sex with bisexual male	1	1	16	4
Sex with person with hemophilia	0	0	2	0
Sex with HIV-infected transfusion recipient	0	0	0	0
Sex with HIV-infected person, risk factor not specified	21	30	130	30
Receipt of blood transfusion, blood components, or tissue	0	0	1	0
Other/risk factor not reported or identified	24	35	109	25
Total	**69**	**100**	**435**	**100**
Asian[c]				
Injection drug use	7	4	19	4
Hemophilia/coagulation disorder	1	1	2	0
High-risk heterosexual contact[b]	88	54	235	47
Sex with injection drug user	6	4	17	3
Sex with bisexual male	4	2	12	2
Sex with person with hemophilia	0	0	0	0
Sex with HIV-infected transfusion recipient	7	4	7	1
Sex with HIV-infected person, risk factor not specified	71	44	199	40
Receipt of blood transfusion, blood components, or tissue	3	2	7	1
Other/risk factor not reported or identified	63	39	233	47
Total	**162**	**100**	**496**	**100**
Black/African American				
Injection drug use	894	11	7,781	14
Hemophilia/coagulation disorder	2	0	36	0
High-risk heterosexual contact[b]	3,561	44	26,378	46
Sex with injection drug user	358	4	3,660	6
Sex with bisexual male	123	2	1,357	2
Sex with person with hemophilia	8	0	75	0
Sex with HIV-infected transfusion recipient	18	0	138	0
Sex with HIV-infected person, risk factor not specified	3,054	38	21,148	37
Receipt of blood transfusion, blood components, or tissue	40	0	325	1
Other/risk factor not reported or identified	3,622	45	22,212	39
Total	**8,119**	**100**	**56,732**	**100**

TABLE 4.2

Reported cases of HIV infection for female adults and adolescents, by transmission category and race/ethnicity, 2007 and cumulative [CONTINUED]

[47 states, the District of Columbia, and 5 U.S. dependent areas with confidential name-based HIV infection reporting]

Transmission category	2007		Cumulative[a]	
	No.	%	No.	%
Hispanic/Latino[d]				
Injection drug use	375	13	2,578	18
Hemophilia/coagulation disorder	2	0	13	0
High-risk heterosexual contact[b]	1,470	53	7,587	52
Sex with injection drug user	233	8	1,519	10
Sex with bisexual male	63	2	323	2
Sex with person with hemophilia	1	0	12	0
Sex with HIV-infected transfusion recipient	15	1	53	0
Sex with HIV-infected person, risk factor not specified	1,158	41	5,680	39
Receipt of blood transfusion, blood components, or tissue	7	0	56	0
Other/risk factor not reported or identified	941	34	4,374	30
Total	**2,795**	**100**	**14,608**	**100**
Native Hawaiian/other Pacific Islander				
Injection drug use	3	16	9	18
Hemophilia/coagulation disorder	0	0	0	0
High-risk heterosexual contact[b]	13	68	28	56
Sex with injection drug user	3	16	5	10
Sex with bisexual male	0	0	4	8
Sex with person with hemophilia	0	0	0	0
Sex with HIV-infected transfusion recipient	0	0	0	0
Sex with HIV-infected person, risk factor not specified	10	53	19	38
Receipt of blood transfusion, blood components, or tissue	0	0	0	0
Other/risk factor not reported or identified	3	16	13	26
Total	**19**	**100**	**50**	**100**
White				
Injection drug use	733	25	4,819	26
Hemophilia/coagulation disorder	3	0	26	0
High-risk heterosexual contact[b]	1,326	45	8,644	46
Sex with injection drug user	246	8	2,024	11
Sex with bisexual male	105	4	756	4
Sex with person with hemophilia	6	0	116	1
Sex with HIV-infected transfusion recipient	14	0	78	0
Sex with HIV-infected person, risk factor not specified	955	32	5,670	30
Receipt of blood transfusion, blood components, or tissue	17	1	150	1
Other/risk factor not reported or identified	892	30	5,041	27
Total	**2,971**	**100**	**18,680**	**100**

or Pacific Islander men, and 1% of Asian-American men were infected solely via IDU.

WOMEN AND AIDS

The proportion of women among AIDS sufferers increased steadily, from a reported 7% in 1985 to 23% in 1999. (See Figure 4.3.) During 2000 there were about 10,000 American women with AIDS, and since then the number has not varied significantly. By 2007 female adults and adolescents accounted for 27% of AIDS cases.

Nearly half of the 201,205 cumulative 1981–2007 cases of AIDS among females were associated either directly or indirectly with IDU. (See Table 3.5 in Chapter 3.) Of those 96,416 cases, 69,591 cases (72%) occurred among female IDUs and another 26,825 cases (28%) were among women who reported sexual contact with male IDUs.

The racial and ethnic differences among women with AIDS and their children are striking. Even though African-American and Hispanic women made up 14% and 11%, respectively, of all women in the United States in

TABLE 4.2

Reported cases of HIV infection for female adults and adolescents, by transmission category and race/ethnicity, 2007 and cumulative [CONTINUED]

[47 states, the District of Columbia, and 5 U.S. dependent areas with confidential name-based HIV infection reporting]

Transmission category	2007 No.	%	Cumulative[a] No.	%
Total				
Injection drug use	2,041	14	15,509	17
Hemophilia/coagulation disorder	8	0	79	0
High-risk heterosexual contact[b]	6,528	46	43,517	47
Sex with injection drug user	863	6	7,353	8
Sex with bisexual male	299	2	2,491	3
Sex with person with hemophilia	15	0	207	0
Sex with HIV-infected transfusion recipient	54	0	276	0
Sex with HIV-infected person, risk factor not specified	5,297	37	33,190	36
Receipt of blood transfusion, blood components, or tissue	71	0	545	1
Other/risk factor not reported or identified	5,578	39	32,354	35
Total	**14,226[e]**	**100**	**92,004[f]**	**100**

[a]From the beginning of the epidemic through 2007.
[b]Heterosexual contact with a person known to have, or to be at high risk for, HIV infection.
[c]Includes Asian/Pacific Islander legacy cases (see Technical Notes).
[d]Hispanics/Latinos can be of any race.
[e]Includes 91 females of unknown race or multiple races.
[f]Includes 1,003 females of unknown race or multiple races.

SOURCE: "Table 24. Reported Cases of HIV Infection (not AIDS) for Female Adults and Adolescents, by Transmission Category and Race/Ethnicity, 2007 and Cumulative—47 States, the District of Columbia, and U.S. Dependent Areas with Confidential Name-Based HIV Infection Reporting," in *HIV/AIDS Surveillance Report, 2007*, vol. 19, Centers for Disease Control and Prevention, 2009, http://www.cdc.gov/hiv/topics/surveillance/resources/reports/2007report/pdf/table24.pdf (accessed June 22, 2009)

2007, they accounted for 79% (120,148 and 38,340, respectively) of all U.S. women (201,205) diagnosed with AIDS since 1981. (See Table 3.11 in Chapter 3.) The estimated number of AIDS cases diagnosed in females in 2007 was roughly the same for Hispanic (1,452) and white females (1,600); however, the rate for Hispanic females (8.9) was nearly five times as high as the rate for white females (1.8). (See Table 4.3.)

Women can infect their unborn children with HIV in the course of pregnancy, during delivery, or by breast-feeding after birth. The 48% decrease in the number of women who gave birth to HIV-infected babies during the 1990s was largely attributable to the introduction of the antiretroviral drug zidovudine (ZDV; previously called azidothymidine). Women of childbearing age can be tested for HIV perinatally (before and during pregnancy), and, if they are positive, have the option of receiving ZDV to prevent transmitting the virus to their unborn children.

According to the CDC (December 12, 2008, http://www.cdc.gov/hiv/topics/perinatal/1test2lives/default.htm), 91% of all AIDS cases among children in the United States

result from perinatal transmission. The CDC notes that "antiretroviral therapy during pregnancy can reduce the transmission rate to 2% or less. The transmission rate is 25% without treatment."

Along with antiretroviral therapy, which lowers the mother's viral load to undetectable levels, deliveries via elective cesarean section (the surgical delivery of a baby) rather than vaginal births may also help reduce mother-to-child transmission. States with HIV case surveillance data are better able to direct resources (e.g., targeted public health education programs, health professionals, and pre-natal care) aimed at eliminating prenatal (before birth) transmission of HIV.

HIV/AIDS in Women in Small Towns and Rural Areas

Most HIV/AIDS cases occur among women who live in large metropolitan areas with populations of greater than 500,000. However, the number of HIV/AIDS cases is increasing in rural areas, especially through heterosexual transmission. Figure 4.4 reveals that in 2007 the highest rates of AIDS were reported in the District of Columbia (90.2 cases per 100,000 people), the U.S. Virgin Islands (27.2), Maryland (22.2), New York (17.7), and Florida (17) and the lowest rates were reported by states in the Midwest. Because many women live in states that do not have HIV/AIDS surveillance, it is likely that there are many who have not been tested. As a result, the numbers of women with HIV/AIDS may be underestimated.

Sexually Transmitted Diseases

Prevention, identification, and prompt treatment of STDs are vitally important for the health of young women. Most HIV/AIDS cases in young women are spread through heterosexual sex. Women accounted for 90,229 of the 142,852 total cumulative cases spread through heterosexual sex (representing 63% of such cases, while men accounted for only 43% of cases spread this way), and the increase in STDs parallels that of HIV/AIDS. (See Table 3.5 in Chapter 3.) For instance, the geographic areas with the highest numbers of cases of syphilis and gonorrhea have the highest incidence of cases of HIV/AIDS among women of childbearing age.

In "The Role of STD Detection and Treatment in HIV Prevention—CDC Fact Sheet" (April 10, 2008, http://www.cdc.gov/std/hiv/STDFact-STD&HIV.htm), the CDC explains that women with STDs are "at least two to five times more likely than uninfected [women] to acquire HIV infection if they are exposed to the virus through sexual contact" because they have an increased number of HIV target cells (CD4+ T cells) present in their cervical secretions. These cells facilitate the entrance of HIV into the body. Furthermore, women with STDs are more likely to shed HIV in both ulcer-forming and inflammatory genital

FIGURE 4.3

Estimated number and percentages of AIDS cases among female adults and adolescents, 1985–2007

[United States and dependent areas]

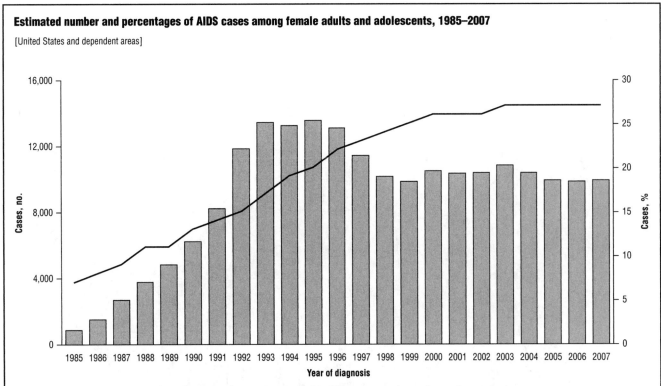

Year of diagnosis

Notes: Data have been adjusted for reporting delays. Bars indicate number of cases. Line indicates percent of cases diagnosed among females.

SOURCE: "Slide 1. Estimated Number and Percentages of AIDS Cases among Female Adults and Adolescents 1985–2007—United States and Dependent Areas," in *HIV/AIDS Surveillance in Women*, Centers for Disease Control and Prevention, May 5, 2009, http://www.cdc.gov/hiv/topics/surveillance/resources/slides/women/slides/Women1.pdf (accessed June 22, 2009)

TABLE 4.3

Estimated numbers of AIDS cases and rates for female adults and adolescents, by race/ethnicity, 2007

[50 states and Washington D.C.]

Race/ethnicity	Cases	Rate (Cases per 100,000 population)
American Indian/Alaska Native	46	5.0
Asian[a]	93	1.6
Black/African American	6,243	39.8
Hispanic/Latino[b]	1,452	8.9
Native Hawaiian/other Pacific Islander	12	7.1
White	1,600	1.8
Total[c]	**9,579**	**7.5**

Note: Data have been adjusted for reporting delays.
[a]Includes Asian and Pacific Islander legacy cases.
[b]Hispanics/Latinos can be of any race.
[c]Includes 132 female adults and adolescents of unknown race or multiple races.

SOURCE: "Slide 2. Estimated Number of AIDS Cases and Rates for Female Adults and Adolescents, by Race/Ethnicity 2007—50 States and DC," in *HIV/AIDS Surveillance in Women*, Centers for Disease Control and Prevention, May 5, 2009, http://www.cdc.gov/hiv/topics/surveillance/resources/slides/women/slides/Women2.pdf (accessed June 22, 2009)

secretions. They are also more likely to shed HIV in greater amounts than people infected with HIV alone, which contributes to the spread of HIV. By treating an STD, the shedding of HIV on sexual contact is lessened, which in turn reduces the spread of HIV infection.

MSM SEXUAL CONTACT

MSM is still the major risk category for HIV infection, although the increase in the number of cases has slowed steadily over the past few years. Epidemiologists (public health researchers who analyze the extent and types of illnesses in a population and the factors that influence their distribution) believe that HIV/AIDS among MSM may have peaked in 1992.

In 2000, 44,467 adult and adolescent males whose only stated mode of exposure to HIV was through MSM contact made up 46% of the 97,712 cumulative male adult and adolescent HIV infection cases. In 2001 the percentage had fallen slightly, to 43%. However, the actual number of cases attributable to MSM had risen to 52,139 out of a cumulative total of 120,868. In 2007, 129,915 reported cases of HIV infection were attributable to MSM, representing 54% of the cumulative total of 239,760 cases. (See Table 4.1.)

As in previous years, in 2007 MSM contact was the overwhelming mode of exposure and transmission for white males with or without IDU (16,652 of 20,661, or 81%, of cases in white males in 2007). It was also cumulatively the highest percentage of mode of transmission (76,061

FIGURE 4.4

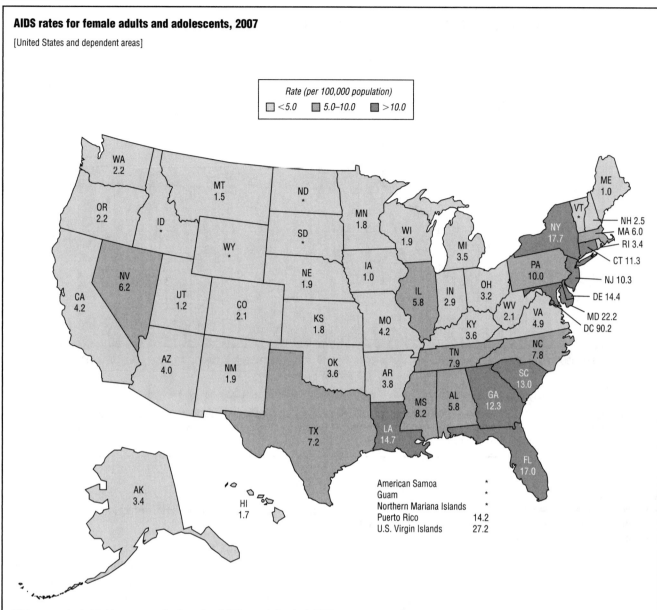

AIDS rates for female adults and adolescents, 2007

[United States and dependent areas]

Rate (per 100,000 population)
☐ <5.0   ◻ 5.0–10.0   ◼ >10.0

American Samoa	*
Guam	*
Northern Mariana Islands	*
Puerto Rico	14.2
U.S. Virgin Islands	27.2

*Rates were not calculated for areas reporting fewer than 5 AIDS cases in females in 2007.

SOURCE: "Slide 4. AIDS Rates for Female Adults and Adolescents Reported in 2007—United States and Dependent Areas," in *HIV/AIDS Surveillance in Women*, Centers for Disease Control and Prevention, May 5, 2009, http://www.cdc.gov/hiv/topics/surveillance/resources/slides/women/slides/Women4.pdf (accessed June 22, 2009)

cumulative cases, representing 77% of the cumulative total). (See Table 4.1.) In 2007, 48% of African-American males and 64% of Hispanic males were infected with HIV via MSM contact, with or without IDU. MSM was also the leading mode of HIV exposure for these latter groups. Cumulatively through 2007, 55% of all HIV-infected Hispanic males and 43% of all HIV-infected African-American males had MSM contact, with or without IDU.

PRISONERS AND AIDS

According to Laura M. Maruschak of the Bureau of Justice Statistics, in *HIV in Prisons, 2006* (April 2008, http://www.ojp.usdoj.gov/bjs/pub/pdf/hivp06.pdf), the number of HIV-positive state and federal prisoners has declined each year since 1999, when there were 25,807 infected prisoners. Between 2005 and 2006 the number of HIV-positive inmates in state and federal prisons fell from 22,676 to 21,980; however, HIV/AIDS cases as a percent of the total custody population remained constant at 1.7% for both years. (See Table 4.4.) The rate of HIV/AIDS cases in state and federal prisoners (46 per 10,000 prison inmates) continued to be nearly three times higher than the 2006 case rate in the total U.S. population (17 per 10,000 people). (See Table 4.5.)

Every year since statistics have been gathered, AIDS-related conditions have been the second leading cause of

TABLE 4.4

HIV/AIDS cases among prison inmates, 2004–06

Jurisdiction	Total HIV/AIDS cases[a]			HIV/AIDS cases as a percent of total custody population[b]		
	2006	2005	2004	2006	2005	2004
U.S. total						
Reported[c]	21,980	22,676	22,936	1.7%	1.7%	1.8%
Comparable reporting[d]	21,980	22,202	22,448			
Federal	1,530	1,592	1,680	0.9%	1.0%	1.1%
State	20,450	21,084	21,256	1.8	1.8	1.8
Northeast	**6,099**	**6,456**	**6,646**	**3.6%**	**3.9%**	**4.1%**
Connecticut	423	463	477	2.2	2.6	2.7
Maine	13	10	11	0.6	0.5	0.6
Massachusetts	268	221	215	2.5	2.1	2.2
New Hampshire	16	21	31	0.6	0.9	1.3
New Jersey	612	540	655	2.7	2.3	2.9
New York	4,000	4,440	4,500	6.3	7.0	7.0
Pennsylvania	697	692	693	1.6	1.7	1.7
Rhode Island	58	58	51	1.6	1.7	1.6
Vermont	12	11	13	0.7	0.7	0.9
Midwest	**1,572**	**1,970**	**2,025**	**0.8%**	**0.9%**	**0.9%**
Illinois	/	474	488	/	1.1	1.1
Indiana	/	/	/	/	/	/
Iowa	42	28	32	0.5	0.3	0.4
Kansas	61	34	41	0.7	0.4	0.5
Michigan	490	525	575	1.0	1.1	1.2
Minnesota	47	41	44	0.6	0.5	0.6
Missouri	301	301	294	1.0	1.0	1.0
Nebraska	17	19	20	0.4	0.4	0.5
North Dakota	3	2	6	0.2	0.2	0.5
Ohio	447	410	387	1.0	1.0	0.9
South Dakota	14	14	9	0.4	0.4	0.3
Wisconsin	150	122	129	0.7	0.6	0.6
South	**10,950**	**10,753**	**10,691**	**2.1%**	**2.2%**	**2.1%**
Alabama	297	268	270	1.2	1.1	1.1
Arkansas	98	94	102	0.8	0.8	0.8
Delaware	108	124	149	1.5	1.8	2.2
Florida	3,412	3,396	3,250	4.1	3.9	3.9
Georgia	944	1,042	1,109	1.8	2.1	2.2
Kentucky	104	83	74	0.8	0.7	0.6
Louisiana	525	488	487	2.5	2.5	2.5
Maryland	612	671	792	2.7	3.0	3.4
Mississippi	279	302	254	2.4	2.7	2.2
North Carolina	688	718	647	1.8	/	1.8
Oklahoma	163	136	133	0.9	0.8	0.8
South Carolina	454	489	489	2.0	2.2	2.2
Tennessee	190	210	215	1.3	1.5	1.5
Texas	2,693	2,400	2,405	1.9	1.7	1.7
Virginia	368	330	302	1.3	/	1.0
West Virginia	15	2	13	0.3	0	0.3

death for state prison inmates, behind "illness/natural causes." However, the proportion of deaths attributable to AIDS has declined markedly since 1995. Maruschak notes that out of the total number of inmate deaths in state prisons in 1995, 34.2% of the total were from AIDS. (See Table 4.6.) However, by 2006, 4.6% of inmate deaths in state prisons were from AIDS. This remarkable decline in AIDS-related deaths is also reflected by the statistics in the rate of deaths per 100,000 inmates. In 1995 the death rate in state prisons due to AIDS was 100 per 100,000 inmates. (See Table 4.7.) By 2006 the rate had decreased to 11 per 100,000 inmates. This sharp drop is likely attributable to effective treatment with protease inhibitors and combination antiretroviral therapies.

A similar trend is also apparent when the inmate death figures from federal prisons in 2005 and 2006 are examined. Of the total number of inmate deaths in federal prisons in 2005 (388), 327 (84%) were from natural causes other than AIDS and 27 (7%) were from AIDS. (See Table 4.8.) By the following year, 294 (90%) out of a total of 328 deaths were from natural causes other than AIDS, whereas 12 (4%) were from AIDS.

Geographic Differences

Maruschak indicates that 21,980 U.S. inmates were confirmed as infected with HIV or diagnosed with AIDS in 2006. This represents 1.7% of the custody population at that time—a slight decrease from the 1.8% of inmates

TABLE 4.4

HIV/AIDS cases among prison inmates, 2004–06 [CONTINUED]

Jurisdiction	Total HIV/AIDS cases[a]			HIV/AIDS cases as a percent of total custody population[b]		
	2006	2005	2004	2006	2005	2004
West	**1,829**	**1,905**	**1,894**	**0.7%**	**0.7%**	**0.7%**
Alaska	/	/	/	/	/	/
Arizona	169	152	155	0.6	0.5	0.5
California	1,155	1,249	1,212	0.7	0.7	0.7
Colorado	165	148	185	1.0	0.9	1.1
Hawaii	15	23	15	0.4	0.6	0.4
Idaho	22	26	33	0.5	0.6	0.7
Montana	6	6	5	0.3	0.3	0.2
Nevada	126	124	116	1.0	1.1	1.1
New Mexico	36	25	25	0.5	0.4	0.4
Oregon	/	/	/	/	/	/
Utah	44	38	39	0.9	0.8	0.8
Washington	84	107	102	0.5	0.6	0.6
Wyoming	7	7	7	0.6	0.6	0.6

/Not reported.
[a]Counts published in previous reports may have been revised.
[b]Percentages are based on custody counts, except for New Mexico for which percentages are based on its yearend jurisdiction count.
[c]Percentages exclude inmates in jurisdictions that did not report data.
[d]Excludes data from Illinois, Indiana, Alaska, and Oregon for all 3 years due to incomplete reporting.

SOURCE: Laura M. Maruschak,"Table 1. Inmates in Custody of State or Federal Prison Authorities and Reported to be Positive for the Human Immunodeficiency Virus (HIV) or to Have Confirmed AIDS,2004–2006,"in *HIV in Prisons,2006*,Bureau of Justice Statistics,April 2008 http://www.ojp.usdoj.gov/bjs/pub/pdf/hivp06.pdf (accessed June 22,2009)

TABLE 4.5

Percent of AIDS cases in the general population and among state and federal prisoners, 1999–2006

Yearend	State and federal prisoners	U.S. general population[a]	Ratio[b]
1999	0.58%	0.12%	4.8
2000	0.51	0.13	3.9
2001	0.50	0.14	3.6
2002	0.45	0.14	3.2
2003	0.47	0.15	3.1
2004	0.46	0.15	3.1
2005	0.43	0.16	2.7
2006	0.46	0.17	2.7

[a]Based on persons age 13 or older in 1999 and age 15 or older thereafter. Excludes confirmed AIDS cases reported in state and federal prisons.
[b]Percent of confirmed AIDS cases in prisons divided by percent in the U.S. general population.

SOURCE: Laura M. Maruschak, "Table 4. Percent with Confirmed AIDS among State and Federal Prisoners and the U.S. General Population, 1999–2006," in *HIV in Prisons, 2006*, Bureau of Justice Statistics, April 2008, http://www.ojp.usdoj.gov/bjs/pub/pdf/hivp06.pdf (accessed June 22, 2009)

TABLE 4.6

Percent of AIDS-related deaths among all deaths in state prisons and the U.S. general population, selected years 1995–2006

Year	State prisons[a]	U.S. general population ages 15–54[b]	Ratio[c]
1995	34.2%	12.9%	2.6
2001	10.3	4.3	2.4
2002	9.1	4.1	2.2
2003	8.0	4.2	1.9
2004	5.6	4.3	1.3
2005	5.3	3.8	1.4
2006	4.6	—	:

—Not available.
:Not calculated.
[a]Percentages were based on the number of inmate deaths, excluding those in jurisdictions not reporting AIDS-related deaths.
[b]Excludes deaths reported in state prisons.
[c]Percent of AIDS-related deaths in state prisons divided by percent in the U.S. general population, ages 15–54.

SOURCE: Laura M. Maruschak, "Table 8. Percent of AIDS-Related Deaths among All Deaths in State Prison and the U.S. General Population," in *HIV in Prisons, 2006*, Bureau of Justice Statistics, April 2008, http://www.ojp.usdoj.gov/bjs/pub/pdf/hivp06.pdf (accessed June 22, 2009)

---

known to be HIV infected in 2004. This modest decrease has not been geographically uniform, however. In 2006 New York held nearly a fifth (4,000, or 18%) of all inmates known to be HIV positive or diagnosed with AIDS. (See Table 4.4.) The majority of prisoners with HIV/AIDS were held in four states in 2006: New York (4,000 or 18%), Florida (3,612, or 16%), Texas (2,693, or 12%), and California (1,155, or 5%) held a total of 51% of all HIV-positive inmates.

Gender, Racial, and Age Differences

In 2006 an estimated 21,980 U.S. inmates were infected with HIV or had confirmed cases of AIDS—a small decrease from the previous year's estimate of 22,676 HIV/AIDS cases. (See Table 4.4.) Similarly, the numbers of AIDS-related deaths in state prison decreased slightly—from 185 in 2004, to 176 in 2005, to 155 in 2006. (See Table 4.9.)

TABLE 4.7

Rate of AIDS-related deaths in state prisons and the U.S. general population, selected years 1995–2006

| | Rate per 100,000 persons | | |
| | | U.S. general population | |
Year	State prisons	ages 15–54[a]	Ratio[b]
1995	100	29	3.5
2001	25	9	2.9
2002	22	9	2.6
2003	21	9	2.4
2004	14	9	1.7
2005	13	8	1.7
2006	11	6	1.8

[a]Excludes deaths reported in state prisons.
[b]Rate of deaths in state prisons divided by rate in the U.S. general population, ages 15–54. Calculations based on unrounded rates.

SOURCE: Laura M. Maruschak, "Table 9. Rate of AIDS-Related Deaths in State Prisons and the U.S. General Population," in *HIV in Prisons, 2006*, Bureau of Justice Statistics, April 2008, http://www.ojp.usdoj.gov/bjs/pub/pdf/hivp06.pdf (accessed June 22, 2009)

TABLE 4.8

Inmate deaths in federal prisons by cause, 2005 and 2006

| | Number | | Rate per 100,000 inmates* | |
Cause of death	2006	2005	2006	2005
Total	328	388	172	210
Natural causes other than AIDS	294	327	154	177
AIDS	12	27	6	15
Suicide	12	13	6	7
Accident	2	6	1	3
Execution	0	0	0	0
By another person	8	15	4	8

*Detail may not add to total due to rounding.

SOURCE: Laura M. Maruschak, "Table 6. Inmate Deaths in Federal Prisons by Cause, 2005 and 2006," in *HIV in Prisons, 2006*, Bureau of Justice Statistics, April 2008, http://www.ojp.usdoj.gov/bjs/pub/pdf/hivp06.pdf (accessed June 22, 2009)

TABLE 4.9

Inmate deaths in state prisons by gender, age and race/ethnicity, 2004–06

| | Number of AIDS-related deaths[a] | | | Rate of AIDS-related deaths per 100,000 inmates[b] | | |
Characteristic	2006	2005	2004	2006	2005	2004
State total	155	176	185	11	13	14
Gender						
Male	148	166	176	12	14	15
Female	7	10	9	8	12	11
Age						
19 or younger	1	0	0	5	0	0
20–24	2	0	3	1	0	1
25–34	18	25	26	4	6	6
35–44	62	82	88	16	21	23
45–54	58	55	57	32	31	33
55 or older	14	14	11	22	22	19
Race/Hispanic origin						
White[c]	29	33	46	6	8	11
Black[c]	114	120	122	21	24	24
Hispanic	12	21	11	5	9	5

[a]Estimates of the number of AIDS-related deaths by gender, age, and race/Hispanic origin were made by applying the percentages based on DCRP data to the estimated total number of AIDS-related deaths.
[b]To calculate the rate, the number of state prisoners by age was first estimated by applying the age distribution reported in the 2004 Survey of Inmates in State Correctional Facilities to the 2004–2006 midyear custody counts in NPS-1.
[c]Excludes persons of Hispanic or Latino origin.

SOURCE: Laura M. Maruschak, "Table 7. Profile of Inmates Who Died in State Prisons, 2004–2006," in *HIV in Prisons, 2006*, Bureau of Justice Statistics, April 2008, http://www.ojp.usdoj.gov/bjs/pub/pdf/hivp06.pdf (accessed June 22, 2009)

Male inmates make up the overwhelming majority of HIV-infected or confirmed cases of AIDS among inmates in state and federal prisons. In 2006 an estimated 19,842 male inmates had been diagnosed with HIV infection or AIDS, compared with 2,138 female inmates. (See Table 4.10.) However, as a percent of the female prisoner population, a higher percentage of female prisoners were reported with HIV/AIDS (2.4% as compared with 1.6% of male prisoners). The majorities of both male inmates (18,384, or 93%) and female inmates (2,030, or 95%) were in custody in state prisons, where the percentages of prisoners with HIV/AIDS were higher than those in federal prisons for both males (1.7% and 0.9%, respectively) and females (2.6% and 0.9%, respectively).

The AIDS-related deaths in state prisons occurred largely among males, who accounted for 95% of such deaths in 2006. (See Table 4.9.) The majority of these deaths (114, or 74%) were among African-American inmates. Female inmates accounted for 7 (5%) of the AIDS-related deaths, and 3 (2%) of the deaths occurred among inmates less than 24 years old.

Even though nearly twice as many AIDS-related deaths occurred in state prisons (11 per 100,000 people), compared with AIDS-related deaths in the general population (6 per 100,000 people) in 2006, the gap has narrowed considerably since 1995, when more than three times as many inmate deaths (100 per 100,000 people) than deaths in the general population (29 per 100,000) were attributable to AIDS. (See Table 4.7.)

Drug and Needle Use among Prisoners

Public education campaigns about the "safer" use of drugs and syringes appear to be reducing HIV infection in the general public. However, these measures seem to be having no effect in prisons. Many incarcerated IDUs continue to inject while in prison, often sharing needles because injection equipment is in short supply. Indeed, Ralf Jürgens, Andrew Ball, and Annette Verster note in "Interventions to Reduce HIV Transmission Related to Injecting Drug Use in Prison" (*Lancet Infectious Diseases*, vol. 9, no. 1, January 2009) that most incarcerated IDUs report borrowing

TABLE 4.10

HIV/AIDS among inmates in state and federal prisons by gender, 2006

Jurisdiction	Male HIV cases		Female HIV cases	
	Number	Percent of population	Number	Percent of population
U.S. total				
Estimated[a, b]	19,842		2,138	
Reported[c]	19,809	1.6%	2,135	2.4%
Federal	1,425	0.9%	105	0.9%
State	18,384	1.7	2,030	2.6
Northeast	**5,520**	**3.4%**	**579**	**6.4%**
Connecticut	372	2.1	51	3.7
Maine	11	0.6	2	1.4
Massachusetts	231	2.3	37	4.4
New Hampshire	16	0.6	0	0
New Jersey	534	2.4	78	7.2
New York	3,650	6.0	350	12.2
Pennsylvania	641	1.6	56	2.6
Rhode Island	53	1.5	5.0	2.2
Vermont	12	0.8	0	0
Midwest	**1,397**	**0.8%**	**175**	**1.4%**
Illinois	/	/	/	/
Indiana	/	/	/	/
Iowa	41	0.5	1.0	0.1
Kansas	59	0.7	2	0.3
Michigan	449	0.9	41	1.9
Minnesota	46	0.6	1	0.2
Missouri	202	0.7	99	3.8
Nebraska	17	0.4	0	0
North Dakota	3	0.3	0	0
Ohio	424	1.0	23	0.6
South Dakota	13	0.4	1	0.3
Wisconsin	143	0.7	7	0.5
South	**9,843**	**2.1%**	**1,107**	**3.0%**
Alabama	272	1.2	25	2.0
Arkansas	87	0.7	11	1.1
Delaware	91	1.4	17	3.1
Florida	3,041	3.8	371	7.6
Georgia	874	1.8	70	2.0
Kentucky	83	0.7	21	2.3
Louisiana	484	2.5	41	3.6
Maryland	566	2.6	46	4.3
Mississippi	233	2.4	46	2.9
North Carolina	629	1.8	59	2.2
Oklahoma	154	1.0	9	0.4
South Carolina	411	1.9	43	2.7
Tennessee	173	1.3	17	1.4
Texas	2,409	1.9	284	2.8
Virginia	323	1.2	45	2.0
West Virginia	13	0.3	2	0.5

TABLE 4.10

HIV/AIDS among inmates in state and federal prisons by gender, 2006 [CONTINUED]

Jurisdiction	Male HIV cases		Female HIV cases	
	Number	Percent of population	Number	Percent of population
West	**1,624**	**0.7%**	**169**	**0.8%**
Alaska	/	/	/	/
Arizona	155	0.6	14	0.4
California	1,060	0.7	95	0.8
Colorado	152	1.0	13	0.6
Hawaii	12	0.4	3	0.7
Idaho	22	0.5	0	U
Montana	6	0.4	0	0
Nevada	101	0.9	25	2.2
New Mexico	/	/	/	/
Oregon	/	/	/	/
Utah	38	0.8	6	1.2
Washington	73	0.5	11	0.7
Wyoming	5	0.5	2	1.2

/Not reported.
[a]Includes estimates of the number of inmates with HIV/AIDS by gender for New Mexico.
[b]In states that did not report HIV/AIDS cases by gender, estimates were made by applying to the total the percentages by gender from the most recent year for which data were available. For each year, estimates do not include data from states that did not report sufficient data on HIV/AIDS cases.
[c]Percentages exclude inmates in jurisdictions that did not report HIV/AIDS infection by gender.

SOURCE: Laura M. Maruschak, "Table 2. Inmates in Custody of State or Federal Prison Authorities and Reported to be Positive for the Human Immunodeficiency Virus (HIV) or to Have Confirmed AIDS by Gender, 2006," in *HIV in Prisons, 2006*, Bureau of Justice Statistics, April 2008, http://www.ojp.usdoj.gov/bjs/pub/pdf/hivp06.pdf (accessed June 22, 2009)

Nonetheless, Jürgens, Ball, and Verster observe that prison systems can and should do more to prevent HIV transmission related to IDU. They assert that needle and syringe programs and drug substitution therapy, such as methadone maintenance (the use of methadone as treatment for a person addicted to heroin), sharply reduce the sharing of injecting equipment and the spread of HIV and other bloodborne pathogens.

U.S. Prison Systems Take Action to Prevent HIV Infection

In "Sex, Drugs, Prisons, and HIV" (*New England Journal of Medicine*, vol. 356, no. 2, January 11, 2007), Susan Okie states that the Rhode Island prison system's HIV testing practices are highly regarded by U.S. public health experts and are considered to be among the best in the country. Nonetheless, Okie observes that even the Rhode Island program fails to meet international guidelines for reducing the risk of HIV in prisons. The World Health Organization and the Joint United Nations Program on HIV/AIDS recommend that prisoners have access to bleach to clean injecting equipment and that drug treatment, methadone maintenance, and needle exchange programs be offered to inmates. Okie notes that in 2007 condoms were provided on a limited basis in just two state prison systems (Vermont and Mississippi) and five county jail systems (New York, Philadelphia, San

syringes while in prison, which makes prisons a high-risk environment for the transmission of HIV.

This is a dilemma for prisons, where syringes and needles are prohibited, as are illegal drugs, and chemicals for disinfecting the illicit needles are not readily available to prisoners. Even though state and federal prison officials in the United States want to stop the spread of HIV among inmates, most cannot keep pace with or stem the flow of illegal drugs into prisons. To minimize the spread of HIV in prisons, countries such as Switzerland and the United Kingdom provide prisoners with disinfectant or clean needles. U.S. officials believe these actions endorse illegal drug use. Instead, they focus on providing treatment and rehabilitation programs for drug-addicted prisoners.

Francisco, Los Angeles, and the District of Columbia). Mary Sylla of the Policy and Advocacy for the Center for Health Justice explains in "HIV Treatment in U.S. Jails and Prisons" (*The Body*, Winter 2008) that as of 2008, there were just a few methadone maintenance programs and no U.S. prison had even tested the feasibility of a needle exchange program.

In 2009 the Georgia state senate passed a bill requiring that inmates receive HIV testing before their release from state prison. The state already required HIV testing before inmates enter the prison system. According to the article "Senate Passes Bill Requiring HIV Testing in Prisons" (Georgia Public Broadcasting News, March 10, 2009), Senator Kasim Reed (1969–), a Democrat, asserts that informing inmates of their HIV status when they are released will help protect the communities to which they are released. Reed opines that "the data suggests that when people know their status, they change their behavior." Senator John F. Douglas (1953–), a Republican, questions the veracity of this statement, observing that "once these people are released from prison,...there is nothing to force them to tell their partner that they have HIV."

HEMOPHILIACS

Hemophilia is a group of genetic disorders in which defects in a number of genes located on the X chromosome disrupt the proper clotting of blood. The most common type of hemophilia—hemophilia A—is a deficiency of a clotting substance designated Factor VIII. Varying severities of hemophilia can occur, depending on the level of Factor VIII present in the patient's plasma. Treatment of hemophilia involves close attention to injury prevention and periodic intravenous administration of Factor VIII concentrates, commonly known as clotting factors.

Because screening for HIV antibodies was not available until 1985, many hemophiliacs were exposed to HIV-contaminated blood and clotting factors before widespread use of screening procedures. National distribution of clotting factor concentrates before 1985 led to a high prevalence of HIV infections among hemophiliacs. The prevalence of HIV infection differs by the type and severity of the coagulation (clotting) disorder.

According to the National Hemophilia Foundation (NHF), in "NHF—Guardian of the Nation's Blood Supply" (2006, http://www.hemophilia.org/blood_safety/index.htm), in the early 1980s about half of all people with hemophilia became infected with HIV through blood products. Many of these people developed AIDS. Even though precise statistics are unavailable, many health officials—such as those cited in *FDA Workshop on Behavior-Based Donor Deferrals in the NAT Era* (March 8, 2006, http://www.fda.gov/downloads/BiologicsBloodVaccines/NewsEvents/WorkshopsMeetings Conferences/TranscriptsMinutes/UCM054430.pdf)—believe that 70% to 90% of the approximately 17,000

Americans with hemophilia A are HIV positive. The 8,000 or so Americans with the less clinically severe hemophilia B most likely have a lower prevalence rate because they required fewer treatments with the clotting factor and, therefore, were less exposed to HIV-contaminated products. According to the CDC, hemophilia A rates may be overrepresented because the studies were performed at hemophilia treatment centers where the more severe hemophilia A cases are likely to be found.

In "Prognostic Factors for All-Cause Mortality among Hemophiliacs Infected with Human Immunodeficiency Virus" (*American Journal of Epidemiology*, vol. 142, no. 3, 1995), Laura S. Diamondstone et al. note that before the 1980s most hemophiliacs died from intracranial hemorrhage (bleeding within the brain). However, by 1995 one-third of all deaths were related to HIV infection and one-fourth were related to hemorrhage. At that time, hemophiliacs often reported that virtually all their fellow hemophiliacs were infected with the virus. Many sexual partners of hemophiliacs also contracted the virus from sexual intercourse. In the case of females, the virus can be passed to their offspring.

Thomas Tencer et al. explain in "Medical Costs and Resource Utilization for Hemophilia Patients with and without HIV or HCV Infection" (*Journal of Managed Care Pharmacy*, vol. 13, no. 9, November–December 2007) that even though the possibility of contracting HIV or the hepatitis C virus was virtually eliminated in the United States, at the close of 2007 about one-third of hemophiliacs were believed to be HIV infected or infected with both HIV and hepatitis C. Coinfected people have been found to have higher rates of illness, death, and utilization of clotting factor.

A Slow Reaction

Concentrated clotting factor, which is derived from human blood obtained from as many as 2,000 donors, became available in the mid-1970s. Its success at stopping bleeding was so dramatic that hemophilia changed from a disease that produced intense pain, disability, and the possibility of premature death to one that allowed sufferers to lead nearly normal lives. Hemophiliacs could infuse clotting factors into their own veins if they felt bleeding was about to start. Patients were advised by their physicians to "infuse early and often."

During the late 1970s and early 1980s some clotting factor concentrates were inadvertently infected with HIV. Even after the first cases of HIV/AIDS appeared in people with hemophilia and the CDC, along with the NHF, identified this new disease as being bloodborne, physicians did not advise their patients to alter their clotting factor treatments. Hemophiliacs were encouraged to continue using their clotting factor because researchers and physicians were not sure there would be a major epidemic.

Anecdotal comments from hemophiliacs indicate that when many of them became infected, primary care doctors were slow to respond and supplied little information. There was no warning to practice safe sex to prevent the spread of HIV. Some hemophiliacs reported receiving more information from gay men's organizations than from their own hematologists (physicians who specialize in diseases and disorders of the blood).

ANGER AND COMPENSATION. Many hemophiliacs feel they are entitled to compensation or, at the very least, assistance in paying the overwhelming medical expenses they incur as a result of HIV infection and AIDS treatment. They maintain that the companies that produced the clotting factors were slow to warn the public about HIV and slow to use heat treatment to eliminate the live virus from the clotting factors (although this procedure has not gained widespread acceptance among scientists as an adequate method to inactivate HIV).

Hemophilia foundations in some countries have convinced government pharmaceutical or insurance companies to compensate HIV-infected hemophiliacs. In "Legal, Financial, and Public Health Consequences of HIV Contamination of Blood and Blood Products in the 1980s and 1990s" (*Annals of Internal Medicine*, vol. 136, no. 4, February 19, 2002), Peter D. Weinberg et al. report that Armour Pharmaceuticals agreed to pay six Canadians $1.5 million each; Germany offered people infected with HIV and those who became ill with AIDS annual compensation; and Switzerland extended annual compensation of $12,216 to people with AIDS. France gave one-time compensation of $87,735 to hemophiliacs at the time they were diagnosed with AIDS due to tainted blood products. During the first decade of the 21st century, more than 20 developed countries had acted to compensate HIV-infected hemophiliacs. In contrast, developing countries continued to grapple with blood-supply safety issues.

In 1995 the U.S. Supreme Court refused to hear a class action suit brought by hemophiliacs against a pharmaceutical company and other blood-product manufacturers (*Barton v. American Red Cross*, 826 F. Supp. 412 and 826 F. Supp. 407, append 43 F. 3rd 678, certiorari denied 116 S. Ct. 84). Regardless, some companies have reached out-of-court settlements with affected people. For example, according to the article "4 Drug Companies Ordered to Pay Hemophiliacs" (*New York Times*, May 8, 1997), in 1997 four manufacturers of blood clotting products were ordered by a federal judge to pay approximately $670 million to settle cases on behalf of more than 6,000 hemophiliacs infected in the United States during the early 1980s. The settlement compensated each infected hemophiliac with an estimated $100,000 payment.

The NHF explains in "Ricky Ray Program Office Set to Close" (2005, http://www.hemophilia.org/NHFWeb/MainPgs/MainNHF.aspx?menuid=117&contentid=360) that the international catastrophe of HIV/AIDS in the hemophilia community was recognized by the U.S. federal government in 1998 with passage of the Ricky Ray Hemophilia Relief Fund Act, named for a Florida boy with hemophilia who died from HIV/AIDS. According to the NHF, the act provided "payments of $100,000 to individuals with hemophilia who were treated with HIV-contaminated clotting factor products between July 1, 1982, and December 31, 1987. Spouses and children who contracted HIV from these individuals, as well as specified family survivors were also eligible for compassionate payment." Under section 101(d) of the Act, the Trust Fund terminated on November 12, 2003, though payments for petitions received before that date continued to be paid for almost two years after that date. When the program closed in October 2005, it had paid over $559 million to more than 7,171 eligible individuals and survivors.

CHAPTER 5
CHILDREN, ADOLESCENTS, AND HIV/AIDS

HIV/AIDS IN CHILDREN—DIFFERENT FROM HIV/AIDS IN ADULTS

HIV causes AIDS in both adults and children. The virus attacks and damages the immune and central nervous systems of all infected people. However, the development and course of the disease in children differs considerably from its progression in adults.

Before the use of highly active antiretroviral therapy (HAART) and early intervention strategies, there were two patterns of HIV progression among children. The first pattern, which is called severe immunodeficiency, is apparent as recurring serious infections or encephalopathy (any of various diseases of the brain). The National Institute of Allergy and Infectious Diseases (NIAID) reports in the fact sheet "HIV Infection in Infants and Children" (July 2004, http://www.niaid.nih.gov/factsheets/hivchildren.htm) that severe immunodeficiency develops in 20% of infected infants during their first year of life. The second pattern of HIV progression, which occurs in the other 80% infected children, is more gradual and is similar to the development and progression of the disease observed in adults.

HIV nucleic acid detection tests can detect the presence of HIV in nearly all infants aged one month and older. Before the development of these tests, detecting HIV infection, especially in babies, was difficult. This is because the earlier tests involved the detection of antibodies formed by the infant in response to HIV. However, infants have often not developed the full capacity to produce antibodies at the time of testing. Furthermore, HIV-infected mothers may transmit antibodies alone, without the virus, to their babies. In the latter instance, infants with positive results from antibody tests at birth may later test negative, indicating that the mother transmitted the HIV antibodies to the baby, but not the virus itself.

In adults, symptoms of fully developed AIDS include the presence of opportunistic infections (OIs) that may or may not be accompanied by rare forms of several types of cancers. The OIs or the cancers can ultimately prove to be the cause of death. The most common diseases associated with AIDS in adults are *Pneumocystis carinii* pneumonia (PCP) and Kaposi's sarcoma. The latter is a normally rare skin carcinoma that can spread to internal organs. Many adult AIDS patients have one or both of these conditions. Other disorders found in adult AIDS patients are lymphomas (lymph gland cancers), prolonged diarrhea causing severe dehydration, weight loss, and central nervous system infections that can lead to dementia.

Among infants and children, the disease is characterized by wasting syndrome, the failure to thrive, and unusually severe bacterial infections. Except for PCP, children with symptomatic HIV infection rarely develop the same OIs that adults contract. Though adults and children with HIV may both suffer from chronic or recurrent diarrhea, its dehydrating effect may be particularly debilitating and life-threatening to children. Instead of other symptoms common to adults, children are plagued with recurrent bacterial infections such as severe forms of conjunctivitis (pink eye), ear infections, and tonsillitis and persistent or recurrent oral thrush (an infection of the mouth or throat caused by the fungus *Candida albicans*). Children may also suffer from enlarged lymph nodes, chronic pneumonia, developmental delays, and neurological abnormalities. Put simply, the immune system of HIV-infected children is destroyed even as it matures.

Whether HIV positive or not, babies born to HIV-infected mothers appear to be predisposed to a variety of heart problems. In "Cardiovascular Status of Infants and Children of Women Infected with HIV-1 (P2C2 HIV): A Cohort Study" (*Lancet*, vol. 360, no. 9330, August 3, 2002), Steven E. Lipshultz et al. examined more than 500 infants born to HIV-positive women. They discovered that the babies suffered from significantly higher rates of abnormalities, such as defects in the heart wall and valve and reduced pumping action. These defects occurred in less than 1% of healthy children whose mothers were not infected with HIV. Lipshultz et al. recognize that HIV alone did not necessarily cause these anomalies. They observe that a mother's alcohol, drug, or nutrition problems can also interfere with fetal heart development.

A CASE DEFINITION FOR CHILDREN

Because data were limited during the first few years of HIV's acknowledged presence in the United States, the Centers for Disease Control and Prevention's (CDC) definition of AIDS did not differentiate between adults and children until 1987, when the classification system was revised. The CDC Division of HIV/AIDS Prevention, National Center for HIV/AIDS, Viral Hepatitis, STD, and TB Prevention updated the pediatric definition in 1994, 1999, and 2008 as more information about HIV and AIDS became available. The 2008 revision, which takes into account new testing technologies, is intended for public health surveillance purposes and not as a guide for clinical diagnosis.

Changes to the case definitions were published by Eileen Schneider et al. of the CDC in "Revised Surveillance Case Definitions for HIV Infection among Adults, Adolescents, and Children Aged <18 Months and for HIV Infection and AIDS among Children Aged 18 Months to <13 Years—United States, 2008" (*Morbidity and Mortality Weekly Report*, vol. 57, no. RR-10, December 5, 2008). No changes were made to the 24 AIDS-defining conditions listed in Table 5.1. However, the 2008 criteria stipulate that:

- Because of the greater uncertainty associated with diagnostic testing for HIV in this population (maternal antibodies from the HIV-infected mother might exist in the infant after birth, possibly affecting HIV diagnostic testing of the infant that occurs soon after birth), children whose illness meets clinical criteria for the AIDS case definition but does not meet laboratory criteria for definitive or presumptive HIV infection are still categorized as HIV infected when the mother has laboratory-confirmed HIV infection.

- For children aged 18 months to less than 13 years, laboratory-confirmed evidence of HIV infection is required to meet the surveillance case definition for HIV infection and AIDS.

- Diagnostic confirmation of an AIDS-defining condition alone, without laboratory-confirmed evidence of HIV infection, is no longer sufficient to classify a child as HIV infected for surveillance purposes.

Table 5.2 presents the criteria for HIV infection in children. These include laboratory criteria such as the results of the screening test for HIV antibodies or detection of HIV using a virologic (nonantibody) test. HIV infection based on confirmed laboratory test results and documented

TABLE 5.1

AIDS-defining conditions

- Bacterial infections, multiple or recurrent[a]
- Candidiasis of bronchi, trachea, or lungs
- Candidiasis of esophagus[b]
- Cervical cancer, invasive[c]
- Coccidioidomycosis, disseminated or extrapulmonary
- Cryptococcosis, extrapulmonary
- Cryptosporidiosis, chronic intestinal (>1 month's duration)
- Cytomegalovirus disease (other than liver, spleen, or nodes), onset at age >1 month
- Cytomegalovirus retinitis (with loss of vision)[b]
- Encephalopathy, HIV related
- Herpes simplex: chronic ulcers (>1 month's duration) or bronchitis, pneumonitis, or esophagitis (onset at age >1 month)
- Histoplasmosis, disseminated or extrapulmonary
- Isosporiasis, chronic intestinal (>1 month's duration)
- Kaposi sarcoma[b]
- Lymphoid interstitial pneumonia or pulmonary lymphoid hyperplasia complexa[a, b]
- Lymphoma, Burkitt (or equivalent term)
- Lymphoma, immunoblastic (or equivalent term)
- Lymphoma, primary, of brain
- *Mycobacterium avium* complex or *mycobacterium kansasii*, disseminated or extrapulmonary[b]
- *Mycobacterium tuberculosis* of any site, pulmonary,[b, c] disseminated,[b] or extrapulmonary[b]
- *Mycobacterium*, other species or unidentified species, disseminated[b] or extrapulmonary[b]
- *Pneumocystis jirovecii* pneumonia[b]
- Pneumonia, recurrent[b, c]
- Progressive multifocal leukoencephalopathy
- *Salmonella* septicemia, recurrent
- Toxoplasmosis of brain, onset at age >1 month[b]
- Wasting syndrome attributed to HIV

[a]Only among children aged <13 years.
[b]Condition that might be diagnosed presumptively.
[c]Only among adults and adolescents aged >13 years.

SOURCE: Eileen Schneider et al. "Appendix A. AIDS-Defining Conditions," in "Revised Surveillance Case Definitions for HIV Infection among Adults, Adolescents, and Children Aged <18 Months and for HIV Infection and AIDS among Children Aged 18 Months to <13 Years—United States, 2008," in *Morbidity and Mortality Weekly Report*, vol. 57, no. RR-10, December 5, 2008, http://www.cdc.gov/mmwr/PDF/rr/rr5710.pdf (accessed June 23, 2009)

in a medical record also meet the criteria for HIV infection. Children aged 18 months to less than 13 years are categorized for surveillance purposes as having AIDS if the criteria for HIV infection are met and at least one of the AIDS-defining conditions listed in Table 5.1 has been documented.

There are three categories of HIV-infected children: those younger than 18 months who were perinatally exposed (acquired the virus from their mother), children older than 18 months with perinatal infection, and infants and children of all ages who acquired the virus through other types of exposure.

Children Younger Than 18 Months

The screening and confirmatory blood tests that accurately diagnose HIV in adults are not reliable for detecting HIV in children younger than 18 months old due to the presence of passively acquired maternal antibodies. Early recognition of HIV infection in infants younger than 18

TABLE 5.2

Surveillance case definitions for HIV infection in children aged 18 months to <13 years, 2008

These 2008 surveillance case definitions of HIV infection and AIDS supersede those published in 1987 and 1999 and apply to all variants of HIV (e.g., HIV-1 or HIV-2). They are intended for public health surveillance only and are not a guide for clinical diagnosis.

The 2008 laboratory criteria for reportable HIV infection among persons aged 18 months to <13 years exclude confirmation of HIV infection through the diagnosis of AIDS-defining conditions alone. Laboratory-confirmed evidence of HIV infection is now required for all reported cases of HIV infection among children aged 18 months to <13 years.

Criteria for HIV infection

Children aged 18 months to <13 years are categorized as HIV infected for surveillance purposes if at least one of laboratory criteria or the other criterion is met.

Laboratory criteria

Positive result from a screening test for HIV antibody (e.g., reactive EIA), confirmed by a positive result from a supplemental test for HIV antibody (e.g., Western blot or indirect immunofluorescence assay).

or

Positive result or a detectable quantity by any of the following HIV virologic (non-antibody) tests:—HIV nucleic acid (DNA or RNA) detection (e.g., PCR)—HIV p24 antigen test, including neutralization assay—HIV isolation (viral culture)

Other criterion (for cases that do not meet laboratory criteria)

HIV infection diagnosed by a physician or qualified medical-care provider based on the laboratory criteria and documented in a medical record. Oral reports of prior laboratory test results are not acceptable.

EIA = enzyme immunoassay. PCR = polymerase chain reaction.

SOURCE: Eileen Schneider et al., "2008 Surveillance Case Definitions for HIV Infection and AIDS among Children Aged 18 Months to <13 Years," in "Revised Surveillance Case Definitions for HIV Infection among Adults, Adolescents, and Children Aged <18 Months and for HIV Infection and AIDS among Children Aged 18 Months to <13 Years—United States, 2008," in *Morbidity and Mortality Weekly Report*, Centers for Disease Control and Prevention, December 5, 2008, http://www.cdc.gov/mmwr/PDF/rr/rr5710.pdf (accessed June 23, 2009)

months is accomplished using polymerase chain reaction (PCR), a test that amplifies the amounts of viral genetic material to detectable levels, by the direct isolation of the HIV virus using viral culture techniques or by the detection of the p24 viral antigen. According to the NIAID, in "HIV Infection in Infants and Children," these tests can identify about 33% of infected babies at birth and 95% at three months of age. Those who are HIV-antibody positive and asymptomatic (without symptoms) without immune abnormalities have an HIV-infection status that cannot be determined unless a virus culture or other antigen-detection test is positive. As with any diagnostic test, the accuracy of detection is not absolute. The test does not detect 100% of people who are HIV positive because low levels of virus may escape detection. This possibility of a "false negative" result means that a negative culture does not necessarily rule out an infection. A small percentage of people who are infected with HIV can produce a negative result during testing.

Infants and children who are known to have been perinatally exposed (in other words, their mother is known to be HIV positive) but who lack one of the diagnostic criteria for HIV infection should be observed further for HIV-related illnesses and tested at regular intervals. The U.S. Public Health Service recommends that all infants of HIV-infected mothers be given the drug zidovudine (ZDV) for six weeks and that HIV-infected mothers be warned about the risks of transmission through breastfeeding. Infants with negative ZDV tests at birth should be retested periodically during the first 18 months of life. Studies suggest that ZDV therapy does not influence the accuracy of virus detection tests and consequently does not delay the diagnosis of HIV infection.

The 2008 criteria for indeterminate HIV infection stipulate that a child aged less than 18 months born to an HIV-infected mother is categorized as having perinatal exposure with an indeterminate HIV infection status if the criteria for infected with HIV and uninfected with HIV are not met. The CDC advises monitoring children with perinatal HIV exposure for potential complications of exposure to antiretroviral medications during the perinatal period and confirming the absence of HIV infection with repeat clinical and laboratory evaluations.

Classification

The 2008 changes in diagnostic criteria did not alter the existing classification system that was developed in 1994 for HIV infection in children less than 18 months or children aged 18 months to less than 13 years old. Table 5.3 shows the three categories of HIV infection that correspond to no evidence of immunological suppression, moderate immunosuppression, and severe suppression as defined by CD4+ T-lymphocyte counts and the percent of total lymphocytes for children less than one year old, one to five years old, and six to 12 years old.

PERINATAL INFECTION

The overwhelming majority (87%) of the cumulative totals of children younger than 13 who have been reported to have HIV infection through 2007 were infected perinatally. (See Table 5.4.) A number of factors are associated with an increased risk of an HIV-positive mother passing the infection to her baby. They include a low CD4+ T cell count, a high viral load (the concentration of the virus in the blood), advanced HIV progression, the presence of a particular HIV protein (p24) in serum, and placental membrane inflammation. Intrapartum (at the time of birth) events resulting in increased exposure of the baby to maternal blood, breastfeeding, low vitamin A levels, premature rupture of membranes, prenatal use of illicit drugs, and premature delivery also increase the risk of mother-to-child transmission. The risk of perinatal transmission also increases when the mother does not know she is infected until late in the course of the illness.

Despite these potential routes of transmission, the number of HIV-infected infants has been declining,

TABLE 5.3

Pediatric human immunodeficiency virus (HIV) classification

Immunologic category	Age of child					
	<12 mos		1–5 yrs		6–12 yrs	
	μL	(%)	μL	(%)	μL	(%)
1: No evidence of suppression	≥1,500	(≥25)	≥1,000	(≥25)	≥500	(≥25)
2: Evidence of moderate suppression	750–1,499	(15–24)	500–999	(15–24)	200–499	(15–24)
3: Severe suppression	<750	(<15)	<500	(<15)	<200	(<15)

μL = microliter.

SOURCE: M. Blake Caldwell et al., "Table 2. Immunologic Categories Based on Age-Specific CD4+T-Lymphocyte Counts and Percent of Total Lymphocytes," in "1994 Revised Classification System for Human Immunodeficiency Virus Infection in Children Less Than 13 Years of Age," *Morbidity and Mortality Weekly Report*, vol. 43, no. RR-12, September 30, 1994, http://www.cdc.gov/mmwr/preview/mmwrhtml/00032890.htm (accessed June 23, 2009)

TABLE 5.4

Reported cases of HIV infection for children <13, by transmission category and sex, 2007 and cumulative

[47 states, the District of Columbia, and 5 U.S. dependent areas with confidential name-based HIV infection reporting]

Transmission category	Males				Females				Total			
	2007		Cumulative[a]		2007		Cumulative[a]		2007		Cumulative[a]	
	No.	%	No.	%	No.	%	No.	%	No.	%	No.	%
Child (<13 yrs at diagnosis)												
Hemophilia/coagulation disorder	7	2	108	4	0	0	1	0	7	1	109	2
Mother with documented HIV infection or 1 of the												
following risk factors	254	81	2,397	85	283	82	2,669	89	537	82	5,066	87
Injection drug use	44	14	556	20	61	18	615	20	105	16	1,171	20
Sex with injection drug user	22	7	226	8	14	4	223	7	36	5	449	8
Sex with bisexual male	2	1	39	1	7	2	38	1	9	1	77	1
Sex with person with hemophilia	0	0	3	0	1	0	9	0	1	0	12	0
Sex with HIV-infected transfusion recipient	0	0	4	0	1	0	5	0	1	0	9	0
Sex with HIV-infected person, risk factor not specified	76	24	600	21	89	26	698	23	165	25	1,298	22
Receipt of blood transfusion, blood components, or tissue	1	0	17	1	0	0	19	1	1	0	36	1
Has HIV infection, risk factor not specified	109	35	952	34	110	32	1,062	35	219	33	2,014	35
Receipt of blood transfusion, blood components, or tissue	1	0	25	1	2	1	25	1	3	0	50	1
Other/risk factor not reported or identified	50	16	290	10	60	17	307	10	110	17	597	10
Subtotal	312	100	2,820	100	345	100	3,002	100	657	100	5,822	100
Total	48,659	100	242,580	100	14,571	100	95,006	100	63,230	100	337,590[b]	100

[a]From the beginning of the epidemic through 2007.
[b]Includes 4 persons of unknown sex.

SOURCE: Adapted from "Table 20. Reported Cases of HIV Infection (not AIDS) by Transmission Category and Sex, 2007 and Cumulative—47 States, the District of Columbia, and 5 U.S. Dependent Areas with Confidential Name-Based HIV Infection Reporting," in *HIV/AIDS Surveillance Report, 2007*, vol. 19, Centers for Disease Control and Prevention, 2009, http://www.cdc.gov/hiv/topics/surveillance/resources/reports/2007report/pdf/table20.pdf (accessed June 22, 2009)

probably as a result of the more widespread use of HAART to prevent pregnant women from passing HIV infection to their offspring. Planned cesarean section delivery (C-section; the surgical delivery of a baby), the presence of neutralizing antibodies in the mother, and timely antiviral drug therapy (such as with ZDV) further reduce the chances of mother-to-infant HIV transmission. In *HIV/AIDS Surveillance Report, 2007* (2009, http://www.cdc.gov/hiv/topics/surveillance/resources/reports/2007report/), the CDC indicates that between 1994 and 2007 there was a downward trend of HIV/AIDS infants born to HIV-infected mothers in the 25 states with confidential name-based HIV infection reporting.

Brenna L. Anderson and Susan Cu-Uvin note in "Pregnancy and Optimal Care of HIV-Infected Patients" (*Clinical Infectious Diseases*, vol. 48, no. 4, February 15, 2009) that there is evidence that planned C-section, with the administration of HAART, prevents some cases of mother-to-child HIV infection. C-section delivery does not expose the baby to potentially HIV-contaminated vaginal tissue.

ZDV

Even without a C-section, drug therapy can be beneficial. Edward M. Connor et al. discuss in "Reduction of Maternal-Infant Transmission of Human Immunodeficiency Virus Type 1 with Zidovudine Treatment" (*New England*

Journal of Medicine, vol. 331, no. 18, November 3, 1994) the results of their study, which was the first examination of perinatal transmission prevention and is considered a landmark study. Connor et al. conducted a randomized, double-blind, placebo-controlled (an inactive substance that does not contain a drug; placebos are used in comparative studies to measure the effectiveness of an experimental drug or regimen) study of antiviral prophylaxis using ZDV. At 18 months there was a dramatic risk reduction—two-thirds (67.5%)—in mother-to-child transmission. HIV transmission occurred in 25.5% of women who had received the placebo, compared with just 8.3% of those who received ZDV.

According to the World Health Organization (WHO), in *Children and AIDS: Second Stocktaking Report* (April 2008, http://www.unicef.org/publications/files/Children AIDS_SecondStocktakingReport.pdf), global efforts to reduce the rate of mother-to-child transmission have seen the most significant gains. In 2004 only 11% of women living with HIV were getting drugs to prevent transmission, but as of 2008, 31% were receiving treatment.

There have been comparable advances in the care of children with HIV/AIDS. In 2005 only 75,000 children were getting antiretroviral drugs, but in 2006 that number rose to 127,300—a 70% increase. But according to the WHO, in *Towards Universal Access: Scaling up Priority HIV/AIDS Interventions in the Health Sector* (September 2009, http://www.who.int/hiv/pub/2009progressreport/en/index.html) though the number of children receiving antiretroviral therapy (ART) has increased significantly in recent years, at the end of 2008 less than 40% of the 730,000 children needing ART in lower- and middle-income countries were receiving it. Infection usually occurs during the last stages of pregnancy, most often during labor and delivery.

New Thinking about How to Prevent Mother-to-Child Transmission

In "Effect of Breastfeeding on Mortality among HIV-Infected Women" (*Lancet*, vol. 357, no. 9269, May 26, 2001), Ruth Nduati et al. report that the WHO recommended in 2000 that HIV-positive mothers should avoid breastfeeding their infants to prevent transmission of the virus. According to Nduati et al., the WHO stipulated that "when replacement feeding is acceptable, feasible, affordable, sustainable and safe, avoidance of all breastfeeding by HIV-infected women is recommended."

Worldwide, this strategy has had mixed results in terms of its feasibility—in terms of the availability of infant formula and safe, uncontaminated water—and the overall health of infants. Hoosen M. Coovadia et al. find in "Mother-to-Child Transmission of HIV-1 Infection during Exclusive Breastfeeding in the First 6 Months of Life: An Intervention Cohort Study" (*Lancet*, vol. 369, no. 9567,

March 31, 2007) that in areas where HIV-infected mothers chose to use formula and breastfeed or to feed their babies formula and soft foods exclusively, there were actually higher rates of mother-to-infant transmission of HIV.

Coovadia et al. indicate that exclusive breastfeeding reduced the risk of HIV transmission by nearly half compared with when formula was given with breast milk, and by more than 10 times compared with when solid foods were also part of the infants' diets. These findings are somewhat surprising. One might expect that the more breast milk the infants consumed, the greater the viral exposure and rate of infection. Coovadia et al. posit several ideas about how exclusive breastfeeding might protect against infection, including:

- Exclusive breastfeeding protects the integrity of the lining of the gastrointestinal tract (the mouth, esophagus, stomach, and intestines), and an intact gastrointestinal tract may prevent the HIV from entering to the blood.

- The consumption of foreign proteins such as cows' milk protein as in formula milk might stimulate the large numbers of immune receptors that ordinarily line the gastrointestinal tract and enable the virus to better adhere to the lining of the gastrointestinal tract and enter into the underlying tissues.

- Exclusive breastfeeding is also associated with a lower amount of HIV virus in the milk, compared with when the mother combines breastfeeding and formula feeding. When mothers supplement their infants' diets with formula, the breast is not entirely emptied and the remaining milk contains higher levels of virus.

- Breast milk naturally contains several substances that can inhibit virus growth. Even though more breast milk will present more virus, the effects may be countered because the infant also ingests more of the substances that inhibit virus growth.

In "Infant Feeding and HIV: Avoiding Transmission Is Not Enough" (*British Medical Journal*, vol. 334, no. 7592, March 10, 2007), Nigel C. Rollins of the Nelson R Mandela School of Medicine in South Africa states that, in view of the results of this research, the WHO changed its recommendations in 2007. The new recommendations suggest that decision making be based on individual circumstances and acknowledge that infant survival, as opposed to simply preventing HIV transmission, should be the goal of infant feeding practices.

According to the WHO, in *HIV Transmission through Breastfeeding: A Review of Available Evidence—An Update from 2001 to 2007* (2008, http://whqlibdoc.who.int/publications/2008/9789241596596_eng.pdf), HIV-infected women are recommended to "breastfeed their infants exclusively for the first six months of life, unless replacement feeding is acceptable, feasible, affordable, sustainable and safe for them and their infants before that time. When those conditions are met, WHO recommends avoidance of all breastfeeding by HIV-infected women."

TREATMENTS FOR CHILDREN

Prescribing drug therapy for children is often more difficult than prescribing for adults because children respond to drugs differently at different ages and because oral medication must have an acceptable taste to ensure that children will take it as prescribed.

In "Approved Antiretroviral Drugs for Pediatric Treatment of HIV Infection" (May 20, 2009, http://www.fda.gov/ForConsumers/ByAudience/ForPatientAdvocates/HIVandAIDSActivities/ucm118951.htm), the U.S. Food and Drug Administration (FDA) lists 28 drugs used to treat pediatric HIV patients. Nine of these, called protease inhibitors (PIs; used alone or in combination with other drugs to combat viral infection) were available for children two to 13 years old. PI compounds act by preventing the reproduction of HIV that is already in the host cells. However, safety and effectiveness had not been established for four of the PIs: tipranavir, saquinavir mesylate (SQV), darunavir, and atazanavir sulfate. The PIs approved for use and deemed safe and effective by the FDA are:

- Amprenavir

- Lopinavir/ritonavir

- Fosamprenavir calcium

- Ritonavir

- Nelfinavir mesylate

Another group of drugs approved for pediatric use are known as nucleoside reverse transcriptase inhibitors (NRTIs). NRTIs, which are structurally similar to a nucleoside constituent of deoxyribonucleic acid (DNA), limit HIV replication by incorporating themselves into a strand of DNA, which causes the chain to end. The NRTIs approved for pediatric use are:

- Lamivudine

- Emtricitabine

- Abacavir

- Zalcitabine and dideoxycytidine

- Zidovudine

- Tenofovir disoproxil fumarate

- Enteric-coated didanosine

- Didanosine and dideoxyinosine

- Tenofovir disoproxil/emtricitabine

- Stavudine

Another group of antiretroviral drugs are known as nonnucleoside reverse transcriptase inhibitors (NNRTIs). NNRTIs slow down the functioning of the enzyme that allows the virus to become a part of the infected cell's nucleus. Three NNRTIs are presently approved for pediatric use:

- Delavirdine

- Efavirenz

- Nevirapine

In March 1996 the Antiviral Drugs Advisory Committee of the FDA approved the use of the compound didanosine for pediatric use. The approval was based on the results of two separate U.S. AIDS Clinical Trials Group pediatric studies (one of which was the largest controlled pediatric trial to date) and an Australian study, all of which found that didanosine delayed the progression of AIDS and was superior to ZDV alone. ZDV, which is given to children and adults, had been the only drug widely recognized to help delay the progress of HIV infection and to reduce the risk of perinatal infection.

The study results generated high expectations for the performance of didanosine in both children and adults. Indeed, the didanosine and combination therapies were so much more effective than ZDV alone that the AIDS Clinical Trials Group prematurely discontinued the ZDV-only therapy portion of the study. As promising as these early reports seemed, the effectiveness of didanosine alone or in combination with ZDV was short-lived because HIV susceptibility to the drugs decreased over time. Thus, even though didanosine is still used, it has not proven to be a major breakthrough in HIV infections as was hoped.

In 1999 a study conducted jointly by the United States and Uganda demonstrated that the perinatal transmission of HIV from mother to child could be reduced by the drug nevirapine. The drug is given to the mother in labor and to the child within three days of birth. Initial study results showed the drug to be safe for both mother and child and relatively inexpensive ($4 per mother/child dose). In 2000 the Elizabeth Glaser Pediatric AIDS Foundation, a nonprofit organization dedicated to promoting and funding worldwide pediatric AIDS research, secured funds to implement this treatment in developing countries that lack health care resources and infrastructure.

By 2003 the administration of nevirapine to hundreds of thousands of pregnant women in Africa demonstrated the therapeutic potential of the drug in slowing the progression of pediatric AIDS. The WHO, governments throughout sub-Saharan Africa, and the U.S. National Institutes of Health have all recommended that nevirapine use be continued to prevent HIV transmission from mothers to infants.

Also in 2003 the drug enfuvirtide was approved for use by children over the age of six. This drug is the first of the fusion inhibitor class of antiretroviral drugs. It acts by inhibiting the fusion of HIV to the host cell membrane.

In late 2007 two additional drugs—maraviroc and raltegravir—joined the FDA-approved list, although neither had, as of September 2009, established that it is safe and effective for children. Maraviroc is an entry inhibitor, meaning that it acts to block a receptor, CCR5, that HIV uses to enter white blood cells. Raltegravir is a HIV integrase strand transfer inhibitor, which means it targets integrase, an HIV enzyme that integrates the viral genetic material into human chromosomes.

HOW MANY CHILDREN ARE INFECTED?

In 2007, 657 children younger than 13 were diagnosed with HIV infection in the United States. (See Table 5.4.) Of the 38,384 AIDS cases reported in 2007, just 87 were diagnosed in children under the age of 13. (See Table 3.5 in Chapter 3.)

In "Estimated Number of Births to HIV+ Women in the US, 2006" (February 4, 2009, http://www.retroconference.org/2009/PDFs/924.pdf), Suzanne K. Whitmore, Xinjian Zhang, and Allan W. Taylor of the CDC estimate that between 8,650 and 8,900 infants were born to HIV-infected women in the United States in 2006. The CDC indicates in *HIV/AIDS Surveillance Report, 2007* that of the 79 pediatric HIV/AIDS cases reported in 2007 by the 25 states with confidential name-based HIV infection reporting, 57 cases (representing 72% of the total) were in African-American children.

Geographic Distribution

The CDC (May 20, 2008, http://www.cdc.gov/hiv/topics/surveillance/resources/slides/epidemiology/slides/EPI-AIDS_19.pdf) reports that among children younger than 13 years of age in 2006, a total of 86 AIDS cases were reported; this was a decrease from 93 in 2005. As in previous years, most (86%) of these cases were acquired perinatally. In 2006 New York (15), Florida (11), Maryland (7), California (6), and Georgia (6) reported the highest numbers of cases. (See Figure 5.1.) Thirty states reported no pediatric AIDS cases in 2006.

In *Scaling up Early Infant Diagnosis and Linkages to Care and Treatment* (January 2009, http://www.uniteforchildren.org/files/Early_Infant_Diagnosis_Briefing_Note_Feb_2009.pdf), the United Nations (UN) Children's Fund observes that without timely, accurate diagnosis and treatment of HIV infection, "about one third of children living with HIV will die in their first year of life and almost 50% by the second year of life." Worldwide, in 2007 just 33% of HIV-infected expectant mothers received retroviral drug treatment to prevent mother-to-child transmission of HIV and only 8% of infants born to HIV-infected mothers were tested within the first two months of their life. As a result, most infants did not receive the timely treatment necessary for survival. Worldwide, in 2007 the deaths of an estimated 270,000 children under the age of 15 were attributable to HIV. The overwhelming majority (90%) of these deaths occurred in sub-Saharan Africa among children less than five years old.

Gene Mutation in Some Babies May Help

A gene mutation that slows the progress of HIV in adults was shown in the late 1990s to help HIV-infected newborns avoid serious AIDS-associated illnesses longer than those who do not have the mutation. Michael Fischereder et al. report in "CC Chemokine Receptor 5 and Renal-Transplant Survival" (*Lancet*, vol. 357, no. 9270, June 2, 2001) that the gene CC chemokine receptor 5 (CCR5) is present in 10% to 15% of whites but is not found in Asian-Americans or African-Americans.

The gene codes for a protein called CCR5. This protein and another one called CXCR4 are located on the surface of a number of human cells. In "Analysis of the Mechanism by Which the Small-Molecule CCR5 Antagonists SCH-351125 and SCH-350581 Inhibit Human Immunodeficiency Virus Type 1 Entry" (*Journal of Virology*, vol. 77, no. 9, May 2003), Fotini Tsamis et al. demonstrate that CCR5 and CXCR4 can be used as receptors by HIV-1 to enter and infect CD4+ T cells, dendritic cells, and macrophages. Furthermore, CCR5 has been shown to be essential for viral transmission and replication during the early phase of the disease, even before symptoms of infection appear. Researchers expect that further investigation of the CCR5 gene will eventually help them develop drugs to prevent or destroy HIV in newborns.

Some researchers, such as Michael Marmor et al., in "Resistance to HIV Infection" (*Journal of Urban Health*, vol. 83, no. 1, January 2006), speculate that because several of the same genetic mutations have been found in both exposed uninfected populations and in long-term nonprogressor populations (people who become infected but do not develop AIDS), a single theory may explain both phenomena—that the genetic traits prevent or hinder HIV-1 entry into cells, which reduces the likelihood of infection and, should infection occur, slows or entirely eliminates the development of serious disease.

According to María Salgado, in "The Role of the Host in Controlling HIV Progression" (*AIDS Reviews*, April–June 2009), new genetic technology and tools enable researchers to explore the impact of the complex interactions between viral and host factors that result in the control of HIV-induced immunodeficiency in some individuals who are long-term nonprogressors. Different genetic markers associated with the host immune system appear to play important roles in the control of HIV progression. These new technologies enable the collection and analysis of vast amounts of information and may help shed light on the precise role of host genetics in HIV disease progression.

FIGURE 5.1

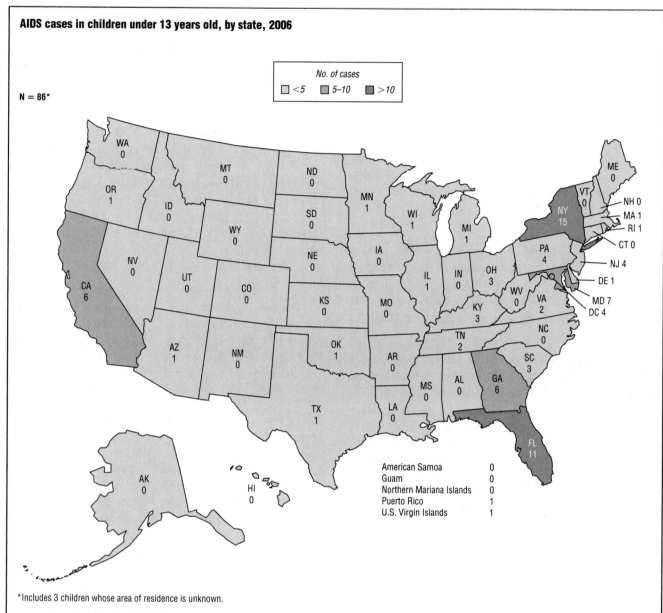

AIDS cases in children under 13 years old, by state, 2006

No. of cases
□ <5   ▨ 5–10   ■ >10

N = 86*

American Samoa	0
Guam	0
Northern Mariana Islands	0
Puerto Rico	1
U.S. Virgin Islands	1

*Includes 3 children whose area of residence is unknown.

SOURCE: "Slide 19. Reported AIDS Cases in Children <13 Years of Age at Diagnosis, 2006—United States and Dependent Areas," in *AIDS Surveillance—General Epidemiology (through 2006)*, Centers for Disease Control and Prevention, May 20, 2008, http://www.cdc.gov/hiv/topics/surveillance/resources/slides/epidemiology/slides/EPI-AIDS_19.pdf (accessed June 24, 2009)

ALL PREGNANT WOMEN SHOULD BE TESTED FOR HIV

When HIV-infected pregnant women know their HIV infection status, they are better able to make informed decisions about antiretroviral therapy to reduce perinatal transmission of HIV to their infants. The U.S. Preventive Services Task Force recommends that all pregnant women be offered HIV counseling and voluntary HIV tests.

In September 2008 the American College of Obstetrics and Gynecology's (ACOG) Committee on Obstetric Practice expanded its recommendations about prenatal and perinatal HIV testing in "ACOG Committee Opinion No. 418: Prenatal and Perinatal Human Immunodeficiency Virus Testing: Expanded Recommendations" (*Obstetrics and Gynecology*, vol. 112, no. 3). The committee recommended that all pregnant women be screened for HIV infection as early as possible during each pregnancy and informed that they will receive an HIV test as part of routine prenatal testing unless they decline or opt-out of HIV screening. Repeat conventional or rapid HIV testing in the third trimester of pregnancy is recommended for:

- Women living in areas with high HIV prevalence rates.

- Women known to be at high risk for acquiring HIV.

- Women who declined testing earlier in pregnancy.

TABLE 5.5

Maternal HIV testing among children with perinatally acquired AIDS, HIV exposure or HIV infection, 2007

Time of maternal HIV test	Perinatally acquired AIDS Population = 73		HIV exposure[a] Population = 2,361		HIV infection[b] Population = 529	
	No.	%	No.	%	No.	%
Before or at birth	28	38	2,240	95	213	40
After birth	29	40	47	2	138	26
Unknown	16	22	74	3	178	34

[a]From 33 areas that report perinatal exposure.
[b]From 53 areas with confidential name-based HIV infection reporting.

SOURCE: "Slide 11. Time of Maternal HIV Testing among Children with Perinatally Acquired AIDS, HIV Exposure or HIV Infection Reported in 2007—United States and Dependent Areas," in *Pediatric HIV/AIDS Surveillance (through 2007)*, Centers for Disease Control and Prevention, May 19, 2009, http://www.cdc.gov/hiv/topics/surveillance/resources/slides/pediatric/slides/pediatric_11.pdf (accessed June 25, 2009)

Of the children who were reported to the CDC in 2007 as being perinatally exposed to HIV (but who had not acquired HIV/AIDS), 95% were born to women who were tested before or at the time of birth. (See Table 5.5.) Of the children who were perinatally HIV infected, only 40% of their mothers were tested before or at the time of birth; of the children diagnosed with AIDS, only 38% were born to mothers tested before or at the time of birth. An additional 26% of mothers who had children reported with HIV infection and 40% of mothers who had children with AIDS were not tested until after the child's birth. These data demonstrate that early testing, which allows the timely ZDV therapy to prevent transmission, can help reduce HIV transmission from mothers to their children.

SURVIVING INTO THEIR TEENS

At the end of 2007, 2,527 children under the age of 13 were reported to be living with HIV infection in the 53 areas (47 states, the District of Columbia, and five U.S. dependent areas) that conducted confidential name-based HIV infection case surveillance in 2007. (See Figure 5.2.) An additional 881 children in these areas were living with AIDS. The states with the greatest numbers of HIV-infected children were New York (662), Florida (282), Texas (237), Georgia (129), Pennsylvania (120), New Jersey (117), and California (93). Even though many HIV-infected children die as infants and toddlers, most infected from birth now survive beyond age five, and it is not uncommon for others to reach their teens.

In "HIV Infection in Infants and Children," the NIAID distinguishes three distinct patterns of disease progression among HIV-infected children. The first group consists of those who display symptoms within their first 18 months following infection. Even with treatment, progression to AIDS in this group is rapid and most children die by age four. Children in the second group experience a less aggressive progression and often have milder or less prolonged symptomatic periods. These children tend to live longer. A third group is a recently emerging group of survivors. These children have grown up with few, if any, symptoms. Researchers are eager to determine precisely why and how these children remain asymptomatic in spite of their infection.

Research indicates that some of the difference in response to HIV is attributable to polymorphisms (common genetic variations). Kumud K. Singh and Stephen Spector find in "Host Genetic Determinants of HIV Infection and Disease Progression in Children" (*Pediatric Research*, January 28, 2009) that HIV-infected children with a specific polymorphism called CCR5-delta32 had half the rate of disease progression compared with children with normal CCR5. They also observe that the most rapid progression of HIV symptoms occurred in children with normal CCR5 plus a polymorphism called 59029-A/A. This particular polymorphism was identified in about 25% of the HIV-infected children studied, representing the genotype that most often accelerated the rate of disease progression in children with normal CCR5. Furthermore, Singh and Spector find that there were some polymorphisms that had an impact in adults but not in children, and some that seemed to have an important impact in children but only a modest impact in adults.

Dealing with Physical and Emotional Problems

When HIV-infected children died in the early years of the AIDS epidemic, they were generally unaware of what was happening to them. In the 21st century, at the Children's Evaluation and Rehabilitation Center of the Albert Einstein College of Medicine of Yeshiva University, school-aged children meet with social workers in a support group to handle the physical and emotional ordeals of growing up with HIV and AIDS. These children are part of the increasing number born with HIV who have survived long enough to realize what it means. They must learn to cope with the physical, psychological, and emotional consequences of HIV/AIDS.

In "Living with 'The Monster'" (*Achieve*, Winter 2009), Raven Lopez writes that HIV-positive children

FIGURE 5.2

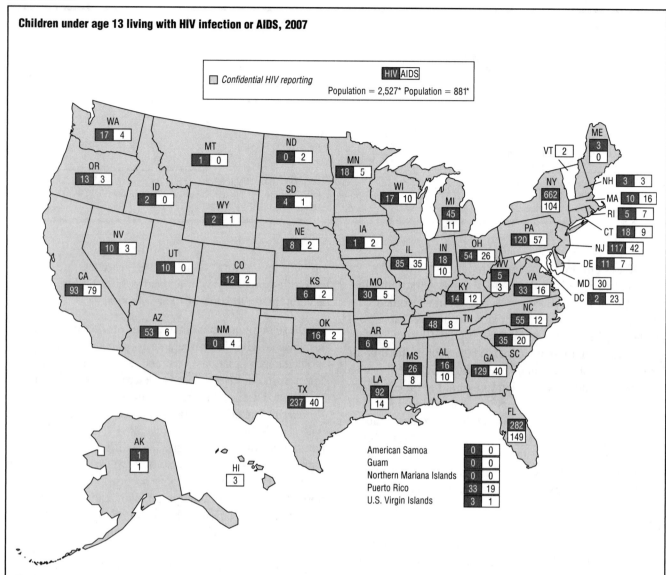

Children under age 13 living with HIV infection or AIDS, 2007

Notes: Data based on person's age as of December 31, 2007.

Data from 53 areas that have had laws or regulations requiring confidential name-based HIV infection reporting.

*Data include children reported with vital status "alive" as of last update.

Totals include persons whose state of residence is unknown or missing. HIV total includes persons reported from areas with confidential name-based HIV infection reporting, who were residents of other areas.

SOURCE: "Slide 6. Children <13 Years of Age Reported to Be Living with HIV Infection (not AIDS) or with AIDS, as of December 2007—United States and Dependent Areas," in *Pediatric HIV/AIDS Surveillance (through 2007)*, Centers for Disease Control and Prevention, May 19, 2009, http://www.cdc.gov/hiv/topics/surveillance/resources/slides/pediatric/slides/pediatric_6.pdf (accessed June 25, 2009)

deal with problems unique to their situation. For example, she recounts being excluded from class trips at school, being shunned and taunted by classmates, and being fearful of disclosing her HIV status to peers.

Lisa Henry-Reid, Lori Wiener, and Ana Garcia observe in "Caring for Youth with HIV" (*Achieve*, Winter 2009) that adolescents with HIV require significant psychological and emotional support because they face unique challenges including:

- Stigma and fear of rejection
- Side effects of HIV drugs

- Coping with a potentially life-threatening illness and an uncertain life span
- Disclosure and transmission
- The impact of loss
- Effectively navigating the health care system

Henry-Reid, Wiener, and Garcia report that adolescents who share their HIV diagnosis with others fare better psychologically and socially than those who do not disclose their HIV status. They assert that HIV-infected adolescents must deal with the normal challenges of adolescence and illness as well as with additional stressors such as poverty, barriers to care and social services, violence, racism, homophobia, broken families, homelessness, and child abuse.

WHO WILL CARE FOR THEM?

The HIV/AIDS pandemic has created many tragedies, including millions of orphans. The UN Joint Program on HIV/AIDS estimates in *2008 Report on the Global AIDS Epidemic* (2008, http://data.unaids.org/pub/GlobalReport/ 2008/jc1510_2008_global_report_pp211_234_en.pdf) that by the end of 2007 there were as many as 15 million orphans due to AIDS worldwide. Nearly 12 million children in sub-Saharan Africa alone had been orphaned due to AIDS.

It is not always possible to find someone to care for an orphan of parents who died of AIDS, particularly if the child also has HIV or AIDS. Some family members may be hesitant to take in the child for fear he or she may spread the infection. In a growing number of cases, however, grandparents (in most cases, grandmothers) are taking these orphans into their homes. This may be a burden on older people who have lost their own children and may feel too old, tired, or impoverished to rear another family. They may also fear that they will die before their grandchildren do, leaving no one to care for them. It is no less difficult for the children who have lost their parents and fear they will probably miss the advantages they would have had with younger parents, such as being able to play more active childhood games.

Older orphans struggle with the rage, shame, and isolation of losing a parent to AIDS. Observers are finding that the AIDS epidemic is creating a class of particularly troubled youth. All children who lose a parent suffer to some degree, but for those whose parents die from AIDS, embarrassment and secrecy often compound the trauma. Teens whose parents became infected as a result of injecting drugs or practicing unsafe sex are often torn between feeling sorry for their parents and blaming them for their illness.

ADOLESCENTS, YOUNG ADULTS, AND HIV/AIDS

Patterns of Infection

The transmission and course of AIDS among adolescents aged 13 to 19 and young adults aged 20 to 24 follow similar patterns to those over the age of 25. From 2004 through 2007 the majority of HIV/AIDS cases reported in male adolescents (87%) and young adults (83%) were attributed to male-to-male sexual contact. (See Table 5.6.) By contrast, female adolescents and young adults became infected through heterosexual contact (88% and 87%, respectively) or injection drug use (11% and 13%, respectively). (See Table 5.7.)

The characteristics of adolescence—a time of development, uncertainty, and a misleading sense of bravado and immortality, often combined with pushing the boundaries of good sense—create the potential for some young people to

TABLE 5.6

HIV/AIDS cases among male adolescents and young adults, by transmission category, 2004–07

Transmission category	13–19 years		20–24 years	
	No.	%	No.	%
Male-to-male sexual contact	3,171	87	10,226	83
Injection drug use	122	3	558	5
Male-to-male sexual contact and injection drug use	130	4	551	4
High-risk heterosexual contact[a]	221	6	910	7
Other/not identified[b]	7	<1	19	<1
Total	**3,651**		**12,264**	

Note: Data include persons with a diagnosis of HIV infection regardless of their AIDS status at diagnosis.
Data from 34 states with confidential name-based HIV infection reporting since at least 2003.
Data have been adjusted for reporting delays and missing risk-factor information.
[a]Heterosexual contact with a person known to have, or to be at high risk for, HIV infection.
[b]Includes hemophilia, blood transfusion, perinatal exposure, and risk factor not reported or not identified.

SOURCE: "Slide 4. Estimated Numbers of HIV/AIDS Cases among Male Adolescents and Young Adults, by Transmission Category 2004–2007—34 States," in *HIV/AIDS Surveillance in Adolescents and Young Adults (through 2007)*, Centers for Disease Control and Prevention, May 14, 2009, http://www.cdc.gov/hiv/topics/surveillance/resources/slides/adolescents/slides/Adolescents_4.pdf (accessed June 25, 2009)

TABLE 5.7

HIV/AIDS cases among female adolescents and young adults, by transmission category, 2004–07

Transmission category	13–19 years		20–24 years	
	No.	%	No.	%
Injection drug use	219	11	555	13
High-risk heterosexual contact[a]	1,694	88	3,846	87
Other/not identified[b]	7	<1	16	<1
Total	**1,920**		**4,417**	

Note: Data include persons with a diagnosis of HIV infection regardless of their AIDS status at diagnosis.
Data from 34 states with confidential name-based HIV infection reporting since at least 2003.
Data have been adjusted for reporting delays and missing risk-factor information.
[a]Heterosexual contact with a person known to have, or to be at high risk for, HIV infection.
[b]Includes hemophilia, blood transfusion, perinatal exposure, and risk factor not reported or not identified.

SOURCE: "Slide 5. Estimated Numbers of HIV/AIDS Cases among Female Adolescents and Young Adults, by Transmission Category 2004–2007—34 States," in *HIV/AIDS Surveillance in Adolescents and Young Adults (through 2007)*, Centers for Disease Control and Prevention, May 14, 2009, http://www.cdc.gov/hiv/topics/surveillance/resources/slides/adolescents/slides/Adolescents_5.pdf (accessed June 25, 2009)

become particularly vulnerable to HIV infection. For many, this is a time of experimentation and risk-taking, often in terms of sexual behavior or use of alcohol and illicit drugs.

Many Adolescents Are Sexually Active

More than one-third of adolescents are sexually active. In *YRBSS: Youth Risk Behavior Surveillance System—National*

Trends in Risk Behaviors (May 2008, http://www.cdc.gov/ HealthyYouth/yrbs/pdf/yrbs07_us_sexual_behaviors_trend .pdf), the National Youth Risk Behavior Survey, which monitors health risk behaviors of adolescents in grades 9 to 12, indicates that in 2007, 35% of high school students reported they were currently sexually active and nearly half (47.8%) said they had had sexual intercourse. (See Table 5.8.)

In 2007 the overwhelming majority (89.5%) of teens said they had been taught in school about AIDS or HIV infection, an increase of about five percentage points since 1991. (See Table 5.8.) Condom use among sexually active teens rose about fifteen percentage points from 1991 to 2007. Among sexually active adolescents surveyed in 2007, nearly two-thirds (61.5%) had used a latex condom during their last sexual intercourse.

SEXUALLY TRANSMITTED DISEASES. Teenagers engaging in sexual activity before becoming sufficiently mature, with ineffective contraceptive methods, have led to record high rates of sexually transmitted diseases (STDs) among heterosexuals. According to the CDC, in *Trends in Reportable Sexually Transmitted Diseases in the United States, 2007* (January 2009, http://www.cdc.gov/ STD/stats07/trends.pdf), 19 million new infections occur each year, almost half of them among young people aged 15 to 24, and many in this group are unaware they are infected.

Even though overall rates of infection for some STDs, such as gonorrhea, declined during the 1990s and leveled off in the first decade of the 21st century, gonorrhea, syphilis, and chlamydia infections among adolescents appeared to be increasing. The CDC notes in "STDs in Adolescents and Young Adults" (January 13, 2009, http:// www.cdc.gov/std/stats07/adol.htm) that in 2007, for the third consecutive year, gonorrhea rates for people 15 to 19 and 20 to 24 years of age increased by 2.1% and 0.7%, respectively. Chlamydia rates for young people aged 15 to 19 and 20 to 24 rose 7.7% and 6.6%, respectively.

The rates of syphilis infection are similar. Rates among 15- to 19-year-old females increased from 1.5 cases per 100,000 population in 2004 to 2.4 cases per 100,000 population in 2007. Among women aged 20 to 24 there were 3.5 cases per 100,000 population in 2007. Among 15- to 19 -year-old males the rate rose from 3 cases per 100,000 population in 2006 to 3.8 cases per 100,000 population in 2007. Men aged 25 to 29 had the highest rates of any age group—14.9 cases per 100,000 population in 2007.

LEADING THE WAY: YOUNG PEOPLE AS AIDS ACTIVISTS AND ORGANIZATIONS THAT HELP YOUNG PATIENTS

Almost since the beginning of the epidemic, children and teenagers have been among the activists campaigning

for HIV/AIDS reforms and awareness of the disease. Their role has been a profoundly personal one. For example, until his death from AIDS on April 8, 1990, Ryan White—an Indiana teenager—generated worldwide attention to the disease and, in particular, to the stigmas and misconceptions surrounding it. White, who contracted the virus during treatment for his hemophilia, was a white, middle-class heterosexual boy, which ran counter to public perception of AIDS at the time as a disease of gay men.

Being expelled from school because of the supposed health risk to other students galvanized White to educate others on the nature of HIV and AIDS. His legacy includes the Ryan White Comprehensive AIDS Resources Emergency Act, the multibillion-dollar program that funds programs to help provide primary health care and support to those living with HIV/AIDS.

The National Association of People with AIDS, founded in 1983, advocates for people, including children, who live with HIV/AIDS. The nonprofit organization—the oldest national AIDS organization in the United States—is a strong advocate for HIV/AIDS social programs and research funding.

The AIDS Alliance for Children, Youth, and Families was established in 1994 to publicize the concerns of women, children, young people, and families who are affected by HIV/AIDS. The nonprofit organization is also a clearinghouse for relevant information and advocates for public policy changes in the areas of HIV/AIDS social welfare and disease prevention.

Metro TeenAIDS focuses on prevention, education, and treatment needs of teenagers. Through its Web site (http://www.metroteenaids.org/) and in-person contact at schools, nightclubs, youth centers, shelters, and on the street, Metro TeenAIDS connects with teenagers in a language that is relevant to them. The intent is to help teenagers protect themselves from the risks of HIV exposure and contamination and in securing medical care for HIV infection and AIDS.

Metro TeenAIDS has been working in conjunction with other youth and AIDS activists groups since 1994 to host annual conferences around the country that focus on educating young people about HIV and AIDS. In 1995 the conference became known as the Ryan White National Youth Conference on HIV and AIDS (RWNYC). In 2001 the first Positive Youth Institute—a one-day gathering specifically focusing on the needs of HIV-positive young people—was held before and in conjunction with the RWNYC. Each year several hundred young people, health care workers, and AIDS activists attend the conference. In February 2009 Metro TeenAIDS (2009, http://metroteen aids.org/?p=185) celebrated 20 years of service to more than 200,000 at-risk and HIV-infected adolescents, families, youth workers, and the community-at-large.

TABLE 5.8

Trends in the prevalence of sexual behaviors of high school students, selected years 1991–2007

	1991	1993	1995	1997	1999	2001	2003	2005	2007	Changes from 1991–2007*	Changes from 2005–2007
Ever had sexual intercourse	54.1 (50.5—57.8)	53.0 (50.2—55.8)	53.1 (48.4—57.7)	48.4 (45.2—51.6)	49.9 (46.1—53.7)	45.6 (43.2—48.1)	46.7 (44.0—49.4)	46.8 (43.4—50.2)	47.8 (45.1—50.6)	Decreased, 1991—2007	No change
Had sexual intercourse with four or more persons during their life	18.7 (16.6—21.0)	18.7 (16.8—20.9)	17.8 (15.2—20.7)	16.0 (14.6—17.5)	16.2 (13.7—19.0)	14.2 (13.0—15.6)	14.4 (12.9—16.1)	14.3 (12.8—15.8)	14.9 (13.4—16.5)	Decreased, 1991—2007	No change
Currently sexually active (Had sexual intercourse with at least one person during the 3 months before the survey.)	37.5 (34.3—40.7)	37.5 (35.4—39.7)	37.9 (34.4—41.5)	34.8 (32.6—37.2)	36.3 (32.7—40.0)	33.4 (31.3—35.5)	34.3 (32.1—36.5)	33.9 (31.4—36.6)	35.0 (32.8—37.2)	Decreased, 1991—2007	No change
Used a condom during last sexual intercourse (Among students who were currently sexually active.)	46.2 (42.8—49.6)	52.8 (50.0—55.6)	54.4 (50.7—58.0)	56.8 (55.2—58.4)	58.0 (53.6—62.3)	57.9 (55.6—60.1)	63.0 (60.5—65.5)	62.8 (60.6—64.9)	61.5 (59.4—63.6)	Increased, 1991—2003 No change, 2003—2007	No change
Used birth control pills before last sexual intercourse (To prevent pregnancy, among students who were currently sexually active.)	20.8 (18.5—23.2)	18.4 (16.3—20.7)	17.4 (15.2—19.8)	16.6 (14.7—18.8)	16.2 (13.6—19.0)	18.2 (16.5—20.0)	17.0 (14.7—19.4)	17.6 (15.1—20.5)	16.0 (14.2—17.9)	No change, 1991—2007	No change
Drank alcohol or used drugs before last sexual intercourse (Among students who were currently sexually active.)	21.6 (18.7—24.8)	21.3 (19.3—23.5)	24.8 (22.1—27.8)	24.7 (22.9—26.7)	24.8 (21.8—28.0)	25.6 (23.8—27.4)	25.4 (23.2—27.8)	23.3 (21.1—25.6)	22.5 (20.7—24.5)	Increased, 1991—2001 Decreased, 2001—2007	No change
Ever taught in school about AIDS or HIV infection	83.3 (80.1—86.0)	86.1 (83.4—88.4)	86.3 (79.0—91.3)	91.5 (90.3—92.5)	90.6 (89.1—91.9)	89.0 (87.6—90.3)	87.9 (85.8—89.7)	87.9 (85.8—89.7)	89.5 (88.1—90.7)	Increased, 1991—1997 Decreased, 1997—2007	No change

*Based on trend analyses using a logistic regression model controlling for sex, race/ethnicity, and grade.

SOURCE: "Trends in the Prevalence of Sexual Behaviors, National YRBS: 1991–2007," in *YRBSS: Youth Risk Behavior Surveillance System—National Trends in Risk Behaviors*, Centers for Disease Control and Prevention, National Center for Chronic Disease Prevention and Health Promotion, Division of Adolescent and School Health, February 17, 2009, http://www.cdc.gov/HealthyYouth/yrbs/pdf/yrbs07_us_sexual_behaviors_trend.pdf (accessed June 25, 2009)

CHAPTER 6

HIV/AIDS COSTS AND TREATMENT

FINANCING HEALTH CARE DELIVERY

Care for HIV/AIDS patients is expensive. Drug treatments, most prominently highly active antiretroviral therapy (HAART), have high per-unit costs. Nonetheless, their introduction in 1996 reduced total health care spending on AIDS by reducing the rate of hospitalization and outpatient care. According to Samuel A. Bozzette et al., in "Expenditures for the Care of HIV-Infected Patients in the Era of Highly Active Antiretroviral Therapy" (*New England Journal of Medicine*, vol. 344, no. 11, March 15, 2001), the average HIV patient incurred costs of about $1,410 per month in 1998. Extended over the full year, a patient's drug treatment for HIV could cost as much as $18,300. People with AIDS could spend up to $77,000 a year on treatment.

Longer survival periods following infection with HIV lead to even greater costs for care and treatment. For example, according to the findings by Bruce R. Schackman et al., in "The Lifetime Cost of Current Human Immunodeficiency Virus Care in the United States" (*Medical Care*, vol. 44, no. 11, November 2006), people with HIV can gain as many as 24.2 extra years of life at a total cost of $618,900 (in 2004 dollars).

This study illustrates the effects of the increasing treatment costs and enhanced survival. Schackman et al. estimate the monthly cost of care at $2,100, with about 70% of costs attributable to medications. This equates to $25,200 a year. In 1998 the average annual cost was $18,300, according to Bozzette et al. The cost increase is not simply a consequence of inflation, because the increased cost of HIV drugs account for much of the difference. Schackman et al. estimate that these costs are $12.1 billion per year.

Some HIV/AIDS patients rely on health insurance to help pay these costs. However, many patients are not insured. Also, many policies exclude or deny coverage to people with preexisting conditions, and, as a result, many HIV-positive people are denied private health insurance.

The article "Policy Facts: Early Treatment for HIV Act" (June 2004, http://www.thebody.com/content/policy/art33771.html) explains that 55% of adults and 90% of children living with HIV/AIDS in the United States have the costs of their treatment paid for by Medicaid. Medicaid is an entitlement program run by the federal and state governments to provide health care insurance to patients younger than 65 who cannot afford to pay for private health insurance. Medicaid eligibility requirements vary from state to state. Generally, however, the program covers people with incomes of less than $700 per month who cannot support themselves financially due to a physical or mental impairment—an impairment that is expected to last at least one year or result in death. The operation of Medicaid programs also varies widely by jurisdiction. Many states supplement federal funding with their own funds, and each state determines its eligibility criteria and benefits—the number and type of treatments provided through the program.

The toll of HIV/AIDS on the Medicaid program is huge. The Kaiser Family Foundation estimates in the fact sheet "U.S. Federal Funding for HIV/AIDS: The President's FY 2010 Budget Request" (May 2009, http://www.kff.org/hivaids/upload/7029-05.pdf) that the federal contribution to Medicaid for HIV/AIDS care rose from $3.6 billion in fiscal year (FY) 2006 to $4.7 billion in FY 2010.

Medicare, the federal health insurance program for adults aged 65 and older and younger adults with permanent disabilities, accounts for approximately a quarter of federal spending on HIV/AIDS care in the United States. The Kaiser Family Foundation projects that Medicare spending for HIV/AIDS will grow from $3.9 billion in FY 2006 to $5.1 billion in FY 2010.

A Reverse in Federal Policy

In early 1997 the administration of President Bill Clinton (1946–) announced that it hoped to expand Medicaid to cover all low-income HIV-infected people. The administration wanted to give low-income HIV-positive people access to HAART drugs that slow the onset of AIDS. By the end of the year, however, the administration announced that it could not follow through because such a nationwide plan would increase government spending. Both the Clinton administration and the administration of George W. Bush (1946–) forbade the federal government and states to change the Medicaid rules if that change would increase spending over a five-year period. As of September 2009, only patients who had been diagnosed with full-blown AIDS, not those who were HIV positive, were covered by Medicaid.

Throughout 2009 efforts were under way to extend Medicaid benefits to cover people with HIV before they develop AIDS. In "Court Orders Medicaid Coverage for Low-Income HIV Patients" (*American Medical News*, January 12, 2009), Amy Lynn Sorrel reports that at the close of 2008 a California court found that California had deprived thousands of HIV-positive patients through Medi-Cal (the California state Medicaid program) and ordered the state to provide coverage for these patients. In March 2009 Representatives Eliot L. Engel (1947–; D-NY), Ileana Ros-Lehtinen (1952–; R-FL), and Speaker of the House Nancy Pelosi (1940–; D-CA) reintroduced H.R. 1616, Early Treatment for HIV Act, to allow states to expand Medicaid coverage to low-income HIV-positive people. This act had been introduced in previous congressional sessions, but despite broad bipartisan support it had not been passed into law.

State Programs to Provide Drugs

In the late 1980s state-administered programs were established to help AIDS patients pay for azidothymidine (now called zidovudine [ZDV]), the newest effective drug at the time. The programs give free drugs to AIDS patients who are not poor enough to qualify for Medicaid coverage but who do not have private health insurance coverage or who have used up their prescription drug coverage. The federal government provides two-thirds of the funding for the state programs, and the balance comes mostly from the states. In "Utilization and Spending Trends for Antiretroviral Medications in the U.S. Medicaid Program from 1991 to 2005" (*AIDS Research and Therapy*, vol. 4, no. 1, October 16, 2007), Yonghua Jing et al. report that in 2005 Medicaid spent $1.6 billion for antiretrovirals. (Since 2006, when a new Medicare prescription drug benefit, Part D, went into effect, people eligible for both Medicaid and Medicare have had the cost of their drugs covered by the new benefit.)

Until recently, these drug programs did not attract many participants, primarily because ZDV alone was not effective against the disease. In the late 1990s, however, with the development of a new class of antiretroviral drugs—called protease inhibitors—that reduce the amount of virus in the blood, more patients wanted to take advantage of the programs. (According to the Institute of Medicine, in *Public Financing and Delivery of HIV/AIDS Care: Securing the Legacy of Ryan White* [May 2004], a typical three-drug cocktail—one new protease inhibitor combined with two other HIV/AIDS medications—costs more than $12,000 per year per patient. By 2009 the costs were higher still. For example, according to Jim Edwards, in "Merck CEO Clark Subject of 'Wanted' Poster over Price of HIV Drugs" [September 8, 2009, http://industry.bnet .com/pharma/10004154/merck-ceo-clark-subject-of-wanted-poster-over-price-of-hiv-drugs/], the AIDS Healthcare Foundation stated that a year's supply of the drug raltegravir cost nearly $13,000.)

This growing demand has put a financial strain on the programs, and many states have to ration HIV/AIDS drugs or turn patients away to remain solvent. Some states are making it harder for people to qualify for the programs, and a few are beginning to charge small copayments (a percentage of the total cost that the patient is responsible for paying) to offset the cost of the drugs. Others are attempting to obtain larger price discounts or rebates on drugs in an effort to reduce their costs so they can continue to provide drugs to an expanding population of patients.

The National Alliance of State and Territorial AIDS Directors reports in *National ADAP Monitoring Project Annual Report* (April 2009, http://www.nastad.org/Docs/highlight/200946_7861%20FULL%20REPORT%20v3.pdf) that as of March 2009, 62 people in Indiana, Montana, and Nebraska were on waiting lists for AIDS Drug Assistance Programs (ADAPs). ADAP spending on prescription drugs accounted for nearly 97% of all program expenditures and totaled $1.2 billion in FY 2007. The majority of ADAPs cover all U.S. Food and Drug Administration (FDA) approved antiretroviral drugs and at least half of the medications used to prevent and treat HIV-related opportunistic infections. Many coordinate with public programs—Medicare and Medicaid—as well as private insurance. ADAPs face significant challenges in the form of increasing demand in response to Centers for Disease Control and Prevention (CDC) programs aimed at increasing the number of people who know their HIV status and growing unemployment (resulting in the loss of health insurance), coupled with decreases in state funding as a result of the economic recession that began in 2007 and continued throughout 2009.

AVAILABILITY OF LIFE INSURANCE. In 1997 Guarantee Trust Life Insurance Company, a small midwestern company, began offering life insurance to some HIV-positive people. Richard S. Holson III, the company president, said the company decided to offer the coverage because it believes that many HIV-positive people are otherwise healthy and should be viewed as having a treatable chronic illness rather than a terminal disease. With new treatments available, affected people are living longer.

The policies provide up to $250,000 of coverage and are offered to those who acquired the virus through sexual activity or accidental needle sticks. Applicants must be between the ages of 21 and 49, have previous and current CD4 tests of 400 or greater, and never have been diagnosed with AIDS. Coverage is not offered to people who acquired the disease through injection drug use because drug use increases the company's risks, including the chance that prescribed medications will not be taken. The coverage is expensive: a typical 30-year-old, nonsmoking male who is HIV-positive pays $1,500 per month for the $250,000 policy.

As of 2009, Guarantee Trust Life Insurance Company was the only U.S. firm to offer coverage for people infected with HIV. Many insurance companies explain that they do not single out HIV-positive people but also exclude those with other diseases such as Alzheimer's disease, amyotrophic lateral sclerosis (also known as Lou Gehrig's disease), or cancer.

Changes to the Health Care System

Since the 1960s U.S. government spending on health services has consistently increased. The U.S. Centers for Medicare and Medicaid Services, Office of the Actuary (December 2008, http://www.census.gov/compendia/statab/tables/09s0124.pdf) reports that federal health expenditures rose 477%, from $194 billion in 1990 to an estimated $926 billion in 2010. At the same time health care providers—doctors, hospitals, and other health-related institutions and professions—watched as payments for Medicare, Medicaid, and private insurance coverage, once easily obtained in the 1960s and 1970s, were increasingly restricted and limited. During the 1990s providers also encountered a greater resistance among private insurers to pay. Bureaucratic management, increasing amounts of paperwork to document medical care and claims, and slow reimbursement rates prompted some physicians to stop caring for Medicare/Medicaid patients.

Managed-care plans (also known as managed-care organizations [MCOs]), which control the use of and reimbursement for services in an effort to contain costs, rely heavily on primary care practitioners (general and family physicians). These plans have become the health care providers for increasing numbers of HIV/AIDS patients. Since 2000 many HIV-infected people have enrolled in managed-care plans. This is partly because more companies are only offering employees managed-care plans and partly because government insurance programs are directing Medicaid recipients to such programs.

A MANAGED-CARE PLAN FOR HIV/AIDS PATIENTS: THE TENNESSEE "CENTERS OF EXCELLENCE" PROGRAM. On January 1, 1994, Tennessee withdrew from the federal Medicaid program and began implementing a state health care reform plan called Tennessee Medicaid (TennCare). In May 1998 TennCare introduced a voluntary managed-care plan for its members with HIV or AIDS. The model plan features "Centers of Excellence" providers—practitioners with expertise in the care of HIV/AIDS patients. The providers must agree to adopt and adhere to a clinical protocol (practice and care guidelines) developed by a committee composed of providers, consumers, MCOs, and public health officials. The committee meets up to twice a month to evaluate and recommend new drug therapies as they become available and to inform participating providers about new treatments.

Providers may be individual practitioners with access to needed services or full-service clinics composed of a group of practitioners. There are no financial incentives to participate in the program. However, providers who meet the Centers of Excellence criteria do not have to obtain prior authorization when they prescribe drugs or treatments that fall under the clinical protocols.

The Centers of Excellence program frees MCOs from the clinical and administrative responsibility of keeping close tabs on HIV/AIDS care. It also allows MCOs to remain confident that providers are capable and have access to a wide range of services needed by members. MCO members know that participating providers meet high standards of HIV/AIDS clinical care. Other managed-care plans are developing comparable programs to meet the unique health and social service needs of people living with HIV/AIDS.

TennCare (2009, http://www.tennessee.gov/tenncare/), which provides health care for 1.2 million people with an annual budget of $7 billion a year, has endured criticism since its beginning. Doctors and hospitals have complained that it has been underfunded, forcing them to carry an unfair proportion of the costs. However, in 2009 TennCare (http://www.tn.gov/tenncare/recovery/) reported that it was slated to receive $1.1 billion in additional federal dollars over the nine-quarter-recession adjustment period (October 2008 to December 2010) outlined in the American Recovery and Reinvestment Act.

CHALLENGES FOR THE DELIVERY SYSTEM

HIV/AIDS poses a major challenge to health care institutions, health care professionals, and others who provide direct health care services. Since its emergence and identification, HIV infection has undergone a dramatic transformation—it has gone from being an infectious disease that was an almost certain death sentence to a chronic disease that for many can be managed for decades. Furthermore, unlike most chronic diseases that afflict older Americans, HIV/AIDS affects people of all ages, and young adults are disproportionately affected. The health care system cares for about a million people in the United States suffering from a disease that is still only partly understood. The system must also plan to deliver services to the tens of thousands of people in United States who are HIV positive and will require specialized health care services during the coming years, even though only a small proportion will need intensive medical care at any one time.

The number of indigent people in need of HIV/AIDS care, particularly those who bring the added complications of drug addiction, homelessness, and other socioeconomic problems, has strained public hospitals in particular. Patients in public hospitals are often different from those in private hospitals. They generally seek care later in the course of the disease's progression and are, therefore, sicker. The scarcity of resources—trained personnel, hospital beds, and support services—in the community, combined with inadequate funding and reimbursement for HIV/AIDS care, are significant obstacles to effective health care delivery for poor HIV/AIDS patients.

Office Visits

Some physicians, particularly those who handle many HIV/AIDS patients, have extended their office hours or hired counselors to deal with these patients because their visits are time consuming. In *Patient Characteristics and the Use of Health Care Services by Persons with HIV* (2007, http://www.cdc.gov/nchs/ppt/ahcd/HingLucas_8.ppt), Esther Hing and Christine Lucas of the CDC note that between 2005 and 2006 there were over 2.8 million outpatient visits for HIV.

Hospital Care

The American Hospital Association reports in "Fast Facts on US Hospitals" (April 13, 2009, http://www.aha.org/aha/resource-center/Statistics-and-Studies/fast-facts.html) that in 2007 there were 5,708 hospitals. These hospitals are also feeling the pinch of Medicare rate limits, reduced payments from MCOs, and intense competition from other providers, such as ambulatory surgical centers and hospices. Many are struggling to remain profitable institutions. During the 1970s and 1980s the steady growth of for-profit hospitals lured many privately insured, middle-class patients away from community hospitals, leaving most of the uninsured, sicker patients to seek care from inner-city public hospitals.

Most HIV/AIDS patients are cared for in inner-city public hospitals that are already overburdened with inadequate revenues, staff shortages, lack of referral facilities, and emergency rooms used by many poor neighborhood residents as sources of primary medical care. Many health care professionals praise a model of hospital care pioneered in San Francisco, California. This city was hit hard in the early days of the AIDS epidemic and developed a range of innovative, effective programs in response to acute need during the early 1990s. This model of care

relies on extensive outpatient services and volunteer social support services provided by the well-established and well-organized gay and lesbian community.

Changes in Health Care Delivery

Even though fewer people are acquiring HIV/AIDS, the evolution of HIV care is altering the ways in which health care is delivered. In the late stages of AIDS, most patients require intermittent hospitalization and home health care. Those who are not as severely affected and have symptoms or conditions that once required intravenous therapy (which had to be administered in a hospital or by home health professionals) are now able to self-medicate at home. Many drugs are now available for oral administration in pill or liquid form. These home care and community-based measures lessen the burden on the health care delivery system and make it easier for HIV/AIDS patients to care for themselves.

People with AIDS (PWAs) who receive informal home health care (such as care from friends and family) often use fewer hospital services, perhaps reflecting a greater desire to remain at home. PWAs with strong social support systems and who prefer to remain at home may also be less likely to demand an aggressive approach to treating their illness. Those who receive formal home health care (visits from physicians, nurses, therapists, social workers, case managers, and other paid caregivers) often use more hospital services. This may reflect a greater use of all types of health services by PWAs with weaker social support systems and/or an aggressive approach to treatment by medical professionals.

An AIDS Care Alternative

In an effort to offer uninsured AIDS patients in Atlanta, Georgia, treatment equal to that available to patients with private insurance, Grady Memorial Hospital (2009, http://www.gradyhealthsystem.org/Specialties/specialties_idp.asp) began an outpatient infectious disease program (IDP) in 1993 that includes an HIV/AIDS clinic. Since that time the Grady IDP has provided emergency care, dental services, mental health counseling, social and support services, HIV research and education, and case management. In 2009 it served about 5,000 adults, adolescents, and children. The program also works closely with many local AIDS service organizations, some housed onsite, to meet the complex needs of people living with HIV/AIDS. The Grady IDP (2009, http://hwgf.org/history.html) is the largest publicly funded program of its kind in the eastern United States and is consistently named one of the top three HIV/AIDS outpatient clinics in the country.

Hospice Care

The AIDS epidemic has had a significant impact on hospices. Hospice care, both in the home and in specialized centers, offers care aimed at comfort rather than cure. This includes expert pain relief, along with emotional, psychological, and spiritual support for patients, their families, and friends. Most hospice patients are older adults who suffer from terminal diseases such as cancer and face imminent death.

At the beginning of the AIDS epidemic, patients did not fit well into the hospices of the day. AIDS patients were younger than traditional hospice patients, and the progression of their disease was less predictable than many cancers. Furthermore, as one hospice administrator noted, because many people with AIDS were accustomed to prejudice, they initially mistrusted the motivation and altruism of hospice workers. However, during the first decade of the 21st century home-based hospice programs were designed to meet the needs of AIDS patients, their partners, and families and gained acceptance in the medical community as well as among HIV-infected people and the voluntary social service agencies organized to support them.

HEALTH CARE PROVIDERS

Physicians

There are physicians from many medical specialties—primary care physicians such as family practitioners, internists, and specialists in infectious diseases, pulmonary medicine, and cancer medicine—who care for people infected with HIV or those suffering from AIDS. Physicians who treat AIDS patients often perform a wide variety of services besides providing care to AIDS patients. Many are also AIDS activists and may be involved in developing policies, planning for care needs, and dealing with the media.

One challenge in the training of physicians to treat AIDS patients is that AIDS care requires skills and training in the multitude of conditions known to be part of HIV/AIDS. However, the amount of experience—rather than the kind of training—may be a better predictor of the quality of care the physician is able to deliver.

Mari M. Kitahata et al. claim in the landmark study "Physicians' Experience with the Acquired Immunodeficiency Syndrome as a Factor in Patients' Survival" (New England Journal of Medicine, vol. 334, no. 11, March 14, 1996) that AIDS patients treated by primary care physicians with no previous experience dealing with the disease died more than a year earlier than those whose doctors had treated at least five AIDS patients. The researchers also show that patients had a 43% decrease in relative risk of death at any given time when treated by a physician who had treated other AIDS patients. The difference, according to Kitahata et al., was that the more experienced physicians consulted more frequently with specialists and reported more visits with their AIDS patients.

Since 1996 Kitahata et al.'s findings have been verified by further research, such as William E. Cunningham et al.'s "The Effect of Hospital Experience on Mortality among Patients Hospitalized with Acquired Immunodeficiency Syndrome in California" (American Journal of Medicine, vol. 107, no. 2, August 1999) and Kitahata et al.'s "Primary Care Delivery Is Associated with Greater Physician Experience and Improved Survival among Persons with AIDS" (Journal of General Internal Medicine, vol. 18, no. 2, February 2003).

There is also a continuing debate about the types of physicians who should treat patients with complex chronic medical conditions such as HIV infection. In "Physician Specialization and the Quality of Care for Human Immunodeficiency Virus Infection" (Archives of Internal Medicine, vol. 165, no. 10, May 23, 2005), Bruce E. Landon et al. describe the results of their research to assess the relationship between specialty training and expertise and the quality of care delivered to patients with HIV infection. The investigators looked at 5,247 patients of 177 physicians who responded to a survey. Over four out of 10 (42%) of the physicians were infectious diseases specialists and 58% were general medicine physicians (primary care physicians who are often called generalists). Nearly two-thirds of the generalists (63% of the generalists and 37% overall) considered themselves expert in HIV care. An analysis of the data Landon et al. collected reveals that infectious diseases physicians and generalists who considered themselves expert in HIV care had performed similarly. In contrast, nonexpert generalists delivered lower-quality care. Landon et al. posit that their findings reconfirm the premise that "generalists with appropriate experience and expertise in HIV care can provide high-quality care to patients with this complex chronic illness."

Nurses

The effect of HIV/AIDS on nurses can be more difficult to assess than its effect on doctors. Nurses often have different viewpoints than some physicians about their professional obligations to patients with HIV. As hospital employees, nurses seldom have the option of choosing whether to treat a particular patient (nor do patients have much choice of nurses). Nurses, however, report that caring for HIV/AIDS patients can take an enormous emotional toll because they are often the primary source of continuous physical and emotional care for these patients, who generally require more intensive care and services than other patients.

Nurses, physicians, and other health care professionals must cope with more than simply their fears of contracting the disease from HIV/AIDS patients and keeping abreast of advances in the treatment of the disease. They also face a wide range of emotional issues when caring for these patients, from feelings of failure when treatment is unsuccessful to grief when witnessing the untimely deaths of patients. In "How Caring for Persons with HIV/AIDS

Affects Rural Nurses" (*Issues in Mental Health Nursing*, vol. 30, no. 5, May 2009), Iris L. Mullins of New Mexico State University explains that caring for patients with HIV/AIDS affects nurses in three distinct areas of their personal and professional lives: their personal sense of self as a nurse in practice; their interactions with their family members, friends, and colleagues; and their interactions with patients with HIV/AIDS. Nurses caring for HIV/AIDS patients in rural areas expressed additional concerns including the need for ongoing continued education about the care of people with HIV/AIDS.

Support groups and counselors help many health professionals, especially hospice workers, to share and understand these feelings so that they are better able to care for HIV/AIDS patients and their families.

CDC Guidelines

In response to an incident in which five patients acquired HIV from David J. Acer (1949–1990), a Florida dentist, the CDC addressed occupational exposure to bloodborne pathogens in "Recommendations for Preventing Transmission of Human Immunodeficiency Virus and Hepatitis B Virus to Patients during Exposure-Prone Invasive Procedures" (*Morbidity and Mortality Weekly Report*, vol. 40, RR-8, July 12, 1991). The updated guidelines were intended to prevent the accidental spread of the infection from health care providers to patients and from patients to health care workers. The recommendations stressed the careful and consistent use, with all patients, of standard infection control procedures for bloodborne agents—the so-called universal precautions—that were published by the CDC in 1987.

The CDC guidelines also recommended that HIV-infected health care workers stop performing exposure-prone invasive procedures and that professional medical and dental groups draw up lists of exposure-prone procedures for their disciplines. The CDC recommended that HIV-infected health care workers consult with a panel of experts to determine which, if any, limits should be placed on their medical practices and further advised practitioners to inform patients of their HIV-infection status before performing medical procedures.

The CDC guidelines resulted in some unforeseen consequences. Professional groups, hospital attorneys, state courts, legislatures, and Congress reacted with alarm to a perception of dangers to patients posed by HIV-infected health care professionals totally out of proportion to the largely theoretical risk. Adelisa L. Panlilio et al. of the CDC note in "Updated U.S. Public Health Service Guidelines for the Management of Occupational Exposures to HIV and Recommendations for Postexposure Prophylaxis" (*Morbidity and Mortality Weekly Report*, vol. 54, RR-9, September 30, 2005) that the average risk of HIV infection after skin contact with HIV-infected blood is estimated to

be about 0.3%, and the risk for transmission is even lower from contact with body fluids or tissues other than blood. In "Surveillance of Occupationally Acquired HIV/AIDS in Healthcare Personnel, as of December 2006" (September 2007, http://www.cdc.gov/ncidod/dhqp/bp_hcp_w_hiv.html), the CDC states that 57 documented cases had been reported from 1981 until 2006 (though no documented cases were reported from 2000 until 2006), and it was possible that an 140 additional cases of HIV infection were linked to occupational exposures.

According to Panlilio et al., the CDC recommends that the following procedures and philosophies would best serve patients and health care workers:

- The universal and meticulous use of well-understood infection-control procedures, particularly those developed from the study of hepatitis B—another bloodborne infection that is 100 times more infectious and 10 times more common in health professionals—should be applied in all health care settings, whether hospital, office, or home based.

- Operative or other invasive procedures, in which injury to health care professionals occurs with any frequency, should be discontinued or modified to the greatest extent possible. This involves developing new instruments and investigating new operative techniques.

- All health care professionals should consider being tested for HIV. However, an HIV-positive result should not justify restricting the practice of health care professionals.

Should Doctors Tell Patients?

Since 1991 the American College of Surgeons (ACS), the nation's largest professional organization of surgeons, has refused to draw up a list of procedures that might pose a high risk of transmitting HIV from doctor to patient. The group maintains that because not a single documented case of surgeon-to-patient transmission has been established, there is no scientific basis for suggesting that a particular surgical procedure increases the risk of viral transmission. The ACS also notes that surgical patients are at greater risk for other surgery-related infections than for HIV, even from an HIV-infected physician.

Panlilio et al. note that the CDC guidelines instruct HIV-infected health care workers to avoid contact with patients that could potentially bring the worker's blood into contact with a patient's body cavities or mucous membranes.

HEALTH CARE WORKERS AND INFECTION
Health Care Workers with HIV and AIDS

In "Surveillance of Occupationally Acquired HIV/AIDS in Healthcare Personnel, as of December 2006," the CDC indicates that as of 2006 it was aware of only 57 documented cases of health care workers other than surgeons in the United States who had become infected with HIV as a result of occupational exposures. The breakdown of those who were infected was as follows:

- Nurses (24)
- Clinical laboratory workers (16)
- Nonsurgical physicians (6)
- Nonclinical laboratory technicians (3)
- Housekeeper/maintenance workers (2)
- Surgical technicians (2)
- Dialysis technician (1)
- Embalmer/morgue technician (1)
- Health aide/attendant (1)
- Respiratory therapist (1)

As of 2006, the CDC was also aware of 140 cases of HIV infection or AIDS possibly linked to occupational exposure among health care workers. These workers had not reported other risk factors for HIV infection. They reported a history of occupational exposure to blood, body fluids, or HIV-infected laboratory material, but they did not document infection after a specific exposure.

The known and possible cases of occupational acquisition of HIV undoubtedly represent an underestimate. There are likely unknown numbers of people who acquired their infection through occupational exposures, although, even in 2009, this is purely conjecture.

According to the National Institute for Occupational Safety and Health, in "Overview of State Needle Safety Legislation" (April 1, 2009, http://www.cdc.gov/niosh/topics/bbp/ndl-law.html), since June 2002, 21 states have enacted needle-safety legislation to safeguard health care workers from bloodborne pathogen (agents that cause disease) exposures. State laws aim to supplement and strengthen the federal standards mandated by the Occupational Safety and Health Administration. Many of the state laws require the creation of a written exposure plan that is periodically reviewed and updated; protocols for safety device identification and selection; logs to document and report injuries with sharp instruments; and strict requirements and training for workers on how to use safety devices.

In "Updated U.S. Public Health Service Guidelines for the Management of Occupational Exposures to HBV, HCV, and HIV and Recommendations for Postexposure Prophylaxis" (*Morbidity and Mortality Weekly Report*, vol. 50, RR-11, June 29, 2001), the U.S. Public Health Service updated the guidelines for treatment to prevent health care workers with occupational exposure to HIV from becoming infected with the virus. Known as postexposure prophylaxis (PEP), the recommendation was that

affected workers be given a four-week regimen of two antiretroviral drugs such as ZDV and lamivudine, with the addition of a third drug for HIV exposures that pose an increased risk of transmission. Another update was issued by Panlilio et al. in September 2005 because since publication of the 2001 update, the FDA had approved new antiretroviral agents, and additional information had become available about the use and safety of PEP. Even though the best strategy to protect health care workers is to avoid exposure to HIV and other bloodborne pathogens, PEP has, as of 2009, proven generally effective in preventing HIV infection in workers who have been exposed.

Risks to Patients

Health care officials are not the only ones worried about HIV transmission in the health care setting. Patients also fear that infected health care workers can transmit the virus to them. In the landmark study "HIV Transmission from Health Care Worker to Patient: What Is the Risk?" (*Annals of Internal Medicine*, vol. 116, no. 10, May 15, 1992), Mary E. Chamberland and David M. Bell develop a model of the risk of HIV transmission to patients and estimate that the risk of a patient becoming infected by an HIV-positive surgeon during a single operation is anywhere from 1 out of 42,000 to 1 out of 420,000. This risk is considerably less than the risks associated with many other medical procedures.

The CDC indicates in "HIV and Its Transmission" (July 1999, http://www.cdc.gov/hiv/resources/factsheets/PDF/transmission.pdf) that of more than 22,000 patients of 63 HIV-infected health care workers, no documented evidence has been found that links HIV infection to medical or dental care, except for the five patients of Acer in 1990. Medical researchers have tried without success to determine how Acer infected his patients and whether the exposure was accidental or deliberate. One theory is that he did not properly sterilize his dental tools; another is that he accidentally cut his finger or jabbed himself with a hypodermic needle, did not notice it, and bled into the patients' mouths. Before his death in 1990, Acer denied intentionally exposing his patients.

In 1990 Rudolph Almarez (1949–1990), a Baltimore, Maryland, breast surgeon who performed operations on as many as 2,000 patients, died from AIDS. The nature of his death stirred up such concern that shortly after he died a Baltimore law firm solicited clients to seek legal advice, regardless of whether they were infected. The law firm told clients that they might be reimbursed for the emotional distress they now suffered if they sued the hospital where Almarez had practiced. Two separate legal complaints—*Rossi v. Almarez* (Baltimore City Cir. Ct. No. 90344028 CL123396, May 23, 1991) and *Faya v. Almarez*, Baltimore City Cir. Ct. No. 90345011 CL12345g, May 23, 1991)—based on the fear of HIV exposure were dismissed by a Baltimore judge. The judge further stated that there were no allegations that Almarez had not followed recommended safety procedures or that any accident had taken place during surgery. None of the patients alleged infection from Almarez. A later study failed to find any HIV-positive patients among those Almarez had treated.

WHAT DOES IT COST TO TREAT HIV/AIDS PATIENTS?

The Kaiser Family Foundation states in the fact sheet "U.S. Federal Funding for HIV/AIDS: The President's FY 2010 Budget Request" (May 2009, http://www.kff.org/hivaids/upload/7029-05.pdf) that in FY 2009 federal government spending for domestic and global HIV-related activities totaled $24.8 billion. President Barack Obama's (1961–) federal budget request for 2010 included an estimated $25.9 billion—$19.4 billion for domestic programs and $6.5 billion for global initiatives and activities. Federal funding has increased significantly throughout the course of the epidemic, and the 2010 federal budget for domestic programs and research represented a 4.7% increase over 2009. Much of the federal funding for HIV/AIDS care, as opposed to other assistance such as housing, was for Medicaid and Medicare programs, which were budgeted for 6.8% and 6.3% increases in funding, respectively.

HIV/AIDS-related costs are expected to increase in response to the rising costs of hospitalization, home care, insurance premiums and copayments, physician services, and pharmaceutical drugs. In 2000 certain drugs (including didanosine and ritonavir) rose substantially in price. Growing concern about rising drug prices led to a self-imposed price freeze by some manufacturers in 2002. However, in February 2003 Roche Pharmaceuticals announced that the price for its formulation of enfuvirtide, at the time the most expensive AIDS treatment on the market, would more than double in Europe. Despite the rising cost of drug treatment, at the 2005 United Nations World Summit the world's leaders pledged to try to achieve universal access to treatment by 2010.

Regardless, some HIV/AIDS care-related expenses have actually been reduced by relocating services from the hospital to a variety of outpatient settings. Examples of cost-saving services include outpatient transfusions and outpatient treatment for opportunistic infections such as *Pneumocystis carinii* pneumonia and cryptococcal meningitis. Increased volunteer-based social service programs that enable patients to be cared for at home can also prevent expensive hospital stays.

During 2009 President Obama was working with Congress to pass comprehensive health reform intended to control rising health care costs and ensure choice of physician and high-quality, affordable health care for all Americans. Even though the long-range impact of such sweeping reform on HIV/AIDS care was not yet known in September 2009, universal coverage was intended to ensure that lack of health insurance does not prevent people with HIV/AIDS from obtaining health services.

The Ryan White Comprehensive AIDS Resources Emergency Act

In 1998 the Ryan White Comprehensive AIDS Resources Emergency (CARE) Act was the only federal program providing funds specifically for medical and support services to individuals with HIV and AIDS. The act was named after Ryan White, who died of AIDS in 1990. White was an Indiana teenager with hemophilia who became infected through a blood transfusion. Shunned by his community because many people feared becoming infected through any kind of contact with him, White fought to attend school and attain rights for those infected with HIV/AIDS. White's efforts helped change the way the world treated those with the disease. The CARE Act was signed in 1990 and reauthorized in 1996, 2000, and 2006. The 2006 reauthorization, called the Ryan White HIV/AIDS Treatment Modernization Act, recalculated CARE Act funding formulas to ensure that rural areas experiencing increasing numbers of HIV/AIDS cases would receive increased funding amounts, which in turn decreased funding for urban areas. The change still grants funding priority to urban areas with the highest number of people living with AIDS, while helping midsized cities with emerging needs, which are called transitional grant areas.

The 2006 reauthorization aims to ensure that more money is spent on direct health care for the grantees' client and patient populations. Under the new law, grantees receiving funds under Parts A, B, and C (formerly called Titles I, II, and III) must spend at least 75% of funds on core medical services. Until 2006, there was no stipulated core set of medical services in the statute. The Kaiser Family Foundation explains in *The Ryan White CARE Act: A Side-by-Side Comparison of Prior Law to the Newly Reauthorized CARE Act* (December 2006, http://www.kff.org/hivaids/upload/7531-03.pdf) that core medical services are defined as:

• Outpatient and ambulatory health services

• Pharmaceutical assistance

• Substance abuse outpatient services

• Oral health

• Medical nutritional therapy

• Health insurance premium assistance

• Home health care

• Hospice services

• Mental health services

- Early intervention services
- Medical case management, including treatment adherence services

The remaining funds may be spent on support services, which are defined as services needed to achieve outcomes that affect the HIV-related clinical status of a person with HIV/AIDS. The Kaiser Family Foundation indicates that the law outlines support services as:

- Outreach
- Medical transportation
- Language services
- Respite care for people caring for individuals with HIV/AIDS
- Referrals for health care and other support services

The funds from the Ryan White HIV/AIDS Treatment Modernization Act are appropriated using five formulas. Part A funds eligible metropolitan areas (EMAs) disproportionately affected by HIV/AIDS and transitional grant areas. Part B funds states to improve the quality, availability, and organization of HIV/AIDS health care and support services. Part C funds early intervention services and ambulatory care. Part D provides family-centered comprehensive care to children, youth, women, and their families and helps improve access to clinical trials and research. Part F encompasses Special Projects of National Significance, which supports the demonstration and evaluation of innovative models of HIV/AIDS care delivery for hard-to-reach populations as well as AIDS Education and Training Centers, dental programs, and the Minority AIDS Initiative.

To qualify for Part A funds, EMAs must have more than 2,000 cumulative AIDS cases reported during the preceding five years and a population of at least 500,000. (The population provision does not apply to any EMA named and funded before FY 1997.) Table 6.1 shows a breakdown by program of Ryan White funding from FYs 2006 to 2008.

Under the Ryan White HIV/AIDS Treatment Modernization Act of 2006, what were previously called Title II funds under the CARE Act are now awarded to state governments under Part B of Title XXVI of the Public Health Service Act. The reauthorized Ryan White law requires that Part B grantees spend 75% of their grant awards on core medical services and that ADAPs maintain a core list and supply of antiretroviral drugs. The states also use Part B funds to contract with service providers for ambulatory (outpatient) health care, insurance coverage, residential and in-home hospice care, transportation to and from appointments, food banks, and home-delivered meals. Part C of Title XXVI of the Public Health Service Act (formerly Title III of the

TABLE 6.1

Ryan White funding, fiscal years 2006–08

[$ = 000's]

Program	Fiscal year 2006	Fiscal year 2007	Fiscal year 2008
Emergency relief (Part A)	$611,581	$603,993	$627,149
HIV care (Part B)	$1,134,596	$1,195,500	$1,195,248
(State formula grants)	(330,972)	(405,954)	(386,748)
(State ADAP)	(789,546)	(789,546)	(808,500)
Early intervention (Part C)	$196,054	$193,721	$198,754
Women, infants, children & youth (Part D)	$72,6960	$71,794	$73,690
AIDS ed training centers (Part F)	$34,700	$34,701	$34,094
Dental reimbursement (Part F)	$13,086	$13,086	$12,857
SPNS (Part F)*			
Total: Ryan White Funding	**$2,062,713**	**$2,112,795**	**$2,141,792**

*Special Projects of National Significance: Normally funded with set-asides from Parts A, B, C, & D. Appropriation Acts have directed that SPNS shall be funded from Department PHS Act evaluation set-asides. The appropriation amounts shown reflect a proportionate redistribution of the $25,000,000 to Parts A, B, C, & D.

SOURCE: "FY2006–FY2008 Appropriations," in "The HIV/AIDS Program: Funding," U.S. Department of Health and Human Services, Health Resources and Services Administration, undated, http://hab.hrsa.gov/reports/funding.htm (accessed July 2, 2009)

CARE Act) funds grants to provide early intervention services and outpatient treatment for low-income, medically underserved people and supports the development of quality HIV primary care programs.

In the press release "HHS to Award $1.79 Billion to Help People Living with HIV/AIDS" (May 14, 2009, http://www.hhs.gov/news/press/2009pres/05/20090514a.html), the Health Resources and Services Administration (HRSA) announces the release of $1.8 billion in grants funded through the Ryan White HIV/AIDS Program. The HRSA explains that

> More than $1.16 billion will be sent to States and Territories under Part B of the Ryan White program, with $780 million of that total earmarked for the AIDS Drug Assistance Program (ADAP).... A total of $590 million will pay for primary care and support services for individuals living with HIV/AIDS under Part A of the Ryan White program. Part A awards are distributed to eligible metropolitan areas (EMAs) with the highest number of people living with HIV/AIDS and to transitional grant areas (TGAs) experiencing increases in HIV/AIDS cases and emerging care needs.... Close to $49 million will fund early intervention services that support medical, nutritional, psychosocial and other treatments for HIV-positive individuals. These grants, awarded under Part C of the program, go to community-based organizations such as health centers and nonprofit providers of primary health care for people living with HIV.

Private Insurance and Medicaid

The financing of HIV/AIDS care is increasingly becoming the responsibility of Medicaid. The greater reliance on Medicaid funding is due in large part to the increase in the number of HIV/AIDS cases among injection drug users and poor people who are unlikely to be covered by private health insurance. In addition, many patients who once had private insurance through their workplace lost their coverage when the illness made them too sick to work, or they lost their job and job-related health benefits during the economic downturn that began at the close of 2007, forcing them to turn to Medicaid and other public programs.

Added to this list are those whose employment or economic status would normally ensure them insurance coverage, but who became virtually ineligible for private health insurance coverage once they tested positive for HIV. Others need assistance because some insurance companies consider HIV infection to be a preexisting condition, making it ineligible for payment of claims. Even insurance companies that do cover HIV treatment often impose caps, limiting coverage to relatively small dollar amounts.

The HIV/AIDS epidemic has prompted private insurers to add an HIV antibody-screening test for people who are not joining insurance programs through groups or employers. According to Cyanne Demchak of Academy-Health, in "Bridging the Gap: The Role of Individual Health Insurance Coverage" (*Changes in Health Care Financing and Organization*, vol. 9, no. 1, February 2006), these individual enrollees—who make up 15% of all people in the insurance market—are required to take medical exams to prove they are insurable.

The National Association of Health Underwriters explains in "Consumer Guide to Individual Health Insurance" (2009, http://www.nahu.org/consumer/individualinsurance.cfm) that in 2009 a person with HIV could be turned down for individual coverage by private insurers in most states. However, several states had developed ways to provide uninsurable people with access to individual health insurance coverage. Thirty-three states provided "coverage to medically uninsurable people through high-risk pools," and another 12 states had other ways of "providing uninsurable people with access to individual coverage."

Death Benefits

Since 1988 an industry has developed that offers dying AIDS patients the opportunity to collect a portion of their life insurance benefits before they die, either to pay for their treatment or to spend as they wish during their remaining time. These viatical (money for necessities given to a person dying or in danger of death) settlements are reached when an insured person sells his or her life insurance policy to an independent insurance company at a reduced or discounted price. This enables the patient to have some cash from the policy while he or she is still alive. After the patient dies, the company that bought the policy is paid the full death benefits. Regulators with the U.S. Securities and Exchange Commission are scrutinizing some practices they believe may victimize AIDS patients.

Some larger companies, such as Prudential, offer policyholders more than 90% of their policy payouts, but only with a physician's certification that they have less than six months to live. Smaller companies usually pay 50% to 80% of the benefit payable at death, although they will pay benefits to people who still have up to five years to live. The longer the policyholders are expected to live, the less the cash disbursement they receive.

Most insurers will not write new life insurance policies for people known to have AIDS. Those that do offer life insurance policies to people infected with HIV or people with AIDS often have stringent requirements and limited benefits. For example, some policies for AIDS patients stipulate that should death occur due to illness during the first two or three years of coverage, then the benefits paid are simply a return of premiums paid plus an annual interest rate. Others offer an initial two- or three-year incremental period; after that initial period full benefits are paid whether death occurs due to accident or to illness.

TREATMENT RESEARCH

Medical and pharmaceutical research to develop and conduct clinical trials of antiretroviral drugs is expensive. According to the National Institutes of Health (NIH), a total of $2.9 billion was allocated for AIDS research in FY 2008, and over $3 billion was budgeted for both FY 2009 and FY 2010 (the FY 2010 budget was $45.2 million higher than the FY 2009 estimate). (See Table 6.2.) However, Doug Trapp reports in "Researchers Decry Flat NIH Budgets, Fear Delays in Treatment Advances" (*American Medical News*, April 9, 2007) that with biomedical research inflation averaging 4% a year since 2004 and with no significant increases in funding for many of its institutes and centers, the NIH has in effect suffered funding cuts since that year.

Decisions about how much is spent to research a particular disease are not based solely on how many people develop the disease or die from it. Rightly or wrongly, economists base the societal value of an individual on his or her earning potential and productivity—the ability to contribute to society as a worker. The bulk of the people who die from heart disease, stroke, and cancer are older adults. Many have retired from the workforce and their potential economic productivity is often minimal. This economic measure of present and future financial productivity should not be misinterpreted as a casting-off of older adults; instead, it is simply an economic measure of present and future financial productivity.

In contrast, AIDS patients are usually much younger and die in their 20s, 30s, and 40s. Until they develop

TABLE 6.2

NIH AIDS research funding by institute and center, fiscal years 2008–10

Institute/center	Fiscal year 2008 actual	Fiscal year 2009 estimate	Fiscal year 2009 Recovery Act[a, b]	Fiscal year 2010 PB	Change fiscal year 2009 estimate/ fiscal year 2010 PB
National Cancer Institute (NCI)	$258,499,000	$265,882,000	$20,000,000	$269,964,000	$4,082,000
National Heart, Lung, and Blood Institute (NHLBI)	65,360,000	66,651,000	9,563,000	66,972,000	321,000
National Institute of Dental and Craniofacial Research (NIDCR)	19,741,000	20,251,000	—	20,251,000	—
National Institute of Diabetes and Digestive and Kidney Diseases (NIDDK)	31,031,000	31,656,000	—	31,031,000	—
National Institute of Neurological Disorders and Stroke (NINDS)	46,451,000	46,531,000	3,500,000	47,027,000	496,000
National Institute of Allergy and Infectious Diseases (NIAID)	1,497,722,000	1,541,074,000	330,986,000	1,566,651,000	25,577,000
National Institute of General Medical Sciences (NIGMS)	54,628,000	56,024,000	7,724,000	56,649,000	625,000
Eunice Kennedy Shriver National Institute of Child Health and Human Development (NICHHD)	138,358,000	142,334,000	227,000	144,402,000	2,068,000
National Eye Institute (NEI)	10,585,000	10,633,000	—	10,631,000	−2,000
National Institute of Environmental Health Sciences (NIEHS)	5,310,000	5,347,000	—	5,347,000	—
National Institute on Aging (NIA)	5,392,000	5,560,000	1,440,000	5,645,000	85,000
National Institute of Arthritis and Musculoskeletal and Skin Diseases (NIAMS)	4,866,000	4,938,000	—	4,938,000	—
National Institute on Deafness and Other Communication Disorders (NIDCD)	900,000	1,284,000	—	1,284,000	—
National Institute of Mental Health (NIMH)	181,153,000	186,665,000	12,714,000	189,586,000	2,921,000
National Institute on Drug Abuse (NIDA)	304,032,000	312,901,000	29,119,000	317,829,000	4,928,000
National Institute on Alcohol Abuse and Alcoholism (NIAAA)	27,017,000	27,797,000	—	28,175,000	378,000
National Institute of Nursing Research (NINR)	12,145,000	12,506,000	—	12,660,000	154,000
National Human Genome Research Institute (NHGRI)	6,855,000	7,048,000	—	7,153,000	105,000
National Institute of Biomedical Imaging and Bioengineering (NIBIB)	1,096,000	1,308,000	—	1,308,000	—
National Center for Research Resources (NCRR)	162,525,000	167,111,000	143,721,000	169,523,000	2,412,000
National Center for Complementary and Alternative Medicine (NCCAM)	2,385,000	2,441,000	—	2,441,000	—
National Center on Minority Health and Health Disparities (NCMHD)	—	—	—	—	—
John E. Fogarty International Center for Advanced Study in the Health Sciences (FIC)	23,138,000	23,799,000	—	24,103,000	304,000
National Library of Medicine (NLM)	7,399,000	7,606,000	—	7,683,000	77,000
Office of the Director (OD)	61,757,000	62,992,000	—	64,241,000	624,000
Buildings and Facilities (B&F)	—	—	—	—	—
Total, NIH	**2,928,345,000**	**3,010,339,000**	**558,994,000**	**3,055,494,000**	**45,155,000**

NIH = National Institutes of Health.

[a]Funds are appropriated from the American Recovery and Reinvestment Act, 2009 (P.L. 111–5) and are available until September 30, 2010.

[b]ARRA funds for AIDS research were determined by each IC and were not allocated by OAR.

SOURCE: "National Institutes of Health Office of AIDS Research Budget Authority by Institute and Center," in *Office of AIDS Research Trans-NIH AIDS Research Budget*, U.S. Department of Health and Human Services, National Institutes of Health, 2009, http://www.oar.nih.gov/budget/pdf/OAR10CJ.pdf (accessed July 2, 2009)

AIDS, the potential productivity of these people, measured in economic terms, is high. The number of work years lost when they die is considerable. Using this economic equation to determine how disease research should be funded, it may be considered economically wise to invest more money to research AIDS because the losses, measured in potential work years rather than in lives, are so much greater.

The primary goals of HIV/AIDS therapy are to prolong life and improve its quality. Even though in the early days of AIDS research a cure for the disease was envisioned, few researchers at the turn of the 21st century realistically expected any drug to cure HIV infection. The bottom-line objective became making the virus less deadly by foiling its efforts to reproduce within the body.

A major obstacle to the discovery of such treatments is the cost of drug research and development. Pharmaceutical manufacturers spend millions of dollars researching and developing new medicines. According to the Pharmaceutical Research and Manufacturers of America (PhRMA), since 1992 U.S. pharmaceutical companies have consistently spent more money each year on research and development (R&D) activities than the annual budget of the NIH. For example, PhRMA (2009, http://www.phrma.org/about_phrma/) reports that in 2008 the estimated pharmaceutical R&D budget was $65.2 billion. By contrast, the U.S. Department of Health and Human Services states in "Fiscal Year 2010 Budget in Brief: National Institutes of Health" (June 4, 2009, http://www.hhs.gov/asrt/ob/docbudget/2010budgetinbriefh.html)

that the entire NIH budget (research and other activities) was $29.4 billion. Furthermore, private-sector spending has been growing faster than government spending since 1995.

In "Glaxo and Pfizer Join Forces to Develop and Market H.I.V. Drugs" (*New York Times*, April 16, 2009), Natasha Singer reports that the pharmaceutical companies GlaxoSmithKline and Pfizer joined together in 2009 to form a specialty company to research, develop, and market HIV treatments. The new company will have 11 HIV drugs, which represent 19% of the market, and will compete with Gilead Sciences, the leading company in the development of HIV drugs, which had sales of $4.3 billion in 2008. HIV drug sales are a staggering $7.2 billion annually in the United States and $12.3 billion worldwide.

PhRMA explains in *Pharmaceutical Industry Profile 2009* (April 2009, http://www.phrma.org/files/PhRMA% 202009%20Profile%20FINAL.pdf) that a pharmaceutical manufacturer must cover the cost not only of R&D for the approximately two out of 10 drugs that succeed but also for many of the drugs—eight out of 10—that fail to make it to the marketplace. Because of this cost, once a new drug receives FDA approval, its manufacturer ordinarily holds a patent or gains exclusivity rights, which guarantee it will be the sole marketer for a specified time (usually from three to 20 years) to recoup its investment. During this time the drug is priced much higher than if other manufacturers were allowed to compete by producing generic versions of the same drug. In contrast to the original manufacturer, the generic manufacturer does not have to pay for the successes and failures that occurred in the drug development pathway or pursue the complicated, time-consuming process of seeking FDA approval. The producer of generic drugs has the formula and must simply manufacture the drugs properly. Because of the lower cost of the generic drug after the original patent or exclusivity period has expired, competition among pharmaceutical manufacturers generally lowers the price. HIV/AIDS drugs are granted seven years of exclusivity under legislation aimed at encouraging research and promoting development of new treatments.

The issue of patent protection for HIV/AIDS drugs is understandably contentious. Pharmaceutical manufacturers and others argue that patent protection is necessary to allow for the financial investments necessary to breed innovation. However, to those directly affected by HIV/ AIDS, and those governments or health care systems that provide care, the enormous costs can be infuriating, especially with the knowledge that generic drugs carrying a lower price tag are possible. The need for less expensive HIV/AIDS drugs is especially urgent in the developing world.

Indeed, reflecting this urgency, a November 2002 meeting of the World Trade Organization (WTO) adopted a resolution affirming the right of WTO member countries to do whatever they deem necessary to protect public health, including overriding pharmaceutical patents. For example, in May 2003 the Zimbabwean government declared a national emergency for six months over the HIV/AIDS pandemic (worldwide epidemic), enabling it to purchase and make available generic versions of HIV/ AIDS drugs that were still under patent protection. Before this declaration, the passage of the Kenya Industrial Property Bill of 2001 allowed the importation and production of more affordable medicines for HIV/AIDS in that country.

In "Access to AIDS Medicines Stumbles on Trade Rules" (May 2006, http://www.who.int/bulletin/volumes/ 84/5/news10506/en/index.html), the World Health Organization (WHO) states that despite the fact that international trade laws exist to assist developing countries to obtain life-saving drugs at affordable prices, few countries are taking advantage of this increased availability. The WHO asserts that political pressures and bureaucratic red tape confound many countries' efforts to access AIDS medicines. Even though many countries have improved access to first-line drugs, second-line antiretroviral drugs (used to combat drug resistance and for patients who experience intolerable side effects from first-line treatments) and newer formulations continue to be prohibitively expensive.

FDA-APPROVED DRUGS

The first drug thought to delay symptoms was ZDV. Even though initially promising, ZDV's effects were found to be temporary at best. Several other drugs worked using the same mechanism of action as ZDV—exclusion of HIV from the host chromosome. A newer class of drugs called protease inhibitors (PIs) appears to keep HIV already in the host cells from reproducing. PIs block the ability of HIV to mature and infect new cells by suppressing a protein enzyme of the virus, called protease, which is crucial to the progression of HIV. In "Treatment with Indinavir, Zidovudine, and Lamivudine in Adults with Human Immunodeficiency Virus Infection and Prior Antiretroviral Therapy" (*New England Journal of Medicine*, vol. 337, no. 11, September 11, 1997), Roy M. Gulick et al. indicate that a combination of indinavir, zidovudine, and lamivudine reduces the viral load and CD4 cell count. In the researchers' study, the changes in the viral load and the CD4 cell count lasted for as long as 52 weeks and the drug regimen was generally well tolerated.

Even if the effectiveness of PIs proves to be transient, they improve patients' prospects simply by creating more roadblocks for HIV, which mutates so rapidly that it becomes resistant to most drugs when the drugs are used alone. Even if a cure is never found, new and better drugs used in various combinations have helped transform HIV infection from a certain death sentence to a chronic but manageable disease, much like diabetes.

The cost, however, is high. When PIs are combined with ZDV or any of the other commonly used antiretroviral drugs, such as lamivudine, zalcitabine, didanosine, or stavudine, the AIDS Treatment Activists Coalition reports in "ADAP Emergency!" (September 2002, http://www.thebody.com/content/art13230.html) that the cost in 2002 was approximately $18,000 per year.

Robert Steinbrook indicates in "HIV Infection—A New Drug and New Costs" (*New England Journal of Medicine*, vol. 348, no. 22, May 2003) that by 2003 the cost of many PIs rose to $10,000 to $12,000 for a year's supply. AVERT, an international AIDS charity, observes in "Reducing the Price of HIV/AIDS Treatment" (September 10, 2009, http://www.avert.org/generic.htm) that at a cost of $10,000 to $15,000 per person per year, "these antiretroviral drugs (ARVs) [are] far too expensive for the majority of HIV infected people in resource poor countries."

In *Curing HIV: What It Means and Why It Must be Done* (September 2008, http://www.projectinform.org/info/ppt/0908_usca.pdf), Martin Delaney observes that lifetime treatment costs are high. He calculates an annual cost of treatment as $16,000 and multiplies it by 50 years, because treatment is lifelong, for a lifetime total of $800,000 in drug treatment costs alone. Delaney's estimates do not even consider cost increases over time.

Types of Antiretroviral Agents

The FDA notes in "Antiretroviral Drugs Used in the Treatment of HIV Infection" (May 20, 2009, http://www.fda.gov/oashi/aids/virals.html) that it approves seven classes of antiretroviral agents for the treatment of HIV/AIDS.

PROTEASE INHIBITORS. As of May 2009, the FDA had approved the following PIs:

- Amprenavir
- Tipranavir
- Indinavir
- Saquinavir mesylate
- Ritonavir
- Fosamprenavir calcium
- Darunavir
- Atazanavir sulfate
- Nelfinavir mesylate

Drugs formulated with combinations of two or more PIs have also received FDA approval:

- Lopinavir and ritonavir; for use in adult and pediatric patients

- Abacavir, retrovir, and lamivudine in a fixed-dose combination

NUCLEOSIDE REVERSE TRANSCRIPTASE INHIBITORS. Nucleoside reverse transcriptase inhibitors (NRTIs) were among the first compounds shown to be effective against viral infections. Research in the 1970s led to the development of the drug acyclovir, which is still being used to treat herpes infections. The first four anti-HIV drugs to be approved—ZDV, didanosine, dideoxycytosine, and stavudine—were nucleoside analogs.

As their name implies, NRTIs exert their action based on their three-dimensional structure, which mimics the structure of the nucleoside building blocks of deoxyribonucleic acid (DNA). By becoming incorporated into the DNA as the molecule is replicated, the analogs can preserve the structure of DNA but make it impossible for the HIV to use its reverse transcriptase to hijack the host replication machinery to make new viral copies.

As of May 2009, the following NRTIs had received FDA approval for use with HIV/AIDS:

- Lamivudine
- ZDV
- Emtricitabine
- Abacavir
- Zalcitabine (also called dideoxycytidine)
- Tenofovir disoproxil fumarate
- Enteric-coated didanosine
- Didanosine (also called dideoxyinosine)
- Tenofovir disoproxil fumarate
- Stavudine
- Abacavir sulfate

NONNUCLEOSIDE REVERSE TRANSCRIPTASE INHIBITORS. Another class of antiretroviral drugs approved in the late 1990s is nonnucleoside reverse transcriptase inhibitors (NNRTIs). NNRTI compounds slow down the process of the reverse transcriptase enzyme that allows the virus to become part of the infected cell's nucleus. The compounds accomplish this by binding to the viral enzyme, which blocks the ability of the enzyme to function.

As of May 2009, there were four NNRTIs approved for use by the FDA:

- Etravirine
- Delavirdine
- Efavirenz
- Nevirapine

AN ANTIFUSION DRUG. As of May 2009, the FDA had approved the drug enfuvirtide, which interferes with the fusion of HIV with the host cell membrane.

Aggressive Treatment

With new drugs in the anti-HIV/AIDS arsenal, many people with HIV/AIDS who had given up hope of effective treatment returned to clinics and doctors' offices. Even though treatment guidelines previously promoted early intervention with ZDV, recommended treatment now combines PIs with other antiretroviral drugs. Treatment recommendations change rapidly in response to the development of new drugs and clinical trials indicating the effectiveness of different combinations of antiretroviral drugs. Researchers are acting quickly to develop new mixtures of the recently approved and older drugs. Because HIV mutates to resist any drug it faces, including all PIs, researchers find that varying the combination of drugs prescribed can "fool" the virus before it has time to mutate.

In "The Case for More Cautious, Patient-Focused Antiretroviral Therapy" (*Annals of Internal Medicine*, vol. 132, no. 4, February 15, 2000), Keith Henry of Regions Hospital in St. Paul, Minnesota, and the University of Minnesota suggests that overly aggressive antiretroviral therapy in the early stages of the disease may expose patients to unpleasant side effects and cause their systems to build resistance. Henry recommends a more cautious strategy: a long-term, patient-focused approach that includes delaying initial therapy, planned interruptions in drug dose administration, therapy switching, and immune-based therapy. In October 2003 the European Medicines Agency advised doctors not to start HIV patients on the aggressive didanosine-lamivudine-tenovir triple-drug combination, because no compelling improvement had been noted in those receiving the treatment.

Near the end of the first decade of the 21st century, thinking about the timing of treatment of people infected with HIV but without symptoms was beginning to change. Mari M. Kitahata et al. indicate in "Effect of Early versus Deferred Antiretroviral Therapy for HIV on Survival" (*New England Journal of Medicine*, vol. 360, no. 18, April 30, 2009) that starting HIV treatment before the patient's immune system is too badly compromised can dramatically improve survival. The researchers find that, compared with patients who started treatment early, those who delayed therapy increased their odds of dying by either 69% or 94%, depending on the patient's initial CD4 blood cell count.

Patients undergoing therapy with new drugs or drug combinations must be highly disciplined. For instance, indinavir must be taken on an empty stomach, every eight hours, not less than two hours before or after a meal, and with large amounts of water to prevent the development of kidney stones. Patients must also be careful to never

skip doses of indinavir, otherwise HIV will quickly grow immune to its effect. (Indinavir has been found to generate cross-resistance, meaning it made patients resistant to other PIs.) Saquinavir mesylate must be taken in large doses. Ritonavir must be carefully prescribed and administered because it interacts negatively with some antifungals and antibiotics used by AIDS patients. Because there are many minor and serious risks associated with use of these drugs, patients must be closely monitored.

The difficulty of dealing with a complicated regimen of daily medication and maintaining the personal resolve to continue the regimen are ongoing issues for many HIV/AIDS patients. Henry argues that more support should be given to those health care professionals (such as nurses and pharmacists) who educate patients and assist them in maintaining their complicated daily medication schedules.

When effective AIDS drugs were introduced, patients sometimes had to wake up in the middle of the night to take pills, and some treatment regimens consisted of as many as 50 or 60 pills administered several times a day. Even with intense pressure to simplify treatment regimens, pharmaceutical companies remained skeptical about an effective once-a-day pill despite the consensus opinion that it would help more people start, and stick with, treatment. Even as recently as 2005, many combined HIV/AIDS medication regimens were administered two to three times per day. Once-a-day regimens were sought after, but were not available until 2006.

Once-a-Day AIDS Treatment

In July 2006 the FDA approved the first once-a-day AIDS treatment, a combination of efavirenz, tenofovir disoproxil fumarate, and emtricitabine. Even though this new once-a-day drug combination reduces the number of pills a patient must take and as a result improves adherence to treatment, it is probably not the sole drug an AIDS patient needs. Many patients also require additional prescription medications to support their immune systems and help them resist infection.

THE DISCOVERY OF AN HIV-RESISTANT GENE

In August 1996 scientists working independently at the Aaron Diamond AIDS Research Center in New York City and the Free University of Brussels, Belgium, announced that some white people have genes that may protect them from HIV, regardless of how many times they are exposed to the virus. The researchers hope their findings will lead to new HIV/AIDS therapies or to the development of drugs or vaccines to prevent HIV infection.

The researchers discovered that a gene called CCR5 is associated with HIV resistance. The gene codes for a protein called CC chemokine receptor 5 (CCR5) that is located on the surface of host cells including macrophages, monocytes, and T cells. HIV exploits this protein by using it as a receptor to bind to, and subsequently infect, cells such as T cells. The CCR5 mutation blocks the manufacture of CCR5. Thus, HIV loses its surface target and cannot invade the immune system.

Subsequent studies conducted in the United States found that one out of 100 people inherits two copies of this gene—one from each parent—and is completely immune to HIV infection. One out of five people with only one copy of the CCR5 gene can become infected, but remains healthy two to three years longer than those without the altered gene. This may be because these people have half as many CCR5 receptors as normal, which limits or slows the spread of the virus.

According to Michael Fischereder et al., in "CC Chemokine Receptor 5 and Renal-Transplant Survival" (*Lancet*, vol. 357, no. 9270, June 2, 2001), the gene is most common in white Americans (10% to 15% of the population). It is rarely found in African-Americans and almost never in Asian-Americans, perhaps reflecting the origins of the mutation.

Certain populations appear to be resistant to HIV because they lack or have a mutated form of the CCR5 receptor. Most populations that carry the mutant CCR5 gene come from Europe, and there are indications that the mutation arose only about 700 years ago. For a mutation to be sustained in a population at a rate of 10%, there must be some benefit bestowed by the mutation. It is likely nothing to do with HIV, because HIV did not appear until the late 20th century.

The exact nature of the selective pressure that caused the appearance of the CCR5 mutation is the subject of considerable debate. The prevailing theory has been that the selective pressure was the bubonic plague; however, new research suggests that smallpox may have been the trigger. Which of these, if either, is true remains to be determined.

Research is also under way to learn more about other genes such as CCR2 that, when expressed dominantly, appears to slow the progression of AIDS. Vijay Kumar et al. confirm in "Genetic Basis of HIV-1 Resistance and Susceptibility: An Approach to Understand Correlation between Human Genes and HIV-1 Infection" (*Indian Journal of Experimental Biology*, vol. 44, no. 9, September 2006) that site-specific mutations in these genes determine the susceptibility or resistance to HIV-1 infection and AIDS. Investigators hope that the study of host genes in relation to HIV-1 infection may speed the development of drug therapies to prevent or cure HIV-1 infection effectively.

RECENT RESEARCH
A Natural Barrier to HIV

Olivier Schwartz of the Pasteur Institute identifies in "Langerhans Cells Lap up HIV-1" (*Nature Medicine*, vol. 13, no. 3, March 2007) a protein that acts as a natural barrier to HIV infection. The protein is called langerin, because it is produced by Langerhans cells, which form a network in the skin and mucosa (the membrane lining the vagina) and were previously thought to promote the spread of HIV. Instead, the Langerhans cells, which line the human genital tract, contain a protein that eats viruses. Langerin scavenges for viruses in the surrounding environment and thereby helps prevent infection. Langerhans cells do not become infected by HIV-1 because they have langerin on their surfaces. It appears that HIV infection occurs when levels of invading HIV are high or if langerin activity is especially weak. In either of these instances, Langerhans cells can become overwhelmed by the virus and infected.

In "Elevated Elafin/Trappin-2 in the Female Genital Tract Is Associated with Protection against HIV Acquisition" (*AIDS*, vol. 23, no. 13, August 24, 2009), Shehzad M. Iqbal et al. identify the protein elafin/trappin-2 as a novel innate immune factor that is strongly associated with HIV resistance. This innate immune factor was found in the mucosal secretions from the genital tracts of HIV-resistant women who are sex workers. Discovery of this factor enhances understanding of natural immunity to HIV infection.

Morning-after Treatment

HIV is classified as a communicable sexually transmitted disease in the United States. Some physicians prescribe the drugs used to treat established infections as "morning-after" pills in an attempt to prevent the transmission of the virus after risky sexual encounters. As of 2009, there was no scientific consensus on the validity of this approach, and the medications were not licensed for this use. Because some forms of HIV are halted by prompt use of the drugs, some doctors believe it is a worthwhile approach. Taryn Young et al. describe the results of a review of the medical literature on PEP in "Antiretroviral Post-exposure Prophylaxis (PEP) for Occupational HIV Exposure" (*Cochrane Database of Systematic Reviews*, 2007) and conclude that "there is no direct evidence to support the use of multi-drug antiretroviral regimens following occupational exposure to HIV. However, due to the success of combination therapies in treating HIV-infected individuals, a combination of antiretroviral drugs should be used for PEP."

This "off-label" use of potent PIs in an attempt to prevent the spread of HIV is controversial. All drugs used in the treatment of HIV have side effects, some of which may be potentially life threatening. Protease inhibitors may cause high blood sugar and diabetes, lipodytrophy (problems with fat metabolism that can result in dangerously high cholesterol levels), and liver problems. Furthermore, some researchers fear that if people believe morning-after treatment will prevent HIV infection, they may stop taking precautions, such as using condoms, to prevent exposure to HIV. Others feel that the treatment is not appropriate as a preventive measure for people exposed to ongoing risk, such as relationships where only one partner is infected, because the drugs are too toxic. Other methods, such as the continued use of condoms, would be much safer.

Finally, postexposure treatment is expensive. The costs of two or three drugs taken for a month, plus laboratory tests and visits to the doctor, may cost more than $1,000. Of course, this is a fraction of the cost for lifetime treatment of HIV infection and certainly money well spent if it prevents a person from acquiring the virus.

In "HIV Postexposure Prophylaxis in the Emergency Department: The Morning after Is Today" (*Annals of Emergency Medicine*, vol. 42, no.5, November 2003), a survey of emergency room physicians, Joshua D. Bamberger of the San Francisco Department of Public Health finds that most physicians believe that offering post-HIV exposure prevention is both feasible and among their responsibilities. Because physicians' confidence about their abilities to assess the need for postexposure prevention varies with exposure type, Bamberger recommends establishing postexposure prevention protocols and providing education to improve their knowledge of prudent postexposure prevention practices.

Charlie Sayer et al. suggest in "Will I? Won't I? Why Do Men Who Have Sex with Men Present for Post-exposure Prophylaxis for Sexual Exposures?" (*Sexually Transmitted Infections*, vol. 85, no. 3, December 15, 2008) that morning-after treatment can save lives. The drugs themselves will save some lives, and the offer of treatment will bring people who are at high risk for acquiring HIV into environments where they can get counseling and care. In San Francisco postexposure treatment is offered to victims of rape as a matter of course. Some doctors feel that if the treatment does not work to prevent the disease, it may work to at least treat it as early as possible. Though there is disagreement about the effectiveness and wisdom of widespread use of postexposure treatment, nearly all researchers and health care providers agree that for sexually active people the best prevention is the use of condoms.

Drugs to Block HIV Infection

In recent years there have been many efforts to develop topical microbicides—preparations to prevent HIV infection. Lawrence K. Altman reports in "Tests of Drug to Block H.I.V. Infection Are Halted over Safety" (*New York Times*, February 1, 2007) that in 2000 a clinical trial revealed that nonoxynol-9, a topical preparation used to prevent pregnancy that initially appeared to help protect against HIV, was unsafe when used to prevent HIV infection. Ironically, participants in the clinical trial developed higher rates of HIV infection, most likely

because the chemical caused an irritation that compromised the mucosa, allowing the virus easier entry. In response to these findings, the clinical trial was halted.

Altman indicates that studies were under way in 2007 to test other topical microbicides because until there is an effective AIDS vaccine, preventing transmission of HIV is an urgent public health priority, especially for women in developing countries, where traditions and cultural norms do not support the use of condoms.

Anita B Garg, Jeremy Nuttall, and Joseph Romano report in "The Future of HIV Microbicides: Challenges and Opportunities" (*Antiviral Chemistry and Chemotherapy*, vol. 19, no. 4, 2009) that as of 2009 a safe and effective microbicide had not yet to been identified; however, ongoing clinical trials of "vaginal gels containing non-specific compounds" had met with some success. One of the potential drawbacks of these gels is that they must be applied close to the time of sexual intercourse to be optimally effective.

IN SEARCH OF A VACCINE

Some pharmaceutical companies claim that the high costs of R&D and the relatively low return on their investments (because the period of patent protection is limited to seven years) leave little financial incentive to develop new HIV/AIDS drugs. The development of such drugs is, for better or worse, an economically driven, rather than strictly humanitarian, enterprise. Similarly, the companies allege that they have little economic motivation to research and develop HIV vaccines. In February 1996 Anthony S. Fauci (1940–), the head of the National Institute for Allergies and Infectious Diseases (NIAID), issued guidelines to promote cooperation between the government and private industry. The plan's goal was to overcome the alleged unfavorable market forces that have caused some companies to abandon research of potential HIV vaccines.

Such vaccine efforts continue. In the press release "HVTN 505 HIV Vaccine Study Begins Enrolling Volunteers" (August 24, 2009, http://www3.niaid.nih.gov/news/newsreleases/2009/HVTN505.htm), the NIAID and the international HIV Vaccine Trials Network announce enrollment in HVTN 505, an exploratory HIV vaccine clinical study.

According to the San Francisco Center for HIV Information (2009, http://chi.ucsf.edu/vaccines/vaccines?page=vc-03-00), as of July 2008, nine vaccine trials were in progress and three additional trials were planned.

The design of the vaccines under trial varies. Some vaccines use a weakened and medically safe version of viruses as a delivery vehicle to carry various HIV genes into the human participants. The hope is that antibody production of the HIV-critical proteins encoded by these

FIGURE 6.1

Recombinant DNA technology and vaccine development

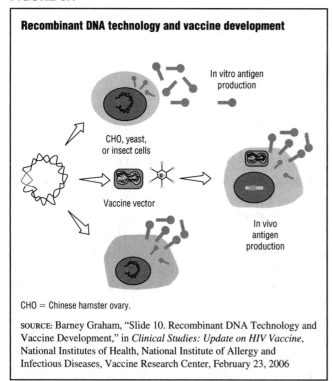

CHO = Chinese hamster ovary.

SOURCE: Barney Graham, "Slide 10. Recombinant DNA Technology and Vaccine Development," in *Clinical Studies: Update on HIV Vaccine*, National Institutes of Health, National Institute of Allergy and Infectious Diseases, Vaccine Research Center, February 23, 2006

genes will occur and that this production will offer protection from HIV infection. Other vaccines use a DNA plasmid to ferry HIV genes into the human participants; the aim again is to stimulate antibody production.

There are experimental design challenges and ethical considerations involved in vaccine trials using human volunteers. Vaccines may be made using recombinant DNA technology—DNA that has been altered by joining genetic material from two different sources. Figure 6.1 shows how recombinant DNA is used to develop vaccines. Even though some recombinant technology uses live attenuated virus (virus that is genetically altered so it is less virulent), this is not feasible with HIV because it would be unwise to create any risk of infection. The challenges are to elicit cell-mediated immune responses against HIV and the need for a balanced immune response consisting of not only cellular immunity but also a broad and strong antibody response that can prevent infection with HIV. Concerning ethical considerations, most volunteers for a vaccine have behaviors that put them at risk for contracting HIV. Some may mistakenly believe that participating in the clinical trial of an experimental vaccine—which may be a vaccine or a placebo (an inactive substance that does not contain a drug)—protects them and, with a false sense of security, they may resume high-risk behaviors.

Despite optimistic projections in the early 1990s that a vaccine would be found in a few years, a considerable number of promising experimental HIV vaccines have proven ineffective against strains of HIV taken from infected people. Researchers reported developing anti-bodies that worked successfully against HIV grown in test tubes, but in every case they failed when used against HIV in human beings. As of September 2009, just one of the candidate vaccines had shown sufficient promise in clinical trials to warrant the investigation necessary to initiate its manufacture, approval, and widespread use.

The First Large-Scale Human Vaccine Trials

In "F.D.A. Authorizes First Full Testing for H.I.V. Vaccine" (*New York Times*, June 4, 1998), Altman indicates that in 1998 the FDA granted permission to VaxGen to conduct the first full-scale test of a vaccine to prevent HIV infection. The VaxGen vaccine—a genetically engineered molecule called AIDSvax—had been found "safe in tests involving 1,200 uninfected volunteers beginning in March 1992 and induced production of antibodies in more than 99 percent of the vaccinated participants." The 1998 test involved 5,000 volunteers in 40 clinics throughout the United States and Canada and 2,500 volunteers in 16 clinics in Thailand.

AIDSvax is made from part of HIV's outer coat, specifically a molecule called gp120. The molecule functions in the attachment of the virus to host cells. The vaccine does not contain the intact virus, only the gp120 protein from two strains of HIV. (Previous vaccines used one strain.) The two strains of the vaccine that were tested in North America were made with strains common in North America. The vaccine used in Thailand contained strains common to that part of the world. Participants in the North American study were men who have sex with men and uninfected partners of HIV-positive people. In Thailand, volunteers were uninfected injection drug users. Two-thirds of the North American volunteers were given the vaccine, and the rest received a placebo. In Thailand, half the group received the vaccine and half were given a placebo. The four-year trial ended in 2002.

The trial results were reported in February 2003. David R. Baker explains in "Vaccine Has No Impact, AIDSVAX's Failure a Blow to Treatment" (*San Francisco Chronicle*, November 13, 2003) that AIDSvax was determined to be a failure, as the comparison of those who received the vaccine versus those receiving a placebo demonstrated a slight reduction in new HIV infections in the vaccine population. Surprisingly, Asian-Americans and African-Americans who received the vaccine displayed a lower rate of infection than their racial counterparts who received the placebo. Considerable debate has arisen concerning these latter observations. Was this a statistical fluke? Or did AIDSvax display demographically specific protection, and if so, why?

Even though health officials and AIDS activists are hopeful, scientists are divided over when and which experimental vaccines should be approved for full-scale testing. Some favor trying any promising vaccine, whereas others advise waiting until the vaccine is completely understood before testing it. The results of the AIDSvax trial could sway this argument toward the latter camp.

One potential problem with AIDSvax, and perhaps a partial explanation of the poor overall results, is that previous tests indicated that it boosted only one part of the immune system—the component of the immune system responsible for antibody production. It is generally believed that a truly effective anti-HIV vaccine must boost another part of the immune system: the killer T cells that destroy virus-infected cells. Some experts consider the vaccine a long shot, but others point out that a failed vaccine does not mean that the experiment failed. Negative results can teach researchers what not to do in the future.

Vaccine Research Center

In 2000 the Dale and Betty Bumpers Vaccine Research Center (VRC, http://www3.niaid.nih.gov/about/organization/vrc/) opened on the NIH campus in Bethesda, Maryland. The facility brings together private companies and federal agencies to research, develop, and produce vaccines. The VRC is not exclusively devoted to HIV research and works to develop vaccines for other diseases.

Johannes F. Scheid et al. report in "Broad Diversity of Neutralizing Antibodies Isolated from Memory B Cells in HIV-Infected Individuals" (*Nature*, vol. 458, no. 7238, March 15, 2009) that they made progress in the development of an AIDS vaccine. The researchers looked at HIV patients who progress very slowly to AIDS because they have a range of neutralizing antibodies that identify and attack the virus. The researchers isolated 433 neutralizing antibodies from the blood of these slow-to-progress HIV patients and uncovered how the antibodies disarm the virus.

Even though most researchers are optimistic that an effective vaccine will be developed, many believe that perfecting a vaccine will take years. Researchers at the VRC believe that more than one vaccine formulation, or a vaccine that works two ways—to boost immunity provided by T cells and to produce antibodies to attach to HIV and mark it for destruction—may be necessary to provide complete protection.

May 15, 2009, marked the 12th annual HIV Vaccine Awareness Day and provided an opportunity to recount the more than two decades of progress in the search for a safe, effective HIV vaccine. In "HIV Vaccine Awareness Day" (May 18, 2009, http://www3.niaid.nih.gov/news/newsreleases/2009/hvad_09.htm), a statement to commemorate the day, Fauci acknowledges disappointing vaccine clinical trial outcomes and describes ongoing research efforts. He emphasizes prevention efforts such as "microbicide gels or creams that can be applied prior to sexual intercourse, and pre-exposure prophylaxis—the use of antiretroviral medicines in people who are not infected with HIV but who are at high risk for infection." He calls for "universal, voluntary HIV testing and treatment for those who test positive," and indicates that "one recent model suggests that such a test-and-treat program could reduce HIV infection rates by 95 percent within 10 years."

On September 24, 2009, the World Health Organization and the Joint United Nations Program on HIV/AIDS heralded the report of promising results of an experimental vaccine that combines two previously unsuccessful ones. A study involving more than 16,000 volunteers in Thailand found that the combination vaccine reduced the risk of becoming infected with AIDS by about one-third of the volunteers. According to Marilyn Marchione and Michael Casey, in "A World First: Vaccine Helps Prevent HIV Infection," (Associated Press, September 24, 2009), Fauci said the results of the study gave him "'cautious optimism about the possibility of improving this result' and developing a more effective AIDS vaccine."

CHAPTER 7
PEOPLE WITH HIV/AIDS

Large numbers of people are afflicted with HIV/AIDS in the United States. An increasing proportion of the population lives with HIV infection. At the end of the first decade of the 21st century, more Americans than ever before are likely to know someone affected by HIV or AIDS. Even people who live in remote geographic areas and do not believe they are personally at risk of acquiring HIV are aware of the epidemic from ongoing public health education campaigns, reports in the media, school health programs, and health and social service agencies dedicated to improving community awareness of HIV/AIDS.

PUBLIC FIGURES WITH HIV/AIDS

Perhaps one of the most famous HIV-infected people in the world is Magic Johnson (1959–), an internationally known former basketball player for the Los Angeles Lakers. When Johnson announced his HIV infection in November 1991, the world was shocked. He had no idea he was infected until he received the results of a routine physical examination for life insurance. Johnson freely admitted that before his marriage he had unprotected sexual contact with many women. He had no idea who transmitted the virus to him. The possibility exists that, however unknowingly, he passed the virus on to one or more subsequent sexual partners, who in turn, passed it on others.

To many, Johnson became a hero for his courage and immediate public acknowledgment of his HIV status. He became an HIV/AIDS spokesperson and began working in prevention programs. In 1991 he started the Magic Johnson Foundation, which seeks to fund and establish community-based education and social and health programs (including HIV/AIDS awareness) in inner-city communities and has given millions of dollars in grants to these causes. He was even named to the President's Commission on AIDS, from which he eventually resigned, frustrated with the lack of progress in HIV/AIDS efforts by the administration of President George H. W. Bush (1924–).

Despite his active, well-publicized efforts to increase awareness and prevention of HIV/AIDS, some people considered Johnson anything but a hero because his highly visible, promiscuous lifestyle sent the wrong message to the millions of young people who admired him.

In September 1992, ten months after Johnson announced his retirement from professional basketball, he indicated that he was returning to basketball on a limited basis. He played on the U.S. "Dream Team" in the 1992 Summer Olympics, assisting the team in its successful bid for a gold medal. Johnson benched himself at the start of the 1993–94 season, when he cut himself in a preseason game, terrifying some of his fellow players. Some players feared infection, whereas others worried that they should not play against Johnson with full force; after all, he was a man with a fatal disease. Johnson retired again but then returned for the end of the 1995–96 season, helping his team reach the play-offs. He retired for a third and final time after that season, but he continues to play basketball with the Magic Johnson All-Stars Team. He shows others, as one observer notes, that HIV infection is not a certain death sentence, but a condition with which one can live.

In 1992 the former tennis star Arthur Ashe (1943–1993) announced that he had become infected with HIV from a blood transfusion in the mid-1980s during a heart bypass operation. His was not a voluntary announcement, but one made necessary when the news media discovered his HIV infection and threatened to announce it before he did. Ashe was reluctant to make his condition public, fearing the effect on his five-year-old daughter. He maintained that because he did not have a public responsibility, he should have been allowed to maintain his privacy. He died of pneumonia, a complication of AIDS, in 1993.

The diver Greg Louganis (1960–) was diagnosed with HIV infection in 1988. The Olympic gold medalist announced his HIV status after the 1992 Summer Olympics, when he hit his head on the diving board during competition.

Even though his injury was not serious, it did result in an open wound. Louganis now competes in dog agility competitions with his dogs and is a published author of two books. He advocates safe sexual practices, because he attributes his HIV infection to unsafe sexual behavior.

Mary Fisher (1948–), a heterosexual and nondrug user who contracted HIV from her husband, stood before her peers at the 1992 Republican National Convention and announced that she was infected with HIV. A former television producer and assistant to President Gerald R. Ford (1913–2006), she said she considered her announcement part of her contribution to the fight against HIV/AIDS. The wealthy and well-educated Fisher was among the first women to publicly dispel the image that still comes to mind when many people think of HIV/AIDS: homosexual, poor, drug addicted, and lacking access to support systems or adequate medical care and housing.

Fisher established the Mary Fisher Clinical AIDS Research and Education Fund at the University of Alabama, Birmingham, in 2000. She is an accomplished artist, public speaker, and author of five books. In 2006 Peter Piot (1949–), the under secretary-general of the United Nations, appointed Fisher to a two-year term as a special representative of the Joint United Nations Program on HIV/AIDS, which Piot directs.

Another sports celebrity who succumbed to AIDS was the National Association of Stock Car Auto Racing (NASCAR) racecar driver Tim Richmond (1955–1989). During his heyday on the NASCAR race circuit in the 1980s, Richmond was one of the circuit's premier drivers. He was also well known for his expensive tastes and playboy lifestyle. Whether his lifestyle contributed to his illness is conjecture. Nonetheless, by the end of the 1986 racing season Richmond had become noticeably ill. He was diagnosed with AIDS that same year. He was able to race again in 1987, but soon thereafter his health deteriorated precipitously. During another attempted comeback in 1988, when his illness was still unpublicized, Richmond faced the hostility and innuendo of his fellow drivers, who, guessing the nature of the illness, speculated about his sexual orientation and the possibility of drug abuse. In response, Richmond filed a defamation of character lawsuit against NASCAR. He subsequently withdrew the lawsuit to avoid making his condition public. Richmond ultimately retired from competitive racing and lived in seclusion with his mother until his death. After his death, as news of his illness and the treatment he received from his fellow drivers and NASCAR became public, many people were outraged at the NASCAR organization, which as of September 2009 had not apologized.

The actor Anthony Perkins (1932–1992), who is best known for his role as Norman Bates in the classic Alfred Hitchcock (1899–1990) film *Psycho* (1960), also died of AIDS. Forever typecast by that performance, Perkins was in fact an accomplished film and stage actor. He was bisexual and had relationships with a number of men, including the dancer Rudolf Nureyev (1938–1993), who also died of AIDS. Shortly before his death in 1992, Perkins commented in a press release about a *National Enquirer* article that revealed his AIDS-positive status by saying, "I have learned more about love, selflessness, and human understanding from the people I have met in this great adventure in the world of AIDS than I ever did in the cutthroat, competitive world in which I spent my life." Perkins's widow, Berry Berenson (1948–2001), was one of the passengers on American Airlines Flight 11, which was hijacked and crashed into the World Trade Center on September 11, 2001.

Another movie star who succumbed to AIDS was Rock Hudson (1925–1985). Indeed, Hudson was the first major U.S. celebrity known to have died from AIDS. His death was especially noteworthy, given his status in the 1950s as the quintessential rugged, all-American male. Despite his many movie roles as a straight man, Hudson was homosexual, a fact that was covered up by movie studios. His 1955 marriage to the studio employee Phyllis Gates (1925–2006), which ended in divorce in 1958, is thought to have been a studio-orchestrated attempt to cover up his sexual orientation. Hudson died at the age of 59.

The African-American rap star Eazy-E (c. 1963–1995) rose to fame as one of the members of the group N.W.A. (Niggaz with Attitude), based in Compton, California. Using money obtained from illegal drug sales, Eazy-E founded Ruthless Records. Soon after, he recruited Ice Cube (1969–), Dr. Dre (1965?–), M.C. Ren (1969–), DJ Yella (1967–), and Arabian Prince (1964–) to form N.W.A. Following the dissolution of N.W.A., Eazy-E went on to have a successful solo career. In 1995 he entered the hospital for treatment of what he thought was asthma. However, he was diagnosed with AIDS and died soon after. Eazy-E is now regarded as one of the influential founders of the style of music known as gangsta rap. Every year, the city of Compton celebrates his life by observing Eazy-E Day.

Another music icon who died of AIDS was Freddie Mercury (1946–1991), the lead vocalist of the British rock band Queen. His more than three-octave vocal range and operatic compositional approach to rock resulted in classic hits such as "Bohemian Rhapsody," "Somebody to Love," and "We Are the Champions." The video made for the 1975 release of "Bohemian Rhapsody" is considered by some music insiders to be one of the decisive influences that spurred the popularity of music videos. Mercury was well known for his extravagance and bisexuality. His diagnosis and deteriorating physical condition were kept private. Indeed, his eventual announcement that he had AIDS was made only one day before his death in 1991.

Elizabeth Glaser (1947–1994), the wife of the actor Paul Michael Glaser (1943–), was galvanized to cofound the Pediatric AIDS Foundation in 1988 (now called the Elizabeth Glaser Pediatric AIDS Foundation), following the discovery that she and her children, Ariel (1981–1988) and Jake (1984–), were all infected with HIV. She originally contracted the virus from contaminated blood administered during pregnancy, but she was unaware of her illness until much later, already having unwittingly passed it to her children. In the ensuing years she became a vocal AIDS activist. The foundation that is her legacy contributes more than $1 million annually to pediatric AIDS research. Ariel died at the age of seven, and Elizabeth died in 1994. Because Jake has a mutation of the CCR5 gene that delays onset by restricting the virus's ability to enter white blood cells, he remains symptom free and no longer takes HIV medication. He and Paul continue to raise money and AIDS awareness through Elizabeth's foundation.

Finally, in a list of examples that is by no means complete, the prolific and influential science-fiction author Isaac Asimov (1920–1992) contracted HIV from infected blood given to him in a transfusion during heart bypass surgery in 1983. He died in 1992 of heart and renal failure that were complications of AIDS.

OLDER PEOPLE WITH HIV/AIDS

In "AIDS among Persons Aged Greater Than or Equal to 50 Years—United States, 1991–1996" (*Morbidity and Mortality Weekly Report*, vol. 47, no. 2, January 23, 1998), the Centers for Disease Control and Prevention (CDC) reports that most older people infected with HIV early in the epidemic were typically infected through contaminated blood or blood products. Through 1989 only 1% of HIV/AIDS cases of people aged 13 to 49 was due to contaminated blood. However, in this same period 6% of cases of people aged 50 to 59, 28% of cases of people aged 60 to 69, and 64% of cases of those aged 70 and older resulted from contaminated blood or blood products.

In 1985 changes introduced to improve the safety of the nation's blood supply, including routine screening of blood donations for HIV, sharply reduced the risk of contracting the virus from contaminated blood or blood products. Subsequently, the proportion of people aged 50 and over who acquired HIV from other types of exposure increased. Even though male-to-male sexual contact and injection drug use remain the primary means by which HIV is transmitted among all age groups in the United States, heterosexual transmission of HIV is steadily increasing in people more than 50 years old.

HIV/AIDS Cases among People Aged 45 and Over

The CDC notes in "HIV/AIDS among Persons Aged 50 and Older" (February 2008, http://www.cdc.gov/Hiv/

TABLE 7.1

AIDS cases by age, 2007 and cumulative

Age (years)	Estimated # of AIDS cases in 2007	Cumulative estimated # of AIDS cases, through 2007*
Under 13	28	9,209
Ages 13–14	80	1,169
Ages 15–19	455	6,089
Ages 20–24	1,927	38,175
Ages 25–29	3,380	120,464
Ages 30–34	4,187	201,906
Ages 35–39	5,888	219,601
Ages 40–44	6,813	177,250
Ages 45–49	5,749	112,896
Ages 50–54	3,636	63,408
Ages 55–59	2,040	34,160
Ages 60–64	980	18,249
Ages 65 or older	800	15,853

*Includes persons with a diagnosis of AIDS from the beginning of the epidemic through 2007.

SOURCE: "AIDS Cases by Age," in *Basic Statistics*, Centers for Disease Control and Prevention, February 26, 2009, http://www.cdc.gov/hiv/topics/surveillance/basic.htm#hivaidsage (accessed July 3, 2009)

topics/over50/resources/factsheets/pdf/over50.pdf) that in 2005, 15% of new HIV/AIDS cases reported in the United States occurred in people over the age of 50. Nearly a quarter (24%) of people living with HIV/AIDS were over the age of 50, up from 17% in 2001. The proportion of adults over the age of 50 with HIV/AIDS is expected to increase as HIV-infected people of all ages live longer as a result of effective drug therapy and other advances in medical treatment.

Through 2007 an estimated 244,566 cases of AIDS in people over the age of 45 had been reported. (See Table 7.1.) Of these reported cases, 112,896 (46% of the cumulative total) were among people aged 45 to 49, 63,408 (26%) were among people aged 50 to 54, 34,160 (14%) were among people aged 55 to 59, 18,249 (7%) were among people aged 60 to 64, and 15,853 (6%) were among people aged 65 and older.

HIV Testing for Those over 50

Many older adults do not seek routine screening for HIV infection because they do not believe they are at risk of acquiring HIV. Among women older than 50, the absence of the risk of pregnancy may lead to a false sense of security and the mistaken belief that they are at less risk for sexually transmitted diseases, including HIV. HIV-infected people aged 50 and over may not be tested promptly for HIV infection. As a result, opportunities to start these patients on therapies to slow the progression of the disease are often lost. The failure to test or the late testing of older patients may be because:

- Physicians are less apt to look for HIV in people of this age group.

- Some opportunistic AIDS illnesses that occur in older people, such as encephalopathy and wasting disease, have similar symptoms to other diseases associated with aging, such as Alzheimer's disease, depression, and malignancies.

It is vitally important to overcome older adults' reluctance to seek testing and other delays to diagnosis because research shows that age speeds the progression of HIV to AIDS and blunts CD4 response to highly active antiretroviral therapy. Equally important is continuing the research to improve the treatment of HIV-infected older adults and the development of effective education programs to prevent infection in this population.

LIVING WITH HIV/AIDS

To gain a more complete view of the impact of HIV/AIDS, it is important to understand the psychosocial and emotional consequences of diagnosis with a potentially fatal disease.

A Frightening Diagnosis

In the introduction to *When Someone Close Has AIDS: Acquired Immunodeficiency Syndrome* (1989), Lewis L. Judd, the former director of the National Institute of Mental Health, writes about the meaning of the diagnosis of AIDS. It means not only a shortened life but also one that is "marred by chronic fatigue, loss of appetite and weight, frequent hospitalizations, AIDS dementia, and debilitating bouts of illness from unusual infections." The person diagnosed with HIV/AIDS also feels anger, confusion, depression, isolation, and hopelessness, which can also affect those around him or her who are often unprepared for the suffering they witness.

Judd explains that people diagnosed with HIV/AIDS need support and reassurance from friends and relatives that they will not be abandoned or isolated. He also recommends that those around HIV/AIDS patients encourage them to pursue hobbies, work as long as they can, and engage in social activities. Judd warns that caring for someone with AIDS is physically and emotionally exhausting and calls for inner strength, as well as the caregivers' coming to terms with their own feelings about the illness.

At the end of the first decade of the 21st century, Judd's advice is still sound. Although no longer a certain death sentence, a diagnosis of HIV may still elicit feelings of fear, confusion, depression, and anger. Furthermore, researchers have identified another reason that people diagnosed with HIV infection require additional emotional support: there is an association between psychosocial stress and HIV disease progression. Yoichi Chida and Kavita Vedhara report in "Adverse Psychosocial Factors Predict Poorer Prognosis in HIV Disease: A Meta-analytic Review of Prospective Investigations" (*Brain, Behavior,*

and Immunity, vol. 23, no. 4, May 2009) the results of a review of 36 articles describing the association between psychosocial factors such as personality types, coping styles, psychological distress, and HIV disease progression. The researchers find a strong relationship between adverse psychosocial factors such as difficulty coping with stress and HIV disease progression.

Coping with Discrimination

Unlike people diagnosed with other terminal or catastrophic illnesses such as cancer or multiple sclerosis, people with HIV/AIDS often confront the social isolation and discrimination that accompany a stigmatized status. Many people continue to mistakenly characterize HIV/AIDS as exclusively a disease of homosexual men and drug users and condemn HIV-infected people for inflicting themselves with the condition. Some still believe that AIDS is divine retribution for an "immoral lifestyle." The fear of unfavorable judgment keeps many infected individuals from disclosing their HIV infection to others, even friends and family. Others simply do not want the pity that is often extended to people with potentially fatal conditions. Still others worry that friends and family, fearing infection, will abandon them.

Under the Americans with Disabilities Act (ADA) of 1990, people infected with HIV and those diagnosed with AIDS are considered disabled and as such are subject to the antidiscrimination provisions of this landmark legislation. As a result, employers may not ask job applicants if they are HIV infected or have AIDS, nor can they require an HIV test of prospective employees. The only exceptions to this provision are those employers who can demonstrate that such questions or testing are job-related and absolutely necessary for the employer to conduct business.

More important, the ADA requires employers to make "reasonable accommodations" for disabled employees. Reasonable accommodation is an adjustment to a job or modification of the responsibilities or work environment that will enable the worker with a disability to gain equal employment opportunity. Examples include flexible work schedules to allow for medical appointments, treatments, and counseling and the provision of additional unpaid leave.

PRESIDENT PROCLAIMS JUNE 2009 AS LESBIAN, GAY, BISEXUAL, AND TRANSGENDER PRIDE MONTH. On June 1, 2009, President Barack Obama (1961–; http://www.white house.gov/the_press_office/Presidential-Proclamation-LG BT-Pride-Month/) issued a proclamation naming June 2009 as Lesbian, Gay, Bisexual, and Transgender (LGBT) Pride Month. He acknowledged the contributions of LGBT Americans and lauded their efforts to spur the nation to respond to the HIV/AIDS epidemic and their role in broadening the United States' response to the HIV/AIDS worldwide. President Obama said, "We must also commit ourselves to fighting the HIV/AIDS epidemic by both reducing the number of HIV infections and providing care and support services to people living with HIV/AIDS across the United States." He also asked "the LGBT community, the Congress, and the American people to work together to promote equal rights for all, regardless of sexual orientation or gender identity."

THE STIGMA OF AIDS. In "A Comparison of HIV Stigma and Discrimination in Five International Sites: The Influence of Care and Treatment Resources in High Prevalence Settings" (*Social Science and Medicine*, vol. 68, no. 12, June 2009), a study designed to examine HIV stigma and discrimination in five high prevalence settings, Suzanne Maman et al. observe that the factors that contribute to HIV stigma and discrimination include the fear of transmission, the fear of suffering and death, and the burden of caring for people with AIDS.

According to Maman et al., the family, access to antiretroviral drugs, and other resources offered some protection against HIV stigma and discrimination. Variation in the availability of health and social services designed to lessen the impact of HIV/AIDS helps explain differences in HIV stigma and discrimination across the settings. The researchers opine that "increasing access to treatment and care resources may function to lower HIV stigma, however, providing services is not enough." They also assert that it is necessary to develop "effective strategies to reduce HIV stigma as treatment and care resources are scaled up in the settings that are most heavily impacted by the HIV epidemic."

More than two decades after the first diagnosis of AIDS and widespread public health and community education efforts to inform people about HIV infection and prevent the spread of HIV, ignorance and misunderstanding of HIV/AIDS persist. Health educators and HIV/AIDS activists stress the importance of intensified, ongoing education to destigmatize people affected by HIV/AIDS and prevent discrimination. Reducing the stigma associated with HIV/AIDS may also encourage individuals to get tested and, for those who are infected, begin treatment as soon as possible.

Because stigma, even among personnel who work with people with HIV/AIDS, persists, efforts to reduce it continue. The HIV/AIDS Stigma Program, which is funded by the Health Resource and Services Administration's HIV/AIDS Bureau, offers training programs that explore the stigma associated with HIV/AIDS. The programs, which are made available to staff employed by agencies and organizations funded by the Ryan White Comprehensive AIDS Resources Emergency Act of 1990, focus on:

- Defining stigma and its origins in society.

- The impact of stigma on an individual's decision-making process and how it deters him or her from seeking HIV testing and counseling services.

- How stigma affects access to care and disclosure of HIV-positive status.

Dealing with Emotions

Not unexpectedly, anger and depression are natural and common reactions to discovering that one is infected with HIV. Experts stress the importance of recognizing and expressing anger and depression; however, if these feelings become all consuming, they can prevent health- and life-improving actions. Many people with HIV/AIDS admit that sharing feelings with friends and family members and participating in support groups ease anguish and help generate more positive attitudes and actions.

Many HIV/AIDS sufferers report that the most difficult thing they had to do after being diagnosed with HIV was to inform people in their present or recent past whom they might have exposed to the virus. If the patient is unable to do this, a physician or public health official can notify present or former sexual partners without revealing the infected person's name.

Early Medication Improves Outlook

The earlier people learn of their infection, the earlier they can begin medical treatment to suppress the virus's destructive growth, delay the onset of AIDS symptoms, and extend life. Along with antiretroviral drugs there are medications that fight the life-threatening opportunistic infections that eventually afflict most people who are HIV infected. Even though these drugs cannot cure HIV infection, they have been shown to keep HIV/AIDS patients healthy and symptom free for increasingly longer periods.

Practicing Good Health Habits

Experts advise HIV-infected people to exercise and maintain a balanced diet with sufficient lean protein. Not only does exercise improve overall fitness and generate a sense of well-being but also it releases endorphins, which are natural substances produced by the brain that boost immunity, reduce stress, and elevate mood. People with HIV/AIDS are advised to avoid smoking, excessive alcohol consumption, and using illegal drugs, all of which can act to depress the immune system.

HOUSING PROBLEMS

The difficulty in finding affordable and appropriate housing can be an acute crisis for people living with HIV/AIDS. HIV-infected people need more than just a safe shelter that provides protection and comfort; they may also require a base from which to receive services, care, and support. Adherence to complicated medical regimens is challenging for many HIV-infected people, but for some homeless people it is nearly impossible.

Some individuals are homeless when they acquire the HIV infection, whereas others lose their homes when they are no longer able to hold jobs or cannot afford to pay for health care and housing costs. The National AIDS Housing Coalition (NAHC) indicates in *Examining the Evidence: The Impact of Housing on HIV Prevention and Care* (2008, http://www.nationalaidshousing.org/PDF/FinalSummit.pdf) that:

- Housing status is a key factor affecting access to care and health behaviors among people with HIV/AIDS—housing assistance reduces HIV health risk behaviors, improves health outcomes, and reduces use of costly emergency and inpatient hospital services.

- Housing remains one of the greatest unmet needs of Americans with HIV/AIDS.

- Even though about 500,000 households affected by HIV/AIDS will require some form of housing assistance during the course of their lives, the federal program Housing Opportunities for Persons with AIDS (HOPWA) serves just 70,000 households per year.

In the fact sheet "HIV/AIDS and Homelessness" (July 2009, http://www.nationalhomeless.org/factsheets/HIV.pdf), the National Coalition for the Homeless (NCH) estimates that in 2006, 3.4% of homeless people were HIV infected. This was nearly nine times higher than the 0.4% of the general population who were HIV infected.

The NCH reconfirms the observation that people living with HIV/AIDS are at a higher risk of becoming homeless. The coalition indicates that one study finds that 50% of people living with HIV/AIDS felt they were at risk of becoming homeless.

The NCH also identifies homeless women and adolescents as at high risk for HIV infection. Homeless women's risk is attributable to high rates of domestic violence and sexual abuse, whereas homeless teens risk infection as a result of sexual exploitation and abuse.

In 1990 the U.S. Department of Housing and Urban Development established a federal program specifically intended to meet the housing needs of people with HIV/AIDS. Congress established the program because the housing resources available at that time were not meeting the needs of people with AIDS, who, because of discrimination, had difficulties obtaining suitable housing and the supportive services that they required. HOPWA was established under the National Affordable Housing Act of 1990. Suzanne Miller notes in "HOPWA Program Continues to Serve People in Need" (*ActionLink Journal*, no. 18, September 2007) that HOPWA began in 1992 and between fiscal years (FYs) 1992 and 2007 Congress had allotted $3.4 billion for the program. FY 2004 funding was $294.8 million, up from $290.1 million in FY 2003. FY 2007 funding of $286 million provided housing assistance for about 67,000.

In "2010 Actual HIV/AIDS Housing Need" (January 2009, http://www.nationalaidshousing.org/PDF/2010needpa-

per.pdf), the NAHC explains that the funding for FY 2009 was estimated at $315 million. It notes in the press release "Flat Funding of $300 Million Proposed for HOPWA in FY2009" (February 5, 2008, http://www.nationalaidshousing.org/PDF/PresBudgetPressrelease_02.05.08.pdf) that this funding provided housing assistance to approximately 70,500 households. The NAHC recommended $360 million in HOPWA funding for FY 2010, which would enable the program to serve twice as many new households as it did in 2008.

SUICIDE

Depression is a common psychiatric problem among patients who are seriously ill with HIV/AIDS. Even though this is a normal grief response, the combination of alienation, hopelessness, guilt, and lack of self-esteem can lead some to contemplate and plan for suicide in search of lost dignity and control. Others counter that the real dignity is in seeing the disease to the end. Those who encourage people with HIV/AIDS to "stick it out" often see the disease as becoming increasingly manageable with drugs and improved treatment techniques.

Several factors make HIV/AIDS patients more likely to commit suicide: They feel they are certain to die sooner than they expected and worry that their deaths will be prolonged as well as emotionally and physically painful. They may also be despondent about the prospects of losing their job, their insurance, or their home. Furthermore, they may be ostracized from society. Researchers find that factors that have a considerable impact on the quality of life include security, family, love, pleasurable activity, and freedom from pain and suffering and from debilitating disease. AIDS patients may lose all these, or they may be consumed by the fear of losing vital capacities and freedoms. For some, suicide seems like a reasonable alternative; it offers an end to pain and suffering, insecurity, self-pity, dependency, and hopelessness.

According to Seth C. Kalichman et al., in "Depression and Thoughts of Suicide among Middle-Aged and Older Persons Living with HIV-AIDS" (*Psychiatric Services*, vol. 51, no. 7, July 2000), 27% of 113 middle-aged and older people with AIDS reported having thought about taking their own life in the previous week. Subjects who contemplated suicide reported higher levels of emotional distress and poorer health-related quality of life than those who had not considered suicide. Those who considered suicide were also more likely to have disclosed their HIV status to the people close to them; regardless, they perceived receiving significantly less social support from friends and family than subjects who reported no thought of suicide. Kalichman et al. conclude, "Persons who are in midlife and older and are living with HIV-AIDS experience significant emotional distress and thoughts of suicide, suggesting a need for targeted interventions to improve mental health and prevent suicide."

Highly active antiretroviral therapy has resulted in people aging with HIV. According to David E. Vance, Linda Moneyham, and Kenneth F. Far of the University of Alabama, Birmingham, in "Suicidal Ideation in Adults Aging with HIV: Neurological and Cognitive Considerations" (*Journal of Psychosocial Nursing*, vol. 46, no. 11, 2008), older adults with HIV are more vulnerable to cognitive declines (impaired thinking and reasoning) than are older adults who are not infected. The researchers posit that stressors such as coping with neurological or cognitive changes associated with aging with HIV may result in increased levels of depression and thoughts of suicide.

The Physician's Role

During the 1990s there were heated debates, voter initiatives, and court decisions about the legalization of physician-assisted suicide. Only two states—Oregon (in 1994) and Washington (in 2008)—have legalized physician-assisted suicide. Oregon and Washington voters determined that the right to end one's own life is intensely personal and should not be forbidden by law. (Even though attempts and acts of suicide are no longer subject to criminal prosecution in the United States, aiding a suicide is considered a criminal offense.)

Both the public and physicians themselves are divided about the issue of physician-assisted suicide. People who support the practice believe that doctors should make their skills available to patients to end anguish and suffering. Those who oppose physician-assisted suicide argue that better end-of-life care—effective pain management, emotional and spiritual support, and widespread education to reduce anxiety about dying—may reduce the frequency of requests for physician-assisted suicide. Opponents also fear that the legal right to assist suicide can be misused or abused and that such abuses might victimize already vulnerable populations.

Some of opponents' worst fears about the practice of euthanasia are confirmed by Diane Martindale in "A Culture of Death" (*Scientific American*, vol. 292, no. 6, June 2005). Martindale describes the research of Russel Ogden, a Canadian graduate student in criminology who interviewed 17 people—social workers, physicians, counselors, nurses, and two priests—about their efforts to help AIDS patients kill themselves. Ogden found that half of the assisted suicides were botched and ultimately resulted in increased suffering and even failed attempts. However, this did not prompt Ogden to renounce the practice of assisted suicide. Instead, he asserted that "without medical supervision and formal regulations, euthanasia is happening in horrific circumstances, similar to back-alley abortions."

CHAPTER 8
TESTING, PREVENTION, AND EDUCATION

HIV TESTING

Voluntary, Not Mandatory

Few issues about the HIV/AIDS epidemic have prompted more controversy than the use of antibody tests to identify people who are infected with HIV. Soon after the enzyme-linked immunosorbent assay test was developed and licensed in 1985, many public health officials supported testing in an attempt to change "undesirable" behaviors that were determining the course of the epidemic (such as unsafe male-to-male sexual contact and injection drug use). Those who favored testing claimed that if a person knew he or she was HIV positive, the infected person would change his or her behavior. Others argued that aggressive public health education and thoughtful counseling would be more productive strategies to achieve the desired results, even if people did not know their HIV status.

In the early years of the epidemic, health care officials in the public and private sectors refrained from advocating mandatory testing; instead, they focused on HIV testing that would be performed by physicians for patients they considered at risk for infection. In 1990 the House of Delegates of the American Medical Association (AMA) voted to declare HIV/AIDS a sexually transmitted disease (STD). This designation allowed physicians more freedom to decide the conditions under which HIV testing should take place.

In the late 1980s, when the research community announced that HIV-infected, symptom-free people could receive early intervention with azidothymidine (now known as zidovudine, or ZDV) to slow the effects of the illness and delay the onset of *Pneumocystis carinii* pneumonia, the debate took another turn. Gay rights advocates, such as the Gay Men's Health Crisis Center in New York, began to encourage those at risk for HIV infection to get tested rather than discouraging testing, as they had previously done. In June 1997 the Gay Men's Health Crisis Center

opened its own testing facility. This service was still available in 2009 as part of the range of care and support services offered by the Michael Palm Center (http://www.gmhc.org/programs/palm_center.html). The center also offered a 12-week "harm reduction program" that was designed to curb risky behaviors such as substance abuse and unprotected sex. The intent of the program was to encourage people to change their risky behavior in a supportive atmosphere of care.

Another controversy surrounding testing concerns reporting HIV-positive patients by name. Every state is required to report AIDS cases. As of 2009, 53 areas—47 states and five dependent areas—had implemented HIV case surveillance using the same confidential system for name-based case reporting for both HIV infection and AIDS, though several states did not implement such reporting until 2006. (See Table 8.1.)

Critics, including the American Civil Liberties Union, assail name reporting as an invasion of privacy that carries social and economic risks. They claim that any benefit that would result from reporting names could not override the negative consequences (such as ostracism and the potential loss of jobs and health insurance) of being classified as infected. They add that name reporting discourages those at risk for HIV from coming forward to seek testing and timely treatment.

As the name-reporting debate subsides, with the overwhelming majority of states acquiescing to federal requirements, there is widespread agreement that testing is most effective if followed by counseling that completely explains the results and their consequences. Furthermore, Bernard M. Branson et al. of the CDC note in "Revised Recommendations for HIV Testing of Adults, Adolescents, and Pregnant Women in Health-Care Settings" (*Morbidity and Mortality Weekly Report*, vol. 55, RR-14, September 22, 2006) that the CDC's 2006 revision of HIV testing guidelines call for routine testing for everyone aged 13 to 64 seen at a physician's office or medical clinic. Routine

TABLE 8.1

Reported cases of HIV infection, by area of residence and age category, 2007 and cumulative

Area of residence (date HIV reporting initiated)	Reported[b]	Diagnosed	Cumulative[a] Adults or adolescents	Cumulative[a] Children (<13 yrs)	Total
Alabama (January 1988)	529	447	6,380	50	6,430
Alaska (February 1999)	27	21	308	2	310
Arizona (January 1987)	771	488	6,329	89	6,418
Arkansas (July 1989)	206	180	2,487	18	2,505
California (April 2006)	17,588	2,687	24,199	195	24,394
Colorado (November 1985)	382	274	6,334	31	6,365
Connecticut (January 2005)[c]	932	259	3,178	109	3,287
Delaware (February 2006)	480	88	1,270	18	1,288
District of Columbia (November 2006)	1,629	483	1,871	10	1,881
Florida (July 1997)[d]	5,165	3,982	39,393	541	39,934
Georgia (December 2003)	3,204	1,059	11,039	218	11,257
Idaho (June 1986)	39	17	377	5	382
Illinois (January 2006)	3,576	936	9,763	190	9,953
Indiana (July 1988)	406	313	4,260	42	4,302
Iowa (July 1998)	93	82	658	4	662
Kansas (July 1999)	110	79	1,330	16	1,346
Kentucky (October 2004)	414	218	1,631	22	1,653
Louisiana (February 1993)	797	642	8,450	167	8,617
Maine (January 2006)	46	36	420	3	423
Massachusetts (January 2007)	777	181	881	29	910
Michigan (April 1992)	623	498	6,996	133	7,129
Minnesota (October 1985)	289	224	3,550	40	3,590
Mississippi (August 1988)	471	411	4,892	61	4,953
Missouri (October 1987)	460	353	5,239	54	5,293
Montana (September 2006)	92	5	118	2	120
Nebraska (September 1995)	78	52	716	11	727
Nevada (February 1992)	369	299	3,827	28	3,855
New Hampshire (January 2005)	52	32	509	9	518
New Jersey (January 1992)	1,571	693	18,297	314	18,611
New Mexico (January 1998)	92	80	997	4	1,001
New York (June 2000)	5,197	2,836	45,786	1,765	47,551
North Carolina (February 1990)	1,746	1,465	15,325	154	15,479
North Dakota (January 1988)	9	3	88	2	90
Ohio (June 1990)	852	600	8,760	112	8,872
Oklahoma (June 1988)	199	172	2,449	29	2,478
Oregon (April 2006)	1,477	134	1,565	27	1,592
Pennsylvania (October 2002)[e]	3,694	1,007	12,162	243	12,405
Rhode Island (July 2006)	130	67	146	5	151
South Carolina (February 1986)	542	451	7,147	94	7,241
South Dakota (January 1988)	17	16	226	6	232
Tennessee (January 1992)	841	708	7,602	92	7,694
Texas (January 1999)[f]	3,495	2,507	26,030	430	26,460
Utah (April 1989)	92	73	953	14	967
Virginia (July 1989)	823	560	10,790	97	10,887
Washington (March 2006)	620	386	4,423	42	4,465
West Virginia (January 1989)	55	50	689	8	697
Wisconsin (November 1985)	220	181	2,593	30	2,623
Wyoming (June 1989)	15	12	103	2	105
Subtotal	**61,292**	**26,347**	**322,536**	**5,567**	**328,103**

HIV tests in physicians' offices and clinics no longer require the pretest counseling that was a requisite part of all HIV testing before the revised guidelines.

Rates of HIV Testing among Men Who Have Sex with Men

In 2003 the CDC, in cooperation with 25 state and local health departments, launched the National HIV Behavioral Surveillance System (NHBS). The NHBS considers people at risk for HIV infection and surveys the three populations at highest risk for HIV in the United States—men who have sex with men (MSM), injection drug users (IDUs), and high-risk heterosexuals—and collects information from them.

The most recent NHBS for which data have been analyzed covers the period from November 2003 to April 2005, during which more than 10,000 MSM were surveyed. Travis Sanchez et al. of the CDC indicate in "Human Immunodeficiency Virus (HIV) Risk, Prevention, and Testing Behaviors—United States, National HIV Behavioral Surveillance System: Men Who Have Sex with Men, November 2003–April 2005" (*Morbidity and Mortality Weekly Report*, vol. 55, no. SS-6, July 7, 2006, http://www .cdc.gov/mmwr/PDF/ss/ss5506.pdf) that the overwhelming majority (92%) reported ever having an HIV test and 77% had been tested in the 12 months preceding the survey. Table 8.2 shows that more than half had been tested in a physician's office (36%) or a clinic or community health center (26%).

TABLE 8.1

Reported cases of HIV infection, by area of residence and age category, 2007 and cumulative [CONTINUED]

Area of residence (date HIV reporting initiated)	Reported[b]	Diagnosed	Cumulative[a] Adults or adolescents	Cumulative[a] Children (<13 yrs)	Cumulative[a] Total
U.S. dependent areas					
American Samoa (August 2001)	0	0	1	0	1
Guam (March 2000)	1	1	67	0	67
Northern Mariana Islands (October 2001)	0	0	7	0	7
Puerto Rico (January 2003)	1,450	580	6,693	108	6,801
U.S. Virgin Islands (December 1998)	20	17	253	7	260
Persons reported from areas with confidential name-based HIV infection reporting but who were residents of other areas	151	54	1,016	87	1,103
Total[g]	**63,230**	**27,126**	**331,768**	**5,822**	**337,590**

Note: Includes data from 47 states, the District of Columbia, and 5 U.S. dependent areas with confidential name-based HIV infection reporting as of December 2007.

[a]From the beginning of the epidemic through 2007.

[b]Cases of HIV infection (not AIDS) reported in 2007 include cases diagnosed during earlier years.

[c]Beginning in 1992, Connecticut had name-based HIV reporting for cases in children only. From January 2002 through December 2004, Connecticut had name-or code-based HIV reporting for cases in adolescents and adults. As of January 2005, Connecticut has name-based reporting of all cases of HIV infection.

[d]Florida has confidential name-based HIV infection reporting for only the diagnoses made during July 1997 or later.

[e]On October 18, 2002, Pennsylvania initiated confidential name-based HIV infection reporting in all areas except Philadelphia. Code-based reporting was implemented in Philadelphia in March 2004, and the switch to name-based reporting was made in October 2005.

[f]From February 1994 through December 1998, Texas reported HIV infection in children only.

[g]Includes 1,248 persons reported from areas with confidential name-based HIV infection reporting but whose area of residence is unknown.

SOURCE: "Table 18. Reported and Diagnosed Cases of HIV Infection (not AIDS), by Area of Residence, 2007 and Cumulative—47 States, the District of Columbia and 5 U.S. Dependent Areas with Confidential Name-Based HIV Infection Reporting," in *HIV/AIDS Surveillance Report*, vol. 19, Centers for Disease Control and Prevention, February 2009, http://www.cdc.gov/hiv/topics/surveillance/resources/reports/2007report/pdf/table18.pdf (accessed July 6, 2009)

TABLE 8.2

Most recent testing sites for men who have sex with men and who had HIV tests during the previous 12 months, November 2003–April 2005

Facility type	No.	(%)
Private doctor's office	2,541	(36)
Public health clinic or community health center	1,865	(26)
HIV counseling and testing program	852	(12)
HIV/AIDS* street outreach	309	(4)
Drug treatment program	212	(3)
Hospital (inpatient)	163	(2)
Sexually transmitted disease clinic	107	(2)
Emergency department	103	(2)
HIV/AIDS specialty clinic	88	(1)
Other outpatient clinic	80	(1)
Correctional facility	49	(1)
Other	490	(7)

Notes: Population = 7,057. Numbers might not add to total because of missing data.
*Acquired immunodeficiency syndrome.

SOURCE: Travis Sanchez et al., "Table 3. Number and Percentage of Facility Types Reported As the Most Recent Place of Human Immunodeficiency Virus (HIV) Testing for Those Persons Who Had a Test during the Previous 12 Months—United States, National HIV Behavioral Surveillance System: Men Who Have Sex with Men, November 2003–April 2005," in "Human Immunodeficiency Virus (HIV) Risk, Prevention, and Testing Behaviors—United States, National HIV Behavioral Surveillance System: Men Who Have Sex with Men, November 2003–April 2005," *Morbidity and Morality Weekly Report*, vol. 55, no. SS-6, July 7, 2006, http://www.cdc.gov/mmwr/PDF/ss/ss5506.pdf (accessed July 6, 2009)

Of those who had not been tested during the 12 months preceding the survey, more than half (51%) offered that they "hadn't done anything to get HIV," and 38% cited this as their main reason for not getting tested. (See Table 8.3.) Nearly one-third (30%) said they feared finding out that they were infected and 20% said they did not have time to get tested. Fourteen percent were worried that "someone would find out about the test result," and 13% said they feared discrimination, in the form of losing a job, insurance, family, housing, or friends.

Contact Tracing/Partner Notification

A by-product of testing is contact tracing, or partner notification. When individuals test positive for HIV, health officials ask them to provide, with the promise of anonymity, the names of those with whom they have had sexual contact or shared needles. The CDC asks counselors to inform contacts if the patient is reluctant to do so and strongly endorses contact-tracing programs, but results vary. States struggling under the strain of many HIV/AIDS cases continue to support programs that encourage the infected people to notify partners on their own. Contact-tracing programs in states with fewer HIV/AIDS cases are more likely to contact partners. Many patients who are HIV infected or have AIDS fear that promises of confidentiality will be broken; others fear retribution from those they may have infected.

In "A Systematic Review of HIV Partner Counseling and Referral Services: Client and Provider Attitudes, Preferences, Practices, and Experiences" (*Sexually Transmitted Diseases*, vol. 33, no. 5, May 2006), Warren F. Passin et al. report on their research to improve understanding of client and provider attitudes about, and experiences

TABLE 8.3

Reasons men who have sex with men gave for not being tested for HIV, November 2003–April 2005

Reason reported	A reason[a] No.	A reason[a] (%)	Main reason[b] No.	Main reason[b] (%)
Haven't done anything to get HIV	1,508	(51)	1,143	(38)
Afraid of finding out infected with HIV	888	(30)	546	(18)
Didn't have time	597	(20)	272	(9)
Don't know where to get tested	265	(9)	76	(3)
Afraid of losing job, insurance, family, housing, or friends	372	(13)	74	(2)
Don't like needles	300	(10)	52	(2)
Worried name would be reported to government	352	(12)	38	(1)
Didn't have money or insurance	188	(6)	37	(1)
Worried someone would find out about test result	430	(14)	37	(1)
Couldn't get transportation	75	(3)	12	(<1)
Other	528	(18)	341	(11)

Notes: Population = 2,793.
Includes participants who were never tested for HIV or who were not tested during the preceding 12 months.
[a]Participants were asked to indicate whether each reason had contributed to not being tested for HIV. Participants could report more than one reason.
[b]Participants were asked to indicate which reason was the most important. Numbers might not add to total because of missing data.

SOURCE: Travis Sanchez et al., "Table 4. Number and Percentage of Reasons Reported for Participants Not Being Tested for Human Immunodeficiency Virus (HIV) During the Previous 12 Months—United States, National HIV Behavioral Surveillance System: Men Who Have Sex with Men, November 2003–April 2005," in "Human Immunodeficiency Virus (HIV) Risk, Prevention, and Testing Behaviors—United States, National HIV Behavioral Surveillance System: Men Who Have Sex with Men, November 2003–April 2005," *Morbidity and Morality Weekly Report*, vol 55, no. SS-6, July 7, 2006, http://www.cdc.gov/mmwr/PDF/ss/ss5506.pdf (accessed July 10, 2007)

with, partner notification. They also seek to identify potential negative effects of HIV partner notification on clients such as physical, emotional, or sexual abuse or ending of the relationship with the primary partner as a result of participating in partner notification. The researchers find that clients were willing to self-notify partners and participate in provider notification, and few reported negative effects. In terms of preferences, more clients were willing to provide partner information to a physician (64%) or social worker (62%) than to health department personnel (48%) or a member from the gay community (45%). Passin et al. attribute these preferences to a desire to work with familiar and trusted providers as opposed to seeking assistance from unfamiliar sources or providers whom many clients suspect will not maintain strict confidentiality.

The majority (68% to 98%) of health care providers also favored HIV partner notification, but they did not always refer clients to HIV partner notification programs. Passin et al. conclude, "Considering that clients have positive attitudes toward self- and provider referral, local HIV prevention programs need to ensure that all HIV-positive clients are offered partner notification services. Additional research is needed to assess the potential risks of notifying partners and to identify effective techniques to improve client and provider participation."

INTERNET-BASED PARTNER NOTIFICATION. Because research indicates that a substantial number of new HIV cases and STDs are acquired by MSM who meet new sexual partners on the Internet, health professionals wondered if the same medium could be used to convey information to men, such as in e-mails informing them that they had sex with someone infected with an STD and providing links about the STD and where to get tested for it. In "HIV and STD Status among MSM and Attitudes about Internet Partner Notification for STD Exposure" (*Sexually Transmitted Diseases*, vol. 35, no. 2, February 2008), Matthew J. Mimiaga et al. consider the acceptability and perceived utility of Internet-based partner notification of STD exposure for MSM by HIV status. The researchers find broad acceptance—more than 92% of those surveyed—of Internet partner notification by at-risk MSM, independent of HIV status. The MSM interviewed also expressed a willingness to receive or initiate partner notification-related e-mail.

Rapid Testing

In view of the CDC estimate in the fact sheet "New Estimates of U.S. HIV Prevalence, 2006" (October 2008, http://www.cdc.gov/nchhstp/newsroom/docs/prevalence.pdf) that 21% of HIV-positive individuals in the United States are unaware of their infection, researchers and public health professionals continue to seek more and better ways to increase the number of people who are aware of their HIV status. One way to increase access to HIV testing is through rapid testing, which may be readily performed in a variety of settings such as correctional facilities, military battlefield operations, and worksites where occupational exposures may occur.

Several rapid HIV antibody tests have been approved by the U.S. Food and Drug Administration (FDA) for use in the United States. Table 2.5 in Chapter 2 lists the FDA-approved rapid HIV screening tests and provides their features and prices. The tests contain test strips with HIV antigens. If the blood or sputum they come in contact with contains HIV antibodies, then the antibodies bind to the antigens and a reagent in the test kit creates a color change. The tests are interpreted visually and, like conventional HIV enzyme immunoassays, they are screening tests that require additional testing by a Western blot or immunofluorescent assay to confirm a positive response.

Because rapid HIV testing informs clients with reactive test results that it is highly likely that they are HIV positive, compared with receiving no test result information at the conclusion of a visit where a conventional HIV test specimen is drawn, it is vitally important for health care workers to explain the meaning of preliminary positive results. Counseling for patients who receive rapid HIV testing is somewhat different from conventional testing and involves determining how prepared clients are to receive test results in the same session.

As of 2009, the sale of rapid HIV tests was restricted to clinical laboratories where workers who administer the tests have reviewed and use the instructional materials provided with the tests. The FDA also requires that people tested with the rapid tests receive the informative pamphlet provided with the test.

Home Testing

Home HIV tests were developed in the mid-1980s but were opposed by the FDA and some HIV/AIDS organizations and health care agencies. The FDA was concerned about telephone counseling for those who tested positive, the accuracy of the tests, and confidentiality. In 1996 the FDA reversed its position, deciding that despite its limitations, the benefits of home testing outweigh the risks.

Public health officials explain that many people are afraid of obtaining testing at a physician's office or public clinic because of the associated stigma. Some drug companies suggest that an HIV-antibody test that can be performed at home may be the only way some of these people will learn their HIV status, and argue that more people will then enter treatment and take precautions to prevent spreading the infection.

Some home tests use saliva, which does not require a needle stick, and others use blood samples. When blood is tested, the patient draws a few drops of blood from a fingertip, places it on filter paper, and mails the paper to a company laboratory, which performs the standard HIV assay. If the results are positive, a confirmation test is performed. An HIV test kit called the Home Access Express HIV-1 Test System, manufactured by Home Access Health Corporation, which was approved by the FDA in 1996, was the only HIV home test kit approved by the agency as of 2009. Seven days (or sooner if express service is requested) after Home Access Health receives the test kit, results and counseling are available by calling a 24-hour toll-free number and giving an identification code. Home Access claims an accuracy rate of 99.9%.

Critics of home testing say that news of HIV infection is not as easy to accept as the results of other in-home tests, such as those for pregnancy and cholesterol. They claim that most people cannot properly prepare themselves for the news that they have a life-threatening disease. They advocate the expansion of current testing sites to include mobile vans, sports clubs, and other places that are not exclusively associated with HIV testing, but where in-person counseling could be provided.

Military Practices

The U.S. Department of Defense (DOD) regularly screens all members of the armed services as well as those seeking to join for HIV. The DOD (October 17, 2006, http://www.dtic.mil/whs/directives/corres/rtf/648501x.rtf) policy is to "deny eligibility for military service to individuals with serologic evidence of HIV infection for appointment, enlistment, pre-appointment, or initial entry training for military service." Biannual HIV testing is required of all personnel on active duty, as well as of all members of the reserves and National Guard. In 1995, after two months of debate in Congress, federal legislators scrapped a discharge provision that would have forced the DOD to dismiss members of the military within 6 months of testing positive for HIV. Along with HIV infection, a number of chronic conditions, including cancer, asthma, diabetes, heart disease, or complications of pregnancy, place troops on limited assignment, precluding them from overseas service or combat.

In "DoD Standardizes HIV Test Interval across All Services" (American Forces Press Service, May 21, 2004), Gerry J. Gilmore reports that the HIV infection rate across the military is about two out of every 10,000 service members, which is comparable to or lower than the rate for the U.S. civilian population of the same age. Military personnel serving outside the continental United States who are confirmed as HIV infected are reassigned to the continental United States as quickly as possible. Selected branches of the military, such as the U.S. Army Special Operations Command and Ranger organizations, are completely closed to people infected with HIV.

Pregnant Women and Newborns

The issue of testing newborns has placed the rights of mothers at odds with those of their newborns. States have kept HIV test results anonymous to preserve a mother's right to privacy. Civil libertarians and some groups that represent women, gays, and lesbians support anonymous testing, claiming that attaching names to test results would start local, state, and federal governments down the "slippery slope" of mandatory testing of adults. They also raise further privacy concerns, contending that once names are known, there is no guarantee they will not fall into the hands of employers, insurance companies, and others who might discriminate on the basis of HIV status.

On the contrary, proponents of disclosure claim newborns who test HIV positive could be denied adequate medical care because their parents are unaware of their status. M. Blake Caldwell et al. of the CDC explain in "1994 Revised Classification System for Human Immunodeficiency Virus Infection in Children Less Than 13 Years of Age" (*Morbidity and Mortality Weekly Report*, vol. 43, RR-12, September 30, 1994) that 15% to 30% of the babies who test positive for HIV immediately after birth actually develop the disease. However, if their mothers breastfeed, some may contract the infection from their mother's breast milk.

In May 1996 the U.S. House of Representatives and the U.S. Senate passed bills that would cut off federal money for HIV/AIDS treatment to states that failed to comply with the new disclosure requirements. President Bill Clinton (1946–) signed the Ryan White Comprehensive AIDS Resources Emergency Act Amendments requiring mandatory testing of newborns if too few pregnant women agreed to voluntary testing. In June 1996 New York became the first state to mandate that health officials tell parents the results of HIV tests that the state routinely performs on all newborns. Before June 1996 parents in New York did not receive results unless they requested them, as was still the case in many states in 2009.

NEW JERSEY LEGISLATION MANDATES TESTING OF PREGNANT WOMEN AND SOME NEWBORNS. In June 2007 New Jersey lawmakers approved a bill requiring pregnant women and some newborns—infants born to mothers who have tested positive or those whose HIV status is unknown at the time of birth—to be tested for HIV. The law requires that pregnant women be tested twice for HIV, once early and once late in the pregnancy, unless the mother specifically requests not to be tested.

Supporters of this legislation contend that the requirement for testing will save children's lives. Detractors argue that all infants of HIV-infected mothers test positive for HIV antibodies because they inherit their mother's antibodies. This initial positive result does not necessarily mean the infant is infected. Because it takes several months for the mother's antibodies to clear from the infant, it may be more prudent to test infants when they are between three and six months old to determine their HIV status. According to the Kaiser Family Foundation, in "New Jersey Legislature Approves Bill Requiring Pregnant Women, Some Infants to Receive HIV Tests" (June 25, 2007, http://www.kaisernetwork.org/daily_reports/rep _index.cfm?hint=1&DR_ID=45784), the American Civil Liberties Union and women's health advocacy groups assert that the legislation "deprives women of authority to make medical decisions."

Even though the CDC recommends routine opt-out HIV screening of all pregnant women and newborn testing if the mother's HIV status is unknown, state policies vary. The Kaiser Family Foundation reports in "United States: HIV Testing for Mothers and Newborns" (February 2008, http://www.statehealthfacts.kff.org/profileind.jsp?rgn=1& cat=11&ind=563) that as of February 2008, 22 states had opt-out testing of pregnant women. Opt-out HIV testing is part of routine prenatal care and pregnant women are tested unless they refuse or "opt-out." Thirty states have opt-in HIV testing of pregnant women—an HIV test is not part of routine prenatal care and pregnant women must

specifically request or "opt-in" to receive an HIV test. Ten states require newborn testing when the mother's HIV status is unknown or test results are not available; some states allow parents to refuse the test on religious grounds.

Health Care Workers

There has been a continuing debate over whether health care workers, who, many believe, have an obligation to inform their patients about their own HIV status, should be required to obtain HIV tests. As of 2009, there was no law requiring health care workers to submit to HIV testing, although many employers require it as a condition of employment. They cannot, however, discriminate against health care workers on the basis of their HIV status because like other employees, they are covered by the Americans with Disabilities Act of 1990, the federal law that prohibits discrimination against individuals with disabilities.

According to the CDC, in "Are Health Care Workers at Risk of Getting HIV on the Job?" (January 22, 2007, http:// www.cdc.gov/hiv/resources/qa/qa28.htm), the risk of health care workers becoming infected with HIV on the job is low, especially if they follow prudent safety measures known as universal precautions, which include the use of gloves, goggles, and masks to prevent HIV and other bloodborne infections. The largest risk is posed by accidental needle-stick injuries, but even this risk is less than 1%.

Furthermore, Mitchell J. Schwaber reports in "Investigation of Patients Treated by an HIV-Infected Cardiothoracic Surgeon—Israel, 2007" (*Morbidity and Mortality Weekly Report*, vol. 57, no. 53, January 9, 2009) about an investigation of HIV transmission from a heart surgeon to the surgeon's patients, which found no transmission from the infected surgeon to patients. Schwaber confirms that HIV transmission from health care worker to patient is rare. Reports such as this support the premise that when universal precautions are taken, HIV-infected health care workers pose negligible risk to their patients, especially when they are being treated, because blood infectivity of HIV carriers has been shown to vary as a function of viral load, which can now be reduced to undetectable levels using antiretrovirals.

Testing Policies in U.S. Prisons

Guidelines for the testing of inmates for HIV exist in all 50 states, in the District of Columbia, and in the regulations of the Federal Bureau of Prisons. However, the timing of testing varies. The CDC finds in *HIV Testing Implementation Guidance for Correctional Settings* (January 2009, http://www.cdc.gov/hiv/topics/testing/resources/ guidelines/correctional-settings/pdf/Correctional_Settings _Guidelines.pdf) that in 2006 less than half of the state prison systems and few jails routinely provided prisoners with HIV testing on entry, while in custody, or before release. Federal prisons and 45 states tested inmates if they had HIV-related symptoms, and the federal system and 43 states tested inmates on request. Just 16 states and the federal system tested inmates who were considered to belong to high-risk populations.

The CDC recommends universal opt-out HIV screening in correctional facilities. It states that "voluntary HIV testing is as cost-effective as other screening programs in health care settings in which HIV prevalence is as low as 0.1%. Since many incarcerated populations have a prevalence of diagnosed HIV infection >1%, HIV screening in prisons and jails is a highly cost-effective public health strategy." The CDC acknowledges that some systems face logistical, security, and financial constraints that require alternative options. For these types of situations, the CDC advises several alternative approaches including risk-based screening that routinely offers HIV screening to inmates with HIV risk characteristics such as IDUs, MSM, or inmates diagnosed with another STD.

PREVENTION
Critics Fault Programs' Focus and Funding

The objective of HIV prevention programs is to reduce the number of new cases to as close to zero as possible. All prevention efforts are based on the belief that individuals can be educated in a way that will lead to changes in behavior, which will help bring an end to the spread of HIV/AIDS. However, many AIDS advocacy groups have long been critical of the ways the CDC has communicated this message. In 1987 CDC officials chose to emphasize the universality of AIDS, instead of focusing efforts on those most at risk: MSM and IDUs. According to AIDS advocates, this strategy misdirected the spending of available prevention dollars during the first decade of the epidemic. In 2009, even though the number of infected people outside of these two groups was growing, HIV/AIDS was still largely a threat to MSM, IDUs, their partners, and their children. Most women with HIV/AIDS were IDUs or were sex partners of IDUs.

Steve Sternberg reports in "Obama Administration Putting AIDS 'Back on the Nation's Radar'" (*USA Today*, April 7, 2009) that in April 2009 President Barack Obama (1961–) launched a government-sponsored public health education initiative that will spend $45 million over five years on media messages aimed at reinvigorating interest in, and enthusiasm for HIV/AIDS prevention and testing. The program' focus is the statistic that every 9 and 1/2 minutes someone in the United States is infected with HIV. The campaign will primarily target African-Americans and Latinos, because these communities have an increased risk for HIV/AIDS.

President Obama's (June 27, 2009, http://www.white house.gov/blog/gettested/) commitment to HIV/AIDS awareness and education is longstanding. During a trip to Kenya in August 2006, when he was a senator, he and his wife, Michelle (1964–), had themselves tested for HIV to underscore the importance of getting tested.

CDC Prevention Activities

The CDC's HIV prevention strategy, as described in *Advancing HIV Prevention: New Strategies for a Changing Epidemic* (March 7, 2007, http://www.cdc.gov/hiv/topics/prev_prog/AHP/default.htm), aims to reduce the incidence and prevalence of HIV infection as well as the morbidity (illnesses) and mortality (deaths) that result from HIV infection by working with communities and other partners. The agency's efforts focus on four areas:

- Incorporating HIV testing as a routine part of care in traditional medical settings.

- Implementing new models for diagnosing HIV infection outside medical settings.

- Preventing new infections by working with people diagnosed with HIV and their partners.

- Screening and treating expectant mothers to further decrease mother-to-child HIV transmission.

The prevention strategy capitalizes on new rapid test technologies, interventions that bring people unaware of their HIV status to HIV testing, and behavioral interventions that provide prevention skills to people living with HIV. To carry out its strategy, the CDC works in conjunction with governmental and nongovernmental partners to implement, evaluate, and further develop and strengthen effective HIV prevention efforts nationwide. Along with direct programs and service, the CDC provides financial and technical support for:

- Disease surveillance

- HIV antibody counseling, testing, and referral services

- Street and community outreach

- Risk-reduction counseling

- Prevention case management

- Prevention and treatment of other STDs

- Public information and education

- School-based AIDS education

- International research studies

- Technology transfer systems

- Organizational capacity building

- Program-relevant epidemiological, sociobehavioral, and evaluation research

Figure 8.1 shows how the CDC prevention strategy targets distinct populations—people at risk and people living with HIV—and works in concert to create a comprehensive HIV prevention initiative.

FIGURE 8.1

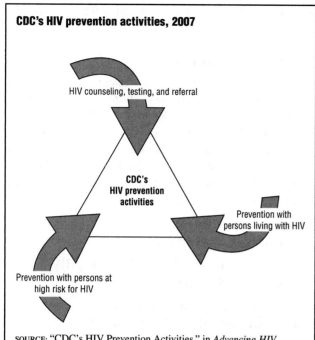

CDC's HIV prevention activities, 2007

CDC's HIV prevention activities

HIV counseling, testing, and referral

Prevention with persons living with HIV

Prevention with persons at high risk for HIV

SOURCE: "CDC's HIV Prevention Activities," in *Advancing HIV Prevention: New Strategies for a Changing Epidemic*, Centers for Disease control and Prevention, Divisions of HIV/AIDS Prevention, March 7, 2007, http://www.cdc.gov/hiv/topics/prev_prog/AHP/resources/brochures/AHP_Brochure.htm (accessed July 6, 2009)

CDC health education and disease prevention efforts continue to emphasize that the most reliable ways to avoid HIV infection or transmitting the virus are by abstaining from sexual intercourse, maintaining a mutually monogamous, long-term relationship with a partner who is uninfected, and/or to refrain from sharing needles and syringes in drug use. Even though seemingly logical, critics contend that the emphasis of the CDC, and of the administration of President George W. Bush (1946–) in particular, on abstinence burdens people with an unrealistic expectation. Critics also point to the insistence on abstinence policies as a condition of U.S. government assistance for other countries' health programs to be an ill-advised foreign policy intrusion.

The CDC states in *Comprehensive HIV Prevention: Essential Components of a Comprehensive Strategy to Prevent Domestic HIV, 2006* (April 2006, http://www.cdc.gov/hiv/resources/reports/comp_hiv_prev/pdf/comp_hiv_prev.pdf) that the HIV prevention strategy has as its overarching goal to "reduce the number of new HIV infections in the U.S. from an estimated 40,000 to 20,000 per year, focusing particularly on eliminating racial and ethnic disparities in new HIV infections." The agency explains that this goal can be achieved by:

- Decreasing the number of people who are at high risk for acquiring or transmitting HIV infection.

- Increasing the number of HIV-infected people who are aware that they are infected.

- Increasing the number of HIV-infected people who have access to prevention services and appropriate care and treatment.

- Improving the ability to monitor the epidemic nationwide, to develop and implement effective HIV prevention interventions, and to evaluate prevention programs.

According to the Kaiser Family Foundation, in the fact sheet "U.S. Federal Funding for HIV/AIDS: The President's FY 2010 Budget Request" (May 2009, http://www.kff.org/hivaids/upload/7029-05.pdf), for fiscal year 2010 the CDC was allocated $950 million for domestic HIV/AIDS prevention activities conducted by the National Center for HIV, STD, and TB Prevention. The total allocation to the CDC for prevention represented a $53 million increase over fiscal year 2009. The increase would be used to fund HIV testing and surveillance and prevention programs targeting at-risk populations.

EDUCATING YOUTH

In "Basic Statistics" (February 26, 2009, http://www.cdc.gov/hiv/topics/surveillance/basic.htm), the CDC estimates that in 2007, 10,678 new cases of HIV/AIDS were reported for people between the ages of 20 and 29. With an average incubation period of 10 years, it is likely that most of these young people were infected while they were teenagers. Because some people begin having sexual relationships and using intravenous drugs at earlier ages, many health officials fear the number of HIV-positive young people will grow.

Most states offer prevention programs for students in public schools. However, youths who are not in school may not have ready access to such programs. Many homeless shelters and local health departments employ roving counselors who seek out these young people to offer prevention information and direct them to health and social service agencies.

Sexual Health Education

Many education programs offer students sufficient information about STDs and HIV/AIDS, but only high-quality education affects behavior. In *Impact of HIV and Sexual Health Education on the Sexual Behavior of Young People: A Review Update* (1997, http://data.unaids.org/Publications/IRC-pub01/JC010-ImpactYoungPeople_en.pdf), the Joint United Nations Program on HIV/AIDS (UNAIDS) concludes that effective sexual education programs should include:

- Focused curricula, clear statements about behavioral goals, a clear picture of the risks of unprotected sex, and ways to avoid it.

- Teaching and practicing communication and negotiation skills.

- Openness in communicating about sex.

- Theories stressing the social nature of learning.

The review's conclusions were still relevant and controversial in 2009. Some people did not agree that information about sexual health or decisions should be offered in public schools, preferring that parents instill their own values in their children. However, others pointed out that some parents never talk to their children about sex and drugs and that school may be the only place a child can get reliable information. According to the Guttmacher Institute, in "Sex and STI/HIV Education" (*State Policies in Brief*, September 1, 2009), 35 states and the District of Columbia required HIV/AIDS prevention education in 2009. Three states—Arizona, Nevada, and Utah—required parental consent for students to receive HIV education. Even though laws vary from state to state, and some allow local school districts to decide on curricula, many of these states have one or more mandates determining the material that may be taught in the programs. The mandates range from requiring age-appropriate materials, to teaching comprehensive sex education programs (advocating contraceptive and condom use), to providing programs in which abstinence from premarital sex is presented as the only 100% effective means of preventing HIV/AIDS.

Federal funding for abstinence-only educational programs was initiated in 1998. Proponents of these programs claim they change attitudes about casual sex, reducing both teen pregnancies and rates of STDs. They also maintain that teaching students about contraceptive and condom use condones, or even encourages, unsafe sexual behavior. Critics of these programs argue that there is no reliable evidence that abstinence-only programs are effective. In addition, they contend that for the five out of 10 teens aged 15 to 19 who do choose to have sex, lack of knowledge about contraception and condom use will only result in continued teen pregnancies, STDs, and HIV infections.

The U.S. Department of Health and Human Services concludes in *Review of Comprehensive Sex Education Curricula* (May 2007, http://www.acf.hhs.gov/programs/fysb/content/docs/comprehensive.pdf) that abstinence-only education is ineffective. The review finds that students given abstinence-only education were no more likely to abstain from sex, that those who had sex did so with a similar number of partners as those who had not received abstinence-only education, and that students first had sex at the same age, independent of the type of education they had received.

In his 2010 budget, President Barack Obama (1961–) eliminated federal funding for abstinence-only education. Sharon Jayson reports in "Obama Budget Cuts Funds for Abstinence-Only Sex Education" (*USA Today*, May 11, 2009) that the 2010 budget "proposes almost $178 million for teen pregnancy prevention, including $110 million for

community-based programs. About 75% of that is for programs proven to have delayed sex and increased contraceptive use or reduced teen pregnancy. The other 25% could be for 'innovative' programs."

CONDOM USE

In June 2000 a workshop organized by the National Institutes of Health in collaboration with the CDC, the FDA, and the U.S. Agency for International Development evaluated published evidence on the effectiveness of latex male condoms in preventing STDs, including HIV. In the fact sheet "Male Latex Condoms and Sexually Transmitted Diseases" (January 23, 2003, http://www.cdc.gov/condom effectiveness/condoms.pdf), the CDC indicates that studies provide compelling evidence that latex condoms are highly effective in protecting against HIV infection when used properly for every act of intercourse. However, the agency warns that "no protective method is 100 percent effective, and condom use cannot guarantee absolute protection against any STD. Furthermore, condoms lubricated with spermicides are no more effective than other lubricated condoms in protecting against the transmission of HIV and other STDs."

Even though latex condom use is still considered a highly effective method of preventing the transmission of HIV and other STDs, the CDC concludes that abstinence or a mutually monogamous, long-term relationship with an uninfected partner is the "surest way to avoid transmission of sexually transmitted diseases."

The CDC analysis of data from Youth Risk Behavior Surveys conducted from 1991 to 2007 finds that U.S. high school students are engaging in fewer HIV-related risk behaviors—decreasing percentages of students reported being sexually active and having had sexual intercourse with four or more people in their life. Condom use increased from 1991 to 2003, but since then has leveled off. Condom use among sexually active students rose from 46.2% in 1991 to 61.5% in 2007. (See Table 5.8 in Chapter 5.).

Other Forms of Protection

In 1993 the FDA approved Reality, a female condom that serves as a mechanical barrier to viruses. The condom is designed for women to protect themselves from STDs, including HIV. It is made of polyurethane (a resin made of two different compounds used in elastic fibers, cushions, and various molded products) and is unlikely to rip or tear. The condom is prelubricated and is intended for use during only one sex act.

The use of female condoms is low. Rebecca Bowers cites in "Status Report on the Female Condom: What Will Increase Use in the U.S.?" (*AIDS Alert*, vol. 23, no. 3, March 2008) the findings of a New York State study—that 69% of women had heard about female condoms but just

2.6% had used one. Bowers describes the development of a new generation of female condoms, which because they may be more comfortable and easier to use, may be better accepted and more widely used. She observes that there is still no commercially available product other than the female condom that women can use to protect themselves from HIV/AIDS.

CIRCUMCISION MAY SLOW THE SPREAD OF HIV

According to the press release "WHO and UNAIDS Announce Recommendations from Expert Consultation on Male Circumcision for HIV Prevention" (March 28, 2007, http://www.who.int/hiv/mediacentre/news68/en/index.html), in 2007 the World Health Organization (WHO) and UNAIDS recommended circumcision as a strategy to prevent heterosexually acquired HIV infection in men. Circumcision, the surgical removal of the foreskin from the penis, has long been thought to reduce men's susceptibility to HIV infection because the skin cells in the foreskin are especially vulnerable to the virus. Kevin De Cock, the director of the WHO HIV/AIDS Department, asserts that "countries with high rates of heterosexual HIV infection and low rates of male circumcision now have an additional intervention which can reduce the risk of HIV infection in heterosexual men. Scaling up male circumcision in such countries will result in immediate benefit to individuals. However, it will be a number of years before we can expect to see an impact on the epidemic from such investment."

According to Meraiah Foley, in "Circumcision Urged in Curbing AIDS Spread" (Associated Press, July 24, 2007), Robert Bailey of the University of Illinois urges government endorsement of circumcision to slow the spread of HIV. Exhorting international agencies to increase funding for circumcision in countries hardest hit by the epidemic, Bailey contends that "circumcision could drive the epidemic to a declining state toward extinction. We must make safe, affordable, voluntary circumcision available now."

Research conducted in Kenya, South Africa, and Uganda demonstrates that circumcision reduces HIV incidence. In "Can Routine Neonatal Circumcision Help Prevent Human Immunodeficiency Virus Transmission in the United States?" (*American Journal of Men's Health*, January 2009), Xiao Xu et al. of the University of Michigan question whether it would be beneficial to implement routine circumcision of newborn males in the United States for HIV prevention. More than half of male newborns in the United States are circumcised at birth. Xu et al. call for "comprehensive cost-effectiveness analysis considering the various elements of HIV transmission in the context of the United States" to determine potential cost, benefit, and risks of recommending universal circumcision as an HIV prevention strategy.

IMPROVING PREVENTION SERVICES

Cynthia M. Lyles et al. of the CDC discuss in "Best-Evidence Interventions: Findings from a Systematic Review of HIV Behavioral Interventions for US Populations at High Risk, 2000–2004" (*American Journal of Public Health*, vol. 97, no. 1, January 2007) the results of a CDC evaluation of behavioral intervention programs to reduce HIV risk. The researchers considered approximately 100 interventions in an effort to identify "best practices" and "best evidence" of efficacy in reducing HIV-related risk behaviors, STDs, or IIIV incidence.

Lyles et al. identify 18 behavioral interventions as demonstrating the best evidence of efficacy. These interventions were based on behavioral change theories or models, most often social cognitive theory or social learning theory. These theories posit that human behavior is the product of a dynamic interplay of personal, behavioral, and environmental influences. They use a variety of strategies and approaches to change behaviors, including providing consequences, in the form of rewards or punishments for specific behaviors, and learning by observation of others. Social cognitive theory proposes that people are most likely to model the behaviors of someone with whom they strongly identify. Both theories have been used successfully to help people develop new health-supporting skills.

Even though the content of the effective interventions varied, all included learning and practicing skills such as condom use and relaxation techniques as well as interpersonal, communication, and decision-making skills. Most of the effective interventions targeted populations disproportionately affected by the HIV/AIDS epidemic and in urgent need of effective prevention programs. Some best-evidence interventions focused on African-American or Hispanic heterosexual women at risk for HIV infection and two targeted African-American youths at high risk. Others aimed to prevent infection in minority drug users and one focused on female IDUs. Still other best-evidence interventions served people living with HIV. Table 8.4 lists the 37 best-evidence interventions—the programs considered to provide the strongest scientific evidence of efficacy—identified through May 2009 and the target populations they aim to serve.

SYRINGE EXCHANGE PROGRAMS

IDUs often share the syringes they use to inject drugs into their body. When an HIV-positive IDU uses a syringe, he or she may contaminate it with HIV-positive blood that can then spread the disease to other IDUs who use that syringe. Syringe exchange programs (SEPs) attempt to prevent the spread of HIV in this manner by encouraging IDUs to bring in their used, unsafe syringes and exchange them for new, safe syringes. The reasoning behind these programs is that if people are going to use drugs, at least

TABLE 8.4

Best-evidence HIV prevention programs, 2009

Program	Risk category	Sex	Race	Interventional level
BART	HR youth	28% M, 72% F	100% AA	GLI
Be Proud! Be Responsible!	HR youth	100% M	100% AA	GLI
Brief Group Counseling	MSM	100% M	100% API	GLI
CHOICES	HS adult	100% F	54% W, 29% AA, 5% AI, 3% H, 3% API, 6% O	GLI
CLEAR (in person)	HIV+, HR youth, DU	78% M, 22% F	42% H, 26% AA, 23% W, 8% O	ILI
Communal Effectance-AIDS Prevention	HS adult	100% F	55% AA, 42% W, 3% O	GLI
Connect	HS adult	50% M, 50% F	55% AA, 39% H, 6% O	ILI, GLI
¡Cuídate!	HR youth	45% M, 55% F	100% H	GLI
EXPLORE	MSM	100% M	72% W, 15% H, 7% AA, 6% O	ILI
Female- & Culturally-Specific Negotiation	HS adult, DU	100% F	100% AA	ILI
Focus on the Future	HS adult	100% M	100% AA	ILI
FOY + ImPACT	HR youth	42% M, 58% F	100% AA	GLI
Healthy Living Project	HIV+	79% M, 21% F	45% AA, 32% W, 15% H, 8% O	ILI
Healthy Relationships	HIV+	70% M, 29% F, 1% transgender	74% AA, 22% W, 4% O	GLI
Health Improvement Project	HS adult	45% M, 54% F	67% W, 21% AA, 12% O	GLI
LIFT	HIV+ w/ CSA	47% M, 53% F	68% AA, 17% H, 10% W, 5% O	GLI
"light"	HS adult	42% M, 58% F	74% AA, 25% H, 1% O	GLI
Modelo de Intervención Psicomédica	DU	89% M, 11% F	100% H	ILI
Personalized Cognitive Risk-Reduction Counseling	MSM	100% M	74% W, 11% H, 6% API, 3% AA, 6% O	ILI
Positive Choice: Interactive Video Doctor	HIV+	79% M, 21% F	50% AA, 29% W, 13% H, 8%, O	ILI
Project FIO (8 session)	HS adult	100% F	73% AA, 17% H, 10% W, 0.3% API	GLI
Project S.A.F.E. (Standard Version)	HS adult	100% F	77% H, 23% AA	ILI, GLI
Project START	HS adult	100% Male	52% AA, 23% W, 14% H, 12% O	ILI
RESPECT				
Brief Counseling (Best Evidence)				
Enhanced Counseling (Promising Evidence)	HS adult	57% M, 43% F	59% AA, 19% H, 16% W, 6% O	ILI
RESPECT Brief Counseling + Booster	HS adult	54% M, 46% F	51% AA, 22% W, 18% H, 9% O	ILI
Safe in the City	HS adult	70% M, 30% F	46% W, 25% H, 18% AA, 11% O	ILI
SHIELD	DU	61% M, 39% F	94% AA, 6% O	GLI
SiHLE	HR youth	100% F	100% AA	GLI
Sisters Saving Sisters	HR youth	100% F	68% AA, 32% H	GLI
Sister-to-Sister: Group Skills-building	HS adult	100% F	100% AA	GLI
Sister-to-Sister: One-on-one Skills-building	HS adult	100% F	100% AA	ILI
STRIVE	HCV+, DU	76% M, 24% F	57% W, 27% H, 7% AA, 10% O	GLI
SUMIT Enhanced Peer-led	HIV+, MSM	100% M	51% W, 23% AA, 17% H, 1% API, 1% AI, 7% O	GLI
VOICES/VOCES	HS adult	60% M, 40% F	62% AA, 38% H	GLI
WiLLOW	HIV+, HS adult	100% F	84% AA, 15% W, 1% O	GLI
Women's Co-Op	HS adult, DU	100% F	100% AA	ILI, GLI
Women's Health Promotion	HS adult	100% F	*Race:* 100% H	GLI

Key: HS = Heterosexual; HIV+ = HIV-positive; HCV+ = Hepatitis C-positive; HR = High-risk; MSM = Men who have sex with men; DU = Drug users; CSA = Childhood sexual abuse; M = Male; F = Female; T = Transgender; W = White; AA = African American; AI = American Indian; H = Hispanic; API = Asian/Pacific Islander; O = Other racial/ethnic group; GLI = group-level intervention; ILI = individual-level intervention; CLI = community-level intervention.

SOURCE: Adapted from "Complete List of All Best-Evidence Interventions," in *2008 Compendium of Evidence-Based HIV Prevention Interventions: Best-Evidence Interventions*, Centers for Disease Control and Prevention, Divisions of HIV/AIDS Prevention, May 7, 2009, http://www.cdc.gov/hiv/topics/research/prs/best-evidence-intervention.htm#completelist (accessed July 6, 2009)

an effort can be made to make sure they do not contract HIV because of it. Proponents of these programs point out that the spread of HIV among IDUs threatens everyone, as people who contract HIV through drug use can then pass it on to their sexual partners and children.

Despite these arguments, SEPs are highly controversial due to their connection to drug use. Some see them as helping IDUs avoid the consequences of their actions, or even providing them with the means to continue their illegal activities. In April 1998, after much debate, the Clinton administration decided not to lift a nine-year-old ban on federal financing for programs to distribute clean needles to drug addicts. This meant that state and local governments that received federal block grants for HIV/AIDS prevention were not permitted to use this money for SEPs. Public health experts and advocates for people

with HIV/AIDS criticized the decision. Later in 1998 Congress considered even more restrictive legislation that would ban indirect federal funding (such as funding for counseling, medical care, or funds dispersed by city or state) to needle exchange agencies. Regardless, in 2000 five U.S. health groups (including the AMA and the American Pharmaceutical Association) spoke out in favor of SEPs and advised state leaders to coordinate efforts to make clean needles easily available to IDUs.

In "Syringe Exchange Programs—United States, 2005" (*Morbidity and Mortality Weekly Report*, vol. 56, no. 44, November 9, 2007), the CDC summarizes a survey of U.S. SEP activities. The survey was conducted in March 2006 by the Beth Israel Medical Center (BIMC) in New York City, with the North American Syringe Exchange Network (NASEN). Questionnaires were mailed to the directors of all

166 SEPs in the United States that were members of NASEN. (Previous surveys contacted 68 SEPs between 1994 and 1995, 101 in 1996, 113 in 1997, 131 in 1998, 154 in 2000, 148 for 2002, and 174 in 2004.) The BIMC contacted SEP directors and conducted telephone interviews based on the questionnaires. The directors responded to questions about the number of syringes exchanged in 2005 through program operations and services.

Of the 166 SEPs, 118 (71%) participated in the survey. SEPs operated in 91 cities in 28 states/territories and the District of Columbia. A majority of the SEPs were located in six states: California (22), New Mexico (17), Washington (15), Wisconsin (10), New York (9), and Connecticut (6).

In 2005, 117 SEPs exchanged 22.5 million syringes (one SEP did not track the number of syringes it exchanged). The 12 largest SEPs (those that traded 500,000 or more syringes) exchanged approximately 11.9 million (53% of all replaced syringes).

Besides exchanged syringes, most SEPs provided other public health and social services. Nearly all SEPs provided alcohol pads (99%), male condoms (97%), and referrals to substance-abuse treatment 102 (86%). Other onsite health care services provided by some SEPs included counseling and testing for HIV (81%) and hepatitis C (56%). Thirty-four (29%) SEPs offered other onsite medical care. Table 8.5 lists the kinds of prevention, screening, medical care, referral, and education services offered by the SEPs.

Helping IDUs Saves Lives

Scott Burris of Temple University observes in "Overview of Syringe Access Interventions" (January 2009, http://saprp.org/knowledgeassets/knowledge_detail.cfm?KAID=15) that because IDU with unsterile needles and syringes remains a major source of HIV infection in the United States, accounting for approximately one-third of AIDS cases, "the US Public Health Service deems one-time-only use of sterile syringes to be essential to reducing rates of transmission among injection drug users (IDUs)." Burris also notes that "despite substantial evidence that expanded syringe access benefits public health without causing other harms, state laws on syringe distribution and possession, law enforcement practices, and actions by the US Congress that limit federal funding for SEPs may be inhibiting the potential of syringe access programs to prevent HIV."

According to the National Institute on Drug Abuse (NIDA), in *Principles of HIV Prevention in Drug-Using Populations* (March 2002, http://drugabuse.gov/PDF/POHP.pdf), until there is an effective vaccine or a cure for AIDS, comprehensive HIV prevention strategies are the most cost-effective and reliable approaches for preventing new HIV infections in IDUs. The NIDA explains that

TABLE 8.5

Supplies and services provided by syringe-exchange programs, 2005

Supplies and services	No.	(%)
Prevention supplies		
Male condoms	115	(97)
Female condoms	98	(83)
Alcohol pads	117	(99)
Bleach	82	(69)
On-site medical screenings and services		
HIV counseling and testing	96	(81)
Hepatitis C counseling and testing	66	(56)
Hepatitis B counseling and testing	44	(37)
Hepatitis A counseling and testing	28	(24)
Hepatitis B vaccination	46	(39)
Hepatitis A vaccination	43	(37)
Sexually transmitted disease (STD) screening	57	(49)
Tuberculosis screening	33	(28)
On-site medical care	34	(29)
Referrals		
Substance-abuse treatment	102	(86)
Education		
HIV/AIDS prevention	116	(98)
Hepatitis A, B, and C prevention	114	(97)
Safer injection practice	113	(96)
Vein care	110	(93)
STD prevention	110	(93)
Abscess prevention	107	(91)
Male condom use	112	(95)
Female condom use	97	(82)

Note: Population = 118

SOURCE: "Table 2. Number and Percentage of Syringe Exchange Programs (SEPs), by Selected Supplies and Services Provided—United States, 2005," in "Syringe Exchange Programs—United States, 2005," *Morbidity and Mortality Weekly Report*, vol. 56, no. 44, November 9, 2007, http://www.cdc.gov/mmwr/preview/mmwrhtml/mm5644a4.htm#top (accessed July 6, 2009)

"comprehensive HIV prevention includes a variety of complementary components—community-based outreach, drug abuse treatment, and sterile syringe access programs—to help drug-using populations increase their protective behaviors and reduce their risks for HIV/AIDS as well as other blood-borne infections."

Furthermore, the CDC asserts in "Update: Syringe Exchange Programs—United States, 2005" that SEPs provide needed access to health and social services to IDUs who would otherwise go unserved. They also safeguard public health by removing syringes that are potentially contaminated with HIV and other bloodborne infections from the community-at-large.

PHYSICIANS SUPPORT ACCESS TO STERILE SYRINGES FOR IDUS. In many states syringe prescription laws effectively block access to sterile syringes for IDUs. Pharmacists may be reluctant to sell syringes to suspected IDUs, and police may take possession of syringes or arrest IDUs who cannot demonstrate a medical need, other than injection drug use of illegal drugs, for the syringes they possess.

These barriers could be eliminated by physician prescription of syringes.

Grace E. Macalino et al. conducted the first national survey of physicians to determine their willingness to prescribe syringes for IDUs and reported the results in "A National Physician Survey on Prescribing Syringes as an HIV Prevention Measure" (*Substance Abuse Treatment, Prevention, and Policy*, vol. 4, no. 1, June 8, 2009). The researchers find that despite the fact that physicians have, in general, never actually prescribed syringes to IDUs, most would consider doing so. Macalino et al. conclude, "The physicians in our study were generally amenable to participating in syringe prescription programs, but physician willingness to act can be supported by better communication of what constitutes evidence-based practice, alleviation of legal concerns, and explicit validation by peers and professional organizations. Requiring substance abuse as a subject in medical training and continuing medical education would also promote better care for IDUs."

Legal Barriers to Federal Funding of SEPs

Despite the preponderance of evidence from myriad sources that SEPs are effective strategies for the prevention of HIV transmission, the federal government, as well as most local and state governments, have not made them legal. They argue that taxpayers should not finance illicit drug use. Since 1988 Congress has passed at least six laws that contain provisions specifically prohibiting or restricting the use of federal funds for SEPs and activities. The Comprehensive Alcohol Abuse, Drug Abuse, and Mental Health Amendments Act of 1988 requires states, as a condition for receiving block grant funds, to agree that funds will not be used "to carry out any program of distributing sterile needles for the hypodermic injection of any illegal drug or bleach for the purpose of cleansing needles for such hypodermic injection."

However, the Community AIDS and Hepatitis Prevention Act (H.R. 179) was introduced in January 2009. The bill aimed to lift the ban on federal funding for SEPs and allow local communities to make their own choices of how to spend federal funds. The bill was referred to the House Energy and Commerce Committee. Even though President Obama expressed support for lifting the ban on federal funding throughout his campaign, as of September 2009, his administration had yet to take action on this issue.

CHAPTER 9
HIV AND AIDS WORLDWIDE

SCOPE OF THE PROBLEM

Few factors have changed global demographics as inalterably as the HIV/AIDS pandemic (worldwide epidemic). According to the Joint United Nations Program on HIV/ AIDS (UNAIDS), in *2008 Report on the Global AIDS Epidemic* (August 2008, http://www.unaids.org/en/Knowle dgeCentre/HIVData/GlobalReport/2008/), an estimated 33 million people were living with HIV in 2007. There were 2.7 million new HIV cases diagnosed and 2 million HIV-related deaths. Sub-Saharan Africa remains the region that has been hardest hit. Even though it has slightly more than 10% of the world's population, 67% of all people living with HIV and 75% of AIDS-related deaths in 2007 occurred in this region.

The HIV/AIDS pandemic is actually many separate epidemics, each with its own distinctive origin and shaped by specific geography and populations. Each epidemic involves different risk behaviors and practices, such as unprotected sex with multiple partners or sharing injection drug equipment. According to UNAIDS, some countries have made tremendous strides in expanding and ensuring access to treatment, but have made little progress in advancing HIV prevention programs, whereas other countries that are now experiencing a reduction in HIV prevalence are not making rapid progress to ensure access to, and availability of, HIV treatment.

UNAIDS indicates that the global percentage of adults living with HIV has leveled off since 2000 and that women continue to account for half of all HIV infections. Outside of sub-Saharan Africa, HIV disproportionately affects injection drug users (IDUs), men who have sex with men (MSM), and sex workers.

To understand the magnitude and consequences of the worldwide AIDS pandemic, the focus should not be on the number of reported AIDS cases, but instead on the number of people infected with HIV (the virus that causes AIDS), most of whom have not yet developed full-blown AIDS.

The HIV incubation period (the interval between the initial HIV infection and the development of AIDS) is estimated to be about seven to 11 years. With an estimated 2.7 million people diagnosed with HIV in 2007 alone, the number of future AIDS cases will continue to increase dramatically.

Global Trends and Projections

Even though public health programs have made impressive progress in eliminating and controlling many infectious diseases, UNAIDS states in *2008 Report on the Global AIDS Epidemic* that HIV/AIDS "remains a global health problem of unprecedented dimensions" and that by 2008 it had already claimed approximately 25 million lives worldwide. This is due to the constantly changing character of the virus and to the complex factors that determine the progression from HIV infection to full-blown AIDS. In addition, medical treatments that can slow the progression of HIV are generally expensive, and as a result have been and continued to be in 2009 inaccessible for many people living in developing countries.

There are, however, some indications that the global HIV pandemic is stabilizing. For example, the total number of new infections had decreased from an estimated 3 million in 2001 to 2.7 million in 2007. According to the Kaiser Family Foundation, in the fact sheet "The Global HIV/ AIDS Epidemic" (April 2009, http://www.kff.org/hivaids/ upload/3030-13.pdf), prevention efforts have effectively reduced HIV prevalence rates in a few countries and the number of people with HIV receiving treatment was 10 times greater in 2007 than it had been in 2002.

In "Projections of Global Mortality and Burden of Disease from 2002 to 2030" (*PLoS Medicine*, vol. 3, no. 11, November 28, 2006), Colin D. Mathers and Dejan Loncar develop three forecasts of future health trends: baseline, optimistic, and pessimistic projections. In the baseline forecast, which assumes that antiretroviral drug use rises to 80% of the population in all regions by 2012, the researchers project that global HIV/AIDS deaths will to rise to 6.5 million in 2030. In the optimistic projection, which assumes heightened prevention activities, there are 3.7 million HIV/AIDS deaths in 2030. In the pessimistic projection, which assumes that antiretroviral therapy will reach 60% by 2012 in all regions except Latin America, where it reaches 70% in 2013, 6.6 million deaths occur in 2030. In the baseline projection, HIV/AIDS is the third leading cause of death worldwide in 2030.

Effect of AIDS on Death Rates

Life expectancy at birth is an important measure for comparing death rates within and between countries over time. UNAIDS indicates in "The AIDS Response: Relationship to Development in Africa" (September 22, 2008, http://www.unaids.org/en/KnowledgeCentre/Resources/Feature Stories/archive/2008/20080922_development_Africa.asp) that in some regions hardest hit by AIDS, such as southern Africa, the number of years one may expect to live has been reduced by more than 20 years, which are comparable to 1950s levels. Other countries now have levels equivalent to those of the early 1990s, and infant survival rates are slipping as well. By contrast, the comparatively smaller HIV pandemic in western Europe has had practically no effect on life expectancy.

Because it occurred a little later than many other HIV epidemics, South Africa's epidemic peaked later than other parts of sub-Saharan Africa, but it has now stabilized. In *2008 Report on the Global AIDS Epidemic*, UNAIDS states that South Africa is still the largest epidemic in the world with an estimated 5.7 million people living with HIV. Furthermore, deaths from all causes in South Africa rose by 87% from 1997 to 2005. Death rates for women aged 20 to 39 years tripled between 1997 and 2005, and for men aged 30 to 44 they more than doubled during the same period, with at least 40% of deaths considered attributable to HIV.

Because HIV/AIDS epidemics differ considerably from country to country, most current mortality estimates, especially in developing countries, do not accurately reflect the impact of AIDS-related mortality. The HIV/AIDS pandemic continues to change the course of demographic events in developing countries, where the impact has been particularly severe. For example, HIV infection has compromised fertility, and in some areas the population growth rate is lower than it would have been without the epidemic.

PATTERNS OF INFECTION

Globally, HIV/AIDS is primarily a sexually transmitted disease (STD) that is transmitted through unprotected sexual intercourse between men and women or MSM. Like some other STDs, HIV infection can also be spread through

blood, blood products, donated organs, semen, or vaginal fluids and perinatally from a pregnant mother to her unborn child. The majority of worldwide cumulative (over the entire time that statistics have been kept) HIV infections in adults are estimated to have been transmitted through heterosexual intercourse, although the relative proportion of infections resulting from heterosexual contact as opposed to MSM varies greatly in different parts of the world.

More than 90% of children with HIV acquired the virus during pregnancy, birth, or via breastfeeding. The balance were infected by contaminated injections, transfusion with infected blood, sexual abuse, or sexual intercourse.

HIV-1 and HIV-2

Francine E. McCutchan of the U.S. Military HIV Research Program in Rockville, Maryland, explains in "Global Epidemiology of HIV" (*Journal of Medical Virology*, vol. 78, no. S1, April 2006) that two types of HIV have been recognized and identified: HIV-1, the predominant worldwide virus, and HIV-2. HIV-1 and HIV-2 show an extraordinary difference in global distribution. In North and South America HIV-1 has reached pandemic proportions among certain risk groups, primarily through MSM and IDU. Some African and Asian countries have also experienced extensive heterosexual transmission of HIV-1. HIV-2 is largely restricted to West Africa, where its relatively low prevalence is largely attributable to heterosexual transmission.

DIFFERENCES IN EPIDEMIOLOGY, INCIDENCE, AND TRANSMISSION. The epidemiological characteristics (factors such as distribution, incidence, and prevalence that determine the presence, extent, or absence of a disease) of HIV-2 are different from those of HIV-1. Perhaps reflecting these differences, the international spread of HIV-2 is quite limited. In the early course of infection, people with HIV-2 are less infectious than those with HIV-1. This is due to the low levels of the virus isolated from the blood of immunodeficient people with HIV-2. Over time, as an individual's immunodeficiency progresses, HIV-2 probably becomes more infectious, but this more infectious period is relatively shorter than for HIV-1 and tends to occur in older individuals.

According to Elizabeth Pádua et al., in "Assessment of Mother-to-Child HIV-1 and HIV-2 Transmission: An AIDS Reference Laboratory Collaborative Study" (*HIV Medicine*, vol. 10, no. 3, March 2009), multiple studies demonstrate evidence that HIV-2 is not frequently transmitted from mother to child. Even though the mechanics of perinatal transmission are not completely understood, advanced immunodeficiency of the mother is certainly a risk factor. Low levels of the virus are not sufficient to transmit to the baby, and higher levels of virus infection in women past childbearing years may explain why perinatal transmission is less frequent. This is the most likely explanation for the observation that HIV-2 infection is so rare in children.

Interactions and HIV Transmission

One of the major concerns of public health officials worldwide is the possible interaction between HIV and other infections. The same risky behaviors that expose individuals to potential HIV infection also expose them to other STDs, such as gonorrhea, syphilis, and chancroid (a genital ulcer). Considerable data suggests that STDs, particularly herpes simplex, chancroid, and syphilis (which all cause ulcerative lesions), promote the transmission of HIV.

In "Herpes Simplex Virus Type 2: Epidemiology and Management Options in Developing Countries" (*Postgraduate Medical Journal*, vol. 84, no. 992, 2008), Gabriela Paz-Bailey et al. observe that genital herpes simplex virus type 2 is highly prevalent worldwide and is an increasingly important cause of genital ulcer disease, which in turn increases the risk of HIV transmission and acquisition. The researchers call for actions "to improve recognition of genital herpes, to prevent its spread and also to prevent its potential to promote HIV transmission in developing countries."

TUBERCULOSIS. HIV infection is recognized as the strongest known risk factor for the development of active tuberculosis (TB), because people with a latent TB infection are more apt to develop the disease once their immune system has been compromised by HIV. According to the World Health Organization (WHO), in *Diagnostics for Tuberculosis: Global Demand and Market Potential* (2006, http://www.who.int/tdr/publications/publications/pdf/tbdi/tbdi.pdf), latent TB infection is believed to be present in one-third of the world's population. People with latent TB have positive TB skin tests but are not sick with TB—they have been infected with *Mycobacterium tuberculosis* at some point in their life but have not developed active TB.

The WHO indicates in "Frequently Asked Questions about TB and HIV" (2009, http://www.who.int/tb/hiv/faq/en/) that people infected with both latent TB and HIV are 50 times more likely to develop active TB each year. An estimated 13 million adults worldwide, primarily in sub-Saharan Africa, have been infected with both HIV and *M. tuberculosis*. Not only are people infected with HIV who test tuberculin-positive more likely to develop TB but also they are likely to develop TB more rapidly than people without HIV infection. An even more disastrous consequence is that half of all people infected with both will develop contagious TB, which they could then spread to any susceptible individual, even those not infected with HIV.

UNAIDS states in *2008 Report on the Global AIDS Epidemic* that TB is the most common opportunistic infection for people living with HIV (including those on antiretroviral

drugs) and a leading cause of death in low- and middle-income countries. Africa is in the throes of the worst TB pandemic since the advent of widespread use of antibiotics. About 22% of TB cases in Africa are among people with HIV and in some countries as many as 70% of people are infected with both TB and HIV. As many as half of children living with HIV in South Africa also have TB.

Highly Drug-Resistant Tuberculosis

In *2008 Report on the Global AIDS Epidemic*, UNAIDS observes that people living with AIDS are twice as likely to have multidrug-resistant tuberculosis (MDR-TB; this type of TB does not respond to two first-line antituberculosis drugs—rifampicin and isoniazid) as people who are not HIV infected. Extensively drug-resistant tuberculosis (XDR-TB; this type of TB does not respond to first- and second-line drug treatment) is associated with extremely high mortality rates in people with HIV.

To a large extent, drug-resistant TB occurs in response to inadequate TB control, poor patient or clinician adherence to TB treatment regimens, poor-quality drugs, or a lack of drug supplies. People living with HIV are particularly vulnerable to developing drug-resistant TB because of their compromised immune systems, which make them more susceptible to infection and more likely to progress to active TB.

XDR-TB has occurred in other locales as well as sub-Saharan Africa. In "Emergence of *Mycobacterium tuberculosis* with Extensive Resistance to Second-Line Drugs—Worldwide, 2000–2004" (*Morbidity and Mortality Weekly Report*, vol. 55, no. 11, March 24, 2006), the WHO and the Centers for Disease Control and Prevention (CDC) report that between 2000 and 2004, 2% of TB cultures performed at 25 reference laboratories met the criteria for XDR-TB and conclude that XDR-TB is present in all regions of the world. Because TB culture and drug sensitivity testing are not performed routinely in many developing countries, the number of people affected and the full extent of the pandemic cannot be accurately measured or projected.

Geographic Differences

In North America and Europe during the 1980s and early 1990s, HIV was transmitted predominantly through unprotected sexual intercourse among MSM and through IDU with contaminated needles. During the late 1990s heterosexual intercourse and IDU became the prevailing modes of HIV transmission in North America and Europe.

In sub-Saharan Africa the overwhelming mode of transmission has been heterosexual intercourse. In this part of the world, transmission through MSM contact or through IDU is slight. Because many women have been infected, rates of perinatal transmission are increasing. UNAIDS reports in *2008 Report on the Global AIDS Epidemic* that the increasing numbers and percentages of HIV-infected pregnant women receiving antiretroviral drugs to prevent mother-to-child transmission of HIV has effectively reduced transmission. For example, there were just 191 HIV diagnoses attributable to perinatal transmission in western Europe in 2006, and in Botswana, where preventing perinatal transmission was established as a priority, the rate of mother-to-child transmission fell to 4%.

The rates of MSM transmission in Latin America are similar to those of Europe and the United States, but IDU is less frequent, whereas heterosexual transmission is considerably higher. In South and Southeast Asia the rapid increase of HIV can be traced to shared contaminated injection equipment and heterosexual intercourse. Almost half of people living with HIV infections in China in 2006 are thought to have been infected as a result of IDU. Similarly, even though most HIV infections in India are occurring because of unprotected heterosexual intercourse, contaminated injection drug equipment is also a significant risk factor for HIV infection in northeast India and in several large cities in India such as Tamil Nadu, where nearly a quarter of IDUs are HIV infected.

The highest national HIV infection levels in Asia continue to be found in Southeast Asia, where combinations of unsafe practices with sex workers and MSM, along with IDU, continue to fuel and maintain the epidemics. Even though the HIV infection rate has peaked and leveled off in other parts of the world, it is escalating in Indonesia, Pakistan, Vietnam, China, and Bangladesh, largely from heterosexual intercourse and through sex workers.

The article "HIV/AIDS Cases Soar in Indonesia: Official" (Agence France-Presse, June 3, 2009) notes that Nafsiah Mboi, the AIDS commissioner in Indonesia, reported in June 2009 that the country's HIV/AIDS cases had nearly tripled from 9,565 in 2005 to 26,632 in March 2009. Mboi also observed that these numbers underestimate Indonesia's epidemic, because 85% of those infected are unaware of their HIV status.

AFRICA

North Africa and the Middle East

Unreliable and often inadequate HIV surveillance systems complicate an accurate assessment of the patterns and trends of the epidemics in many countries in North Africa and the Middle East—especially among high-risk populations. Improved data collection and surveillance in some countries such as Algeria, Iran, Libya, and Morocco show that HIV epidemics do exist across the region and that an epidemic continues in Sudan. In Algeria and Morocco the majority of reported HIV infections are attributable to unprotected sex, and women make up a growing proportion of people living with HIV. In *2008 Report on the Global AIDS Epidemic*, UNAIDS notes that

an estimated 380,000 people were living with HIV in the region, including 40,000 newly infected in 2007.

UNAIDS also observes that transmission via sex workers and IDUs significantly contribute to the epidemic. In Iran between 15% to 23% of male IDUs are thought to be HIV infected, and IDU is considered a major route of transmission in Libya, Tunisia, Algeria, Morocco, and Syria. In addition, in Algeria, Egypt, Lebanon, and Syria about one-third of IDUs are also involved in buying or selling sex, making it difficult to distinguish the transmission route of new HIV infections.

Unparalleled Infection Rates

UNAIDS estimates in *2008 Report on the Global AIDS Epidemic* that 22 million adults and children in sub-Saharan Africa were infected in 2007. The national prevalence rates (the number of cases of the disease present in a specified population at a given time) of HIV infection among adults vary widely. Some West African countries report relatively low rates of infection, whereas others in the southern portion of the continent experience much higher rates. Even though there are indications that some of the HIV epidemics in this region have already peaked and are diminishing, there is actually an equilibrium—in 2007, 5.7 million (15% of people with HIV globally) lived in South Africa and 350,000 or 18% of AIDS global deaths occurred in this region. Similarly, in many countries in southern Africa an equilibrium exists between the number of people newly infected with HIV and the number of people dying of AIDS.

SEVERAL MODES OF TRANSMISSION. Because heterosexual transmission is the predominant mode of transmission in Africa, men and women have been almost equally infected. However, UNAIDS finds in *2008 Report on the Global AIDS Epidemic* that in 2007 more women (60%) than men were infected with HIV, and they were also more likely to be the ones caring for others infected with HIV or suffering from AIDS. Paid sex workers and their customers play a significant role in the spread of HIV in many countries—in West Africa between 20% and 35% of female sex workers were HIV infected. In five African countries—Burkina Faso, Cameroon, Ghana, Kenya, and the United Republic of Tanzania—in two-thirds of HIV-infected couples just one member of the couple was infected.

IDU also contributes to the pandemic in eastern and southern Africa. In Mauritius, IDU was the major source of HIV infection. MSM also fuels the pandemic in sub-Saharan Africa. For example, in Zambia 33% of MSM were HIV infected, and in Mombasa, the second largest city in Kenya, 43% of MSM were HIV infected.

According to UNAIDS, HIV infection rates in pregnant women in Lesotho and Mozambique are increasing, and one out of five adults is living with HIV in some provinces in central and southern Africa.

UNAIDS notes that even though 2007 data confirm that two-thirds of all HIV-infected people live in sub-Saharan Africa, data emerging from Zimbabwe paint a more optimistic picture. Both the incidence and prevalence of HIV infection are declining in Zimbabwe, and the infection levels among pregnant women dropped from 26% in 2001 to 18% in 2006. Similarly, in Botswana HIV prevalence among pregnant teenagers (aged 15 to 19) decreased from 25% in 2001 to 18% in 2006. There are also signs that the pandemic is stabilizing, as measured by the rate of new infections, among women in Malawi and Zambia.

NEW INFECTIONS AMONG TEENS DECLINE. In *South African National HIV Prevalence, Incidence, Behaviour, and Communication Survey, 2008: A Turning Tide among Teenagers?* (June 2009, http://www.mrc.ac.za/pressreleases/2009/sanat.pdf), Olive Shisana et al. find that the number of new infections among teens and young adults are declining despite the fact that the percentages of adolescents and young adults that continue to have multiple sex partners has actually increased. The decline in HIV incidence is almost entirely attributable to increasing condom use—among males aged 15 to 24 condom use rose from 57.1% in 2002 to 87.4% in 2008. More females aged 15 to 24 also reported using condoms—from 46.1% in 2002 to 73.1% in 2008. Condom use among males aged 25 to 49 nearly doubled, and among females in the same age group it tripled.

The increase in condom use is at least in part attributable to heightened awareness resulting from the intensive national HIV communication and education program conducted from 2005 to 2008. About 90% of young people reported seeing or hearing about HIV/AIDS through this communication program, and 80.9% of older adults (aged 50 and older) said they had been reached by the program. Despite the success of the national communication program, serious gaps in knowledge persist. The survey found that knowledge of how to prevent HIV infection actually declined among people aged 15 to 49, from 64.4% in 2005 to 44.8% in 2008.

PAYING THE PRICE FOR YEARS OF EVASION. Even though their country had experienced the ravages of AIDS for about a decade, Kenya's parliament and cabinet did not debate the issue publicly until 1993. Physicians diagnosed the first AIDS cases in 1984, but the government did not issue national statistics until 1986, when it announced one AIDS-related death. The nation's president and vice president regularly warned the public in speeches to avoid infection, and national officials instructed district administrators, including local tribal chiefs, to encourage their people to practice safe sex and limit their partners, but there had been no official statement.

For many Kenyans, the government's belated commitment to dealing with HIV/AIDS came too late. UNAIDS reports in *2008 Report on the Global AIDS Epidemic* that

in 2007 between 1.5 million and 2 million people were living with HIV in Kenya. Even though there has been a decline in the prevalence of HIV infection among adults from between 7.4% and 9.8% in 2001 to between 7.1% and 8.5% in 2007 and fewer AIDS-related deaths, it may not be entirely attributable to prevention efforts and the observation of increased condom use and a smaller proportion of the population with multiple sex partners. Instead, the lower prevalence of HIV infection may reflect the saturation of the infection in the at-risk population, meaning that the peak of the epidemic may have passed or that deaths from AIDS have served to reduce HIV prevalence.

The Kenyan government's reticence and seeming inability to deal with the epidemic came as a surprise to many observers. Kenya has endured an economic decline that many blame on corruption and the collapse of global commodity prices. Nonetheless, Kenya is still one of Africa's wealthiest countries and has remained relatively stable since gaining its independence from Britain in 1963. Many observers thought that if any African country could cope with or even head off an HIV/AIDS epidemic, it would be Kenya.

However, Kenyan officials chose to downplay the threat, lest it frighten away the much-needed tourist dollars. Even though the country did not launch major prevention efforts until 2000, these relatively late efforts seem to have already made an impact on the epidemic in terms of reducing the prevalence of many, though not all, high-risk behaviors. One remaining challenge is that IDU appears to be fueling the country's HIV epidemic.

Besides the risk of IDU as a factor in the transmission of HIV, long-standing social and cultural practices also abet HIV transmission. For example, "wife inheritance," which was once a socially useful tradition, continues to contribute to the spread of HIV/AIDS. In western Kenya, when a woman is widowed, her former husband's family takes care of her and her children. For generations, a brother-in-law or male cousin took her in with his family. Initially, tradition frowned on his having sexual relations with the inherited wife. Eventually, the inheritors began to ignore this restriction and had sex with the widow. If the widow's former husband had died of AIDS, she was likely to be infected and could pass the virus on to her inheritor, who would pass it on to his wife, causing the disease to spread.

UGANDA'S EFFORTS TO REDUCE HIV INFECTION. Scientists think that more than 20 years ago, in the early 1980s, truck drivers first spread HIV in Uganda's Rakai District, which lies along a Lake Victoria trade route to the capital city of Kampala. Because commercial sex is widely available along the trade route, HIV quickly spread throughout Uganda and all of Africa. At one time, Uganda had the world's highest HIV infection rates. By the turn of the 21st century, it was one of only two developing nations (Thailand is the other) where there was nationwide evidence of declining HIV rates in response to strong prevention programs. UNAIDS indicates in *2008 Report on the Global AIDS Epidemic* that these programs, which emphasized changes in sexual behavior, helped reduce the percentage of HIV infection among people aged 15 to 49.

Uganda was the first African country to respond powerfully to its HIV/AIDS epidemic. The government began by gathering religious and traditional leaders, along with representatives of other sectors of society, in an effort to reach agreement that the problem had to be confronted. Prevention efforts targeted specific populations or communities. For example, prevention programs that focused on delaying sex and safe sex practices were presented in schools. Community groups were formed to counsel and support those living with the virus. Condom use was heavily promoted.

Unlike Kenya, Uganda began an aggressive campaign against the spread of HIV/AIDS in the mid-1980s, when it had the highest number of recorded HIV cases in Africa. With virtually every family touched by HIV/AIDS, much of the cultural, religious, and psychological stigma disappeared in Uganda, where HIV infection rates began to decline. Despite a concerted prevention campaign, UNAIDS notes that the steady decline of Uganda's epidemic was beginning to stabilize at 5.4% in 2006. Even though education did prompt behavior changes that in turn resulted in lower HIV prevalence among pregnant women in Kampala and other cities from the early 1990s to the first decade of the 21st century, the decline was also due in part to increased AIDS mortality.

According to UNAIDS, some of these gains may be short lived as sexual practices revert to old ways. For example, the percentage of adults who reported having sex with a person who was neither a spouse or a member of the household rose from 12% of women and 29% of men in 1996 to 16% of women and 36% of men in 2006. Other research cited by UNAIDS presents the finding that one out of five female teenagers (aged 15 to 19) said her "first sexual experience involved force or coercion," and three out of four unmarried female teenagers said they had received gifts or money in exchange for sex, usually from an older man.

Much of the HIV/AIDS epidemic in Kenya and other nations of East Africa has been attributed to the preponderance of wars and political upheaval. It has been commonly assumed that displaced people and refugees are more likely to be HIV infected than people in more stable settings. In *2008 Report on the Global AIDS Epidemic*, UNAIDS refutes this premise, citing a review of HIV literature on displaced people in 8 countries including Uganda that finds no evidence that conflict increases HIV transmission.

There have also been reports of higher than anticipated rates of HIV infection in adults seeking treatment for malaria in Uganda. (Malaria is a serious, infectious disease that is spread by mosquitoes and is most common in tropical climates.) According to UNAIDS, more than 30% of adults treated at district health centers for malaria were also HIV positive. These findings are consistent with reports from other parts of sub-Saharan Africa that malaria is more serious and occurs more frequently in HIV-infected people.

Lisa M. Bebell et al. report in "HIV-1 Infection in Patients Referred for Malaria Blood Smears at Government Health Clinics in Uganda" (*Journal of Acquired Immune Deficiency Syndrome*, vol. 46, no. 5, December 2007) that among Ugandans evaluated for suspected malaria, associations between malaria test results and HIV infection differed between children and adults. In children, HIV was more common among those with negative malaria blood smears, whereas in adults HIV infection was more common among those with positive blood smears. The researchers conclude that the diagnosis of malaria "is a warning sign for HIV infection in adults, because HIV infection likely diminishes acquired antimalarial immunity. In children, malaria is very common, and a negative malaria smear suggests other causes of fever, including HIV-related infections."

EUROPE

Western Europe

Even though HIV in Europe is spread primarily through MSM, IDU is gaining as a mode of transmission. UNAIDS observes in *2008 Report on the Global AIDS Epidemic* that new HIV diagnoses are increasing and that the number of people living with HIV is also growing, primarily because of widespread use of antiretroviral treatment. The largest proportion of new diagnoses—42%—occurred as a result of heterosexual transmission in 2006, and 29% of new HIV infections occurred among MSM. In western Europe MSM are considered at greatest risk of acquiring HIV, especially because of reports of the increasing frequency of high-risk unprotected sex in this population. For example, in Germany the number of new HIV diagnoses among MSM rose by an alarming 96% between 2002 and 2006.

UNAIDS explains that the proportion of new HIV diagnoses in Europe attributable to IDU fell to just 6% in 2006, compared with 18% in the United States and 19% in Canada. In some countries harm-reduction programs, which aim to reduce HIV infection among IDUs, have served to reduce infection attributable to nonsterile needles. For example, in Denmark the number of new HIV diagnoses among IDUs declined by 72% from 2002–2006 and, during the same time period, by 91% in the Netherlands.

SPAIN. Historically, Spain has had the highest number of HIV/AIDS cases per capita in the European Union. The Ministerio de Sanidad y Consumo Centro de Publicaciones reports in *HIV and AIDS in Spain, 2001* (September 2002, http://www.isciii.es/htdocs/pdf/libroing.pdf) that the first case of HIV was reported in Spain in 1981; by the end of 2001, 110,000 to 150,000 people were living with HIV. According to UNAIDS, in (*Epidemiological Fact Sheet on HIV and AIDS, Spain, 2008 Update* (December 2008, http://apps.who.int/globalatlas/predefinedReports/EFS2008/full/EFS2008_ES.pdf), 140,000 adults and children were living with HIV and an estimated 2,300 deaths were attributed to AIDS in 2007.

The article "Spain's War on AIDS Visits the Prado" (*New York Times*, August 27, 1997) explains that drug use in Spain began to increase during the 1970s and 1980s, after the long Francisco Franco (1892–1975) dictatorship ended. Isabel Noguer of the Health Ministry describes this period as a time of heavy heroin use, with addicts sharing infected needles. In 1997 IDUs still made up the highest risk group, whereas unprotected heterosexual relations was the next most common form of transmission. By 2003 HIV prevalence among IDUs declined in cities that had instituted effective long-standing harm-reduction programs. In *2008 Report on the Global AIDS Epidemic*, UNAIDS notes that in 2006 Spain was one of just 8 countries that provided comprehensive harm reduction, which included needle and syringe exchange and treatment programs for IDUs in prisons.

Eastern Europe and Central Asia

The HIV pandemic did not reach eastern Europe until the mid-1990s. According to UNAIDS, in *2008 Report on the Global AIDS Epidemic*, in 1995 only 30,000 out of 450 million people were infected throughout all of eastern Europe; by 1997 about 190,000 adults were infected with HIV. UNAIDS reports that 1.5 million people throughout eastern Europe and central Asia were HIV infected and 110,000 became infected in 2007.

Ukraine and the Russian Federation have been the hardest hit countries in eastern Europe. In Ukraine new HIV cases diagnosed each year more than doubled from 2001 to 2006. The numbers of new HIV cases are also increasing in Azerbaijan, Georgia, Kazakhstan, Kyrgyzstan, the Republic of Moldova, Tajikistan, and Uzbekistan.

Historically, IDU has been the primary source for the spread of the virus. According to UNAIDS, about 62% of new HIV cases in eastern Europe in 2006 were attributable to IDU. The prevalence of HIV infection among IDUs varies in the Russian Federation from a low of 3% in Volgograd to in excess of 70% in Biysk. In Ukraine the percentage of infected IDUs rose from 11% in 2001 to 17% in 2006. As in other regions, there is considerable overlap between IDU and sex workers—as much as 39%

of female sex workers in parts of the Russian Federation were IDUs in 2007.

The region has also seen an increasing proportion of HIV infections in women. In 2006 an estimated 40% of new cases in eastern Europe and central Asia occurred in women. High rates of HIV infection—1% or higher—among pregnant women were reported in Ukraine. These cases most likely result from women infected by sex partners who used injected drugs.

UNAIDS indicates that even though IDU is the "most important mode of HIV transmission" in the region, there are few harm reduction programs in place, and there is very limited access to drug rehabilitation services. Furthermore, because possession of even small amounts of narcotics is harshly punished in many countries in eastern Europe, IDUs are understandably reluctant to participate in needle exchange programs.

UNAIDS describes its method of rating countries in terms of their efforts to ensure equal access to HIV prevention and treatment based on the countries' responses to questions about policies related to women. Eastern Europe and central Asia earned the lowest scores in terms of equitable policies. By contrast, sub-Saharan Africa earned the highest score for policies ensuring gender equality.

ASIA

Asia could eventually overtake Africa as the continent most affected by HIV. The HIV/AIDS pandemic arrived in Asia much later than in the rest of the world. Until the mid-1990s HIV/AIDS was uncommon, but because the average incubation period is approximately 10 years, more people are now beginning to die from the disease. UNAIDS estimates in *2008 Report on the Global AIDS Epidemic* that 5 million Asian adults and children were infected with HIV in 2007. About 380,000 people were newly diagnosed with the infection that year, and the same number of deaths were attributed to AIDS.

Even though Cambodia, Myanmar, and Thailand report declines in HIV prevalence from 2% in 1998 to 0.9% in 2006, Indonesia, Pakistan, Vietnam, Bangladesh, and China all continued to see increasing numbers of people living with HIV.

Thailand

The spread of HIV in Thailand had been almost unprecedented. Thailand's commercial sex industry is notorious, and travel packages based on the availability of sex workers in Thailand are common in Asia (as they are in other countries, including the United States). In the capital city of Bangkok, brothels are found in virtually every neighborhood. Cheewanan Lertpiriyasuwat, Tanarak Plipat, and Richard Jenkins find in "A Survey of Sexual

Risk Behavior for HIV Infection in Nakhonsawan, Thailand, 2001" (*AIDS*, vol. 17, no. 13, September 5, 2003) that in 1990, 20% of all Thai men reported having paid for sex in the previous year. After a military coup in 1991, the transitional government instituted a comprehensive HIV/AIDS education program, which included a media campaign and condom distribution to brothels and massage parlors. Brothels that refused to use condoms were closed down. Even though the anti-HIV program came too late for those infected in the mid- to late 1980s, Thailand recorded a drop in new HIV infections until the late 1990s.

UNAIDS notes in *2008 Report on the Global AIDS Epidemic* that an estimated 610,000 adults and children in Thailand were living with HIV and approximately 30,000 died from AIDS-related illnesses in 2007. Still, the number of new HIV infections has been decreasing—largely in response to national prevention initiatives. Furthermore, Thailand is distinguished in Asia as a country that has succeeded in providing antiretroviral treatment to those in need, including providing antiretroviral therapy to at least 75% of HIV-infected pregnant women to prevent perinatal transmission.

In "National Expansion of Antiretroviral Treatment in Thailand, 2000–2007: Program Scale-up and Patient Outcomes" (*Journal of Acquired Immune Deficiency Syndrome*, vol. 50, no. 5, April 15, 2009), Sanchai Chasombat et al. observe that before 2000 antiretroviral treatment in Thailand was only available in selected research facilities and private hospitals. Beginning in 2000 all government and some private and university hospitals provided treatment. The program was scaled up so that by the end of 2006 an estimated 115,994 patients had begun antiretroviral treatment. As treatment reached more HIV-infected people, the risk of death and AIDS-related death rates began to decline. The researchers conclude that the observed "treatment outcomes in Thailand are encouraging for other resource-limited countries that are also scaling up HIV treatment programs."

Other Southeast Asian Countries

In other parts of Southeast Asia data about the epidemics reveal different patterns.

Cambodia has been the hardest hit country in the region. However, there is evidence that the epidemic is subsiding. UNAIDS finds in *2008 Report on the Global AIDS Epidemic* that in 2007 there were 75,000 adults and children living with HIV, down from 120,000 in 2001. The estimated number of deaths due to AIDS also dropped from 14,000 in 2001 to 6,900 in 2007. The number of people receiving antiretroviral therapy rose more than fivefold from 5,000 in 2004 to 26,664 in 2007. In 2004, 14% of people in need of antiretroviral therapy were receiving it, and just three years later, in 2007, a full two-thirds (67%) of those in need were receiving antiretroviral drugs. Similarly,

the percentage of pregnant women receiving antiretroviral therapy to prevent perinatal transmission rose from 7% in 2004 to 42% in 2007.

In 2005 Cambodia opened public antiretroviral clinics, so the rising percentages of HIV-infected people in treatment reflect increased access to treatment. Not surprisingly, treatment outcomes improved as well. For example, in "Impact of a Public Antiretroviral Program on TB/HIV Mortality: Banteay Meanchey, Cambodia" (*Southeast Asian Journal of Tropical Medicine and Public Health*, vol. 40, no. 1, January 2009), Benjamin Eng et al. compare treatment outcomes of HIV patients newly diagnosed with TB in 2004 (before clinics opened) with outcomes of HIV patients diagnosed in 2005 (after the public clinics opened). They state that "in 2004, 37% of HIV-infected tuberculosis patients died during TB treatment compared with 5% of HIV-uninfected tuberculosis patients. In 2005, 18% of HIV-infected tuberculosis patients died compared with 5% of HIV-uninfected tuberculosis patients."

India

At the International AIDS Conference held in Vancouver, Canada, in July 1996, a United Nations official reported that India had emerged as the country with the most people infected with HIV. This news came as a surprise to many of the conferees because HIV was not detected in India until 1986. According to UNAIDS, in *Epidemiological Fact Sheet on HIV and AIDS, India, 2008 Update* (October 2008, http://apps.who.int/globalatlas/predefinedReports/EFS2008/full/EFS2008_IN.pdf), in 2007 about 2.4 million people in India were HIV positive, down from 2.7 million in 2001.

In *2008 Report on the Global AIDS Epidemic*, UNAIDS notes that there are high rates of infection among IDUs—as high as 24%—in many parts of India. Most HIV infections are attributable to unprotected heterosexual relationships, and there is also overlap of IDU and sex work. Researchers speculate that many women with HIV acquired the virus from their regular partners, who were infected during paid sex. This seems plausible because in cities such as Nepal, 38% of sex-trafficked females were HIV-infected, and as many as half of all sex workers in Mumbai were found to be infected in 2006.

According to Arvind Pandey et al., in "Improved Estimates of India's HIV Burden in 2006" (*Indian Journal of Medical Research*, vol. 129, no. 1, January 2009), India has, historically, been faulted for overestimating its HIV epidemic, which was estimated as about 0.9%, or 5.7 million people, living with HIV/AIDS in 2005. Revised surveillance procedures in 2006 produced dramatically different statistics—India actually had less than half the number of cases of HIV infection—about 2.5 million—than previously estimated. The new number is the result of improved survey methods. The research also reveals some positive progress in combating the epidemic: the HIV-infection rate declined from about 0.5% of the population in 2002 to about 0.4% percent in 2006, and in southern states, where HIV is most prevalent, the infection rates have stabilized or begun to decline.

China

The first HIV case in China was identified in 1985, but the disease did not begin to spread until the early 1990s, when changes in the structure of the economy produced an increase in drug use and prostitution. The U.S. embassy in China indicates in *Flying Blind on a Growing Epidemic: AIDS in China* (April 1997, http://www.csssm.org/English/e5.htm) that the government of China estimated in 1997 that between 100,000 and 300,000 people were living with HIV/AIDS. By the beginning of 1998 this estimate had doubled. In *Epidemiological Fact Sheet on HIV and AIDS, China, 2008 Update* (December 2008, http://apps.who.int/globalatlas/predefinedReports/EFS2008/full/EFS2008_CN.pdf), UNAIDS notes that HIV infections are on the rise in China—in 2007, 700,000 Chinese were estimated to be HIV positive. That same year, an estimated 39,000 deaths were attributed to AIDS.

Almost half of all new HIV infections in 2006 are thought to have resulted because of IDU. As in other countries, HIV transmission and infection in China have migrated from the traditional high-risk populations—sex workers, IDUs, and the overlap of these populations—to the general population, and as a result the number of HIV infections in women is growing. According to UNAIDS, in *2008 Report on the Global AIDS Epidemic*, about 7% of China's epidemic may be attributable to MSM.

UNAIDS observes that China has about 200 million migrant workers, and in 2007 China launched worksite HIV prevention programs that targeted these workers. To reach the estimated 1 million workers who travel outside the country, China offered health education and prevention programs at 420 ports. HIV education was also provided in 10,000 night schools, which served approximately 3 million migrant workers.

According to UNAIDS, China has also intensified its harm reduction activities; by October 2007, 88,000 IDUs were receiving methadone maintenance (drug treatment that involves using methadone, a narcotic drug, as a maintenance drug to help control withdrawal symptoms in people undergoing treatment for opioid addiction) and almost 50,000 IDUs participated in needle exchange programs.

Despite recent efforts to expand and enhance education and prevention efforts, there is consensus that China's HIV programs are still sorely deficient. HIV awareness remains low, and stigma continues to limit access to, and acceptability of, measures to stem the epidemic. Fear, ignorance, and discrimination persist, even among medical professionals. As a result, prevention and treatment programs neither flourish nor succeed. For example, UNAIDS notes that in 2006 less than 25% of HIV-infected pregnant mothers received antiretroviral treatment to prevent mother-to-child transmission of the virus.

LATIN AMERICA

UNAIDS reports in *2008 Report on the Global AIDS Epidemic* that the number of new HIV infections in Latin America is on the decline. In 2007 there were an estimated 140,000 new cases of HIV, and approximately 1.7 million adults and children in Latin America were living with HIV. There were 63,000 AIDS-related deaths in 2007.

The majority of HIV/AIDS cases in Latin America can be traced to MSM transmission. There are high rates of HIV infection among MSM in Montevideo, Uruguay (22%), Peru (18% to 22%), and Buenos Aires, Argentina (14%). Four cities in Bolivia and Quito, Ecuador, have rates of 15%, and some cities in Colombia report rates ranging from 10% to 25%.

In Central America (Belize, Costa Rica, El Salvador, Guatemala, Mexico, and Nicaragua) from 25% to 33% of MSM also have sex with women—and a 2007 survey found that as many as 40% reported having unprotected sex with men and women in the month before the survey.

UNAIDS states that while MSM remains the principal source of transmission, IDU continues to contribute to the pandemic in many countries. For example, in 2006, 12% of IDUs in the capitals of Paraguay and Uruguay were HIV infected.

UNAIDS reports that growing numbers of women are acquiring the virus in Argentina, Brazil, Peru, and Uruguay. In Uruguay, about two-thirds of new cases of HIV were attributable to sexual transmission, primarily heterosexual. As is the case in other regions, many women become infected by their male partners, who acquired the virus through MSM or IDU.

THE CARIBBEAN

In 1982 the first suspected AIDS cases in the Caribbean appeared in Jamaica. UNAIDS indicates in *2008 Report on the Global Epidemic* that since then the pandemic has changed from a mostly homosexual phenomenon to a largely heterosexual one, attributable to unprotected sex between partners and sex workers.

UNAIDS notes that in 2007 an estimated 230,000 adults and children in the Caribbean were living with HIV, and 20,000 had contracted the infection during that year. Even though these numbers reflect a decline in the region's pandemic that is at least in part attributable to behavior changes and improved access to antiretroviral drugs, AIDS remains a leading cause of death among people aged 15 to 44 in the Caribbean and was responsible for 14,000 deaths in 2007.

Unlike other parts of the world, the Caribbean's connection between HIV and IDU is low. However, the traditionally common practice of men (and, more recently, women) having multiple sexual partners and the region's flourishing sex industry are fueling the spread of HIV. In urban areas and tourist centers there are high rates of HIV prevalence among sex workers—in Guyana 31% of female sex workers were infected with HIV and in Jamaica 9% were infected with the virus.

In "From Haiti, a Surprise: Good News about AIDS" (Associated Press, July 6, 2009), Jonathan M. Katz reports that among pregnant women HIV infection rates decreased from 6.2% in the mid-1990s to 3.1% in 2009. Katz observes that coordinated efforts, implemented by two nonprofit groups—Partners in Health and GHESKIO—to ensure widespread antiretroviral drug use, education, and increasing use of condoms as well as the closing of unregulated blood banks, helped stem Haiti's epidemic.

THE MIDDLE EAST AND NORTH AFRICA

UNAIDS states in *2008 Report on the Global Epidemic* that in 2007 an estimated 380,000 adults and children in the Middle East and North Africa were infected with HIV, 40,000 acquired the infection, and 27,000 deaths were due to AIDS-related illnesses. The largest epidemic in the region is in the Sudan. Historically, unreliable reporting and data, especially about high-risk populations, have made it challenging to track and forecast the epidemics in many countries. However, recent efforts to improve surveillance reveal local epidemics in Algeria, Iran, Libya, and Morocco and a more generalized epidemic throughout the Sudan.

In the Sudan the epidemic is attributable to heterosexual transmission of the virus. Here, as in other countries, an increasing number of women are acquiring the virus from husbands or boyfriends who became infected via IDU or from paid sex. In Morocco one-third of women diagnosed with AIDS in 2006 were married.

Even though a combination of factors account for the smaller epidemics in this region, most are attributable to sex workers and IDU. IDU is the principal contributor to the epidemic in Iran, where between 15% and 23% of male IDUs are infected with the virus. IDU also plays a major role in the epidemics in Algeria, Egypt, Lebanon, and Syria. There is also overlap between paid sex and IDU. For example, in Syria 40% of IDUs report never using condoms and 53% said they have sold sex.

CONTROVERSIES

Even though great strides have been made in the treatment of HIV infection and AIDS and in raising public awareness about the nature of the disease and preventing its spread, several issues and controversies continue to hamper the unity of purpose required to effectively combat HIV/AIDS worldwide.

The Cost of Treatment in Developing Countries

Bruce R. Schackman et al. estimate in "The Lifetime Cost of Current Human Immunodeficiency Virus Care in the United States" (*Medical Care*, vol. 44, no. 11, November 2006) that the direct medical care cost for people with HIV, from their diagnosis until death, is an average of about $2,100 per month. Average projected life expectancy for people receiving optimal HIV treatment is 24.2 years, which yields a lifetime cost of $618,900 per person. Even in a wealthy country such as the United States, this is beyond the reach of most Americans. In the developing world, where the annual income may be only several hundred dollars, the cost of treatment cost can prove absolutely prohibitive without government subsidies for HIV treatment.

Cost of Drugs

The high price of HIV/AIDS drugs has been and continues to be a contentious issue. Even though manufacturers froze their prices briefly in 2002, they subsequently began to raise them again. For example, in February 2003 Roche Pharmaceuticals announced that the price of its antiretroviral drug enfuvirtide, which was already the most expensive AIDS treatment on the market, would more than double in price in Europe.

In November 2002 the World Trade Organization (WTO) adopted a resolution affirming that the governments of WTO member countries have the right to take any actions they deem necessary to protect public health, including overriding pharmaceutical patent protections. For example, in May 2003 the government of Zimbabwe declared a national emergency for six months over the HIV/AIDS pandemic, which allowed it to purchase and make available generic versions of HIV/AIDS drugs that were still under patent protection.

Increased availability of generic versions of these lifesaving drugs and the freedom to seek and obtain them at the most competitive prices is seen as a vital step in stemming the HIV/AIDS pandemic in the developing world. In January 2007 the U.S. Department of Health and Human Services and the U.S. Food and Drug Administration issued approval, or tentative approval, for 34 generic antiretroviral drugs, which was an increase from 15 generic drugs in 2005. The availability of these generic drugs enables thousands of additional people to benefit from life-saving treatment.

PRICE REDUCTIONS ON HIV/AIDS DRUGS FOR DEVELOPING COUNTRIES. According to the press release "Clinton Foundation and UNITAID Announce Price Reductions on

16 AIDS Medicines for 66 Developing Countries" (May 8, 2007, http://www.cptech.org/ip/health/aids/2g/clinton-pr058 2007.pdf), the Clinton Foundation HIV/AIDS Initiative (CHAI), which was founded by the former president Bill Clinton (1946–), assists countries to implement large-scale prevention and treatment programs. The foundation works with the governments of 25 countries in Africa, the Caribbean, and Asia and provides technical assistance and human and financial resources to ensure the delivery of quality care and treatment. The foundation also provides access to reduced prices for HIV/AIDS drugs and diagnostics to 66 countries. In total, CHAI represents over 90% of people living with HIV/AIDS in developing countries.

In "What We've Accomplished" (2009, http://www .clintonfoundation.org/what-we-do/clinton-hiv-aids-initi ative/what-we-ve-accomplished), CHAI reports that as of 2009, it had successfully negotiated price reductions for 40 antiretroviral drug formulations and 16 HIV/AIDS diagnostic tests. CHAI's efforts resulted in price reductions of 50% for first-line drug treatment and a 30% reduction for second-line treatment (for people who develop resistance to first-line drugs) as well as a 90% reduction in the price of drugs used to treat children in low-income countries.

UNITAID is an international drug purchase facility established in 2006 by Brazil, France, Chile, Norway, and the United Kingdom. UNITAID is an innovative funding mechanism aimed at speeding access to quality drugs and diagnostics for HIV/AIDS, malaria, and TB in countries where these diseases pose serious threats to the health of their residents.

UNITAID notes in *UNITAID Annual Report 2008* (June 2009, http://www.unitaid.eu/images/news/annual _report_2008_en.pdf) that in 2008, 29 countries and one foundation supported UNITAID as donors. Besides expanding access to, availability, and affordability of antiretroviral drugs, UNITAID's 2009 initiatives included research to develop diagnostic tests to monitor resistance to antiretroviral drugs; investing in sustainable, local food production; and improving the availability of female condoms.

In *Financing the Response to AIDS in Low- and Middle-Income Countries: International Assistance from the G8, European Commission, and Other Donor Governments in 2008* (July 2009, http://data.unaids.org/pub/Presentation/ 2009/20090704_UNAIDS_KFF_G8_CHARTPACK_2009 _en.pdf), UNITAID states that in 2008 it had $349 million in funding. UNITAID not only works in partnership with the Clinton Foundation to supply antiretroviral drugs to the poorest countries but also with the WHO, the United Nations Children's Fund, UNAIDS, the Global Fund to Fight AIDS, Tuberculosis, and Malaria, Roll Back Malaria Partnership, Stop TB Partnership, the Foundation for Innovative New Diagnostics, the HIV/AIDS Initiative, and the Global Drug Facility.

Tying Foreign Policy Aid to Abstinence

Another controversial issue surrounding HIV/AIDS treatment was the U.S. foreign policy initiative in place until 2008—dubbed the President's Emergency Plan for AIDS Relief (PEPFAR)—that tied funding for developing countries to educational programs that stress abstinence as the principal prevention option. The Center for Health and Gender Equity indicates in the fact sheet "U.S. Global AIDS Policy and HIV Prevention" (September 2008, http:// www.genderhealth.org/pubs/globalaids.pdf) that in 2008 PEPFAR eliminated the requirement that 33% of prevention funds be used for abstinence-until-marriage programs.

Abstaining from sexual intercourse does prevent the sexual transmission of HIV, although most experts, who agree that it is not realistic to expect sexual abstinence from many segments of the population, stress that condom use is essential to stop the spread of the disease. Abstinence education is a key component of PEPFAR, although in 2007 the program's prevention strategy was broadened to include "ABC—Abstain, Be faithful, and correct and consistent Condom use," as well as prevention of mother-to-child transmission, activities that focus on blood safety, and interventions aimed at IDUs.

According to Erika Check, in "Criticism Swells against AIDS Program's Abstinence Policy" (*Nature Medicine*, vol. 13, no. 5, May 2007), a panel convened by the U.S. Institute of Medicine (IOM) observed that even though PEPFAR is achieving many of its objectives, some of its policies impede its effectiveness. The IOM, scientists, and public health activists have requested revision of controversial policies that dictate how funds are dispersed, specifically the mandate to emphasize abstinence-until-marriage as the single most important primary prevention program.

PEPFAR was reauthorized by the Tom Lantos and Henry J. Hyde United States Global Leadership against HIV/AIDS, Tuberculosis, and Malaria Reauthorization Act in July 2008. This act extended the program through 2013 and authorized up to $48 billion to wage war against HIV/AIDS, TB, and malaria between fiscal year (FY) 2009 and FY 2013. The reauthorization act still stipulates that "in countries with generalized HIV epidemics, at least half of all money directed towards preventing sexual HIV transmission should be for activities promoting abstinence, delay of sexual debut, monogamy, fidelity, and partner reduction," but it does not mandate abstinence-only education and prevention programs as a requirement for receiving funds.

The launch of PEPFAR significantly increased U.S. spending to support the fight against the global HIV/AIDS pandemic—it has increased from $2.3 billion in FY 2004 to $6.5 billion in FY 2009. (See Table 9.1.) For FY 2010 President Barack Obama (1961–) requested $6.6 billion.

In FY 2008 PEPFAR supported antiretroviral treatment for more than 2 million people in 15 countries in sub-Saharan Africa, Asia, and the Caribbean. (See Table 9.2.)

TABLE 9.1

PEPFAR funding, fiscal years 2004–09

[$ in millions]

Programs	Fiscal year 2004 enacted	Fiscal year 2005 enacted	Fiscal year 2006 enacted	Fiscal year 2007 enacted	Fiscal year 2008 enacted	Fiscal year 2009 enacted	Cumulative total[a]
Bilateral HIV/AIDS programs[b]	1,677	2,278	2,654	3,699	4,979	5,415	20,702
Global fund	547	347	545	724	840	900	3,903
Bilateral TB programs	87	94	91	95	162	175	704
Total PEPFAR (without Malaria)	**2,311**	**2,719**	**3,290**	**4,518**	**5,981**	**6,490**	**25,309**

[a]Includes fiscal year 2004–fiscal year 2009 enacted.
[b]Bilateral HIV/AIDS programs includes funding for bilateral country/regional programs, UNAIDS, International AIDS Vaccine Initiative, Microbicides and National Institutes of Health (NIH) HIV/AIDS research. As of May 2009, the NIH FY 2009 budget allocation for HIV/AIDS research has not been finalized.
PEPFAR = The United States President's Emergency Plan for AIDS Relief

SOURCE: "PEPFAR Funding (FY 2004–FY 2009)," in *Making a Difference: Funding*, The United States President's Emergency Plan for AIDS Relief, May 2009, http://www.pepfar.gov/documents/organization/80161.pdf (accessed July 9, 2009)

TABLE 9.2

Number of people receiving antiretroviral treatment supported by U.S. government interventions, fiscal years 2005–08

	Total number of individuals reached (on antiretroviral treatment)[a, b]			
	Fiscal year 2005	Fiscal year 2006	Fiscal year 2007	Fiscal year 2008
Botswana[c]	37,300	67,500	90,500	111,700
Côte d'Ivoire	11,100	27,600	46,000	50,500
Ethiopia	16,200	40,000	81,800	119,600
Guyana	800	1,600	2,100	2,300
Haiti	4,300	8,000	12,900	17,700
Kenya	44,700	97,800	166,400	229,700
Mozambique	16,200	34,200	78,200	118,000
Namibia	14,300	26,300	43,700	56,100
Nigeria	28,500	67,100[d]	126,400	211,500
Rwanda	15,900	30,000	44,400	59,900
South Africa	93,000	210,300	329,000	549,700
Tanzania	14,700	44,300	96,700	144,100
Uganda	67,500	89,200	106,000	145,000
Vietnam	700	6,600	11,700	24,500
Zambia	36,000	71,500	122,700	167,500
Total	**401,200**	**822,000**	**1,358,500**	**2,007,800**

[a]Numbers reflect totals of downstream (direct) and upstream (indirect) results.
[b]Number of individuals reached through upstream systems strengthening includes those supported through contributions to national, regional and local activities such as training, laboratory support, monitoring and evaluation, logistics and distribution systems, protocol and curriculum development.
[c]Botswana results are attributed to the National HIV Program. Beginning fiscal year 2006, U.S. government (USG) downstream contributions in Botswana are embedded in the upstream numbers, following a consensus reached between the USG and the government of Botswana to report single upstream figures for each relevant indicator.
[d]In Nigeria, it is currently unknown if the government's number of people on treatment accounts for people who are lost to follow up, therefore the total number of people on treatment had been reduced by 15% to account for the estimated attrition.

SOURCE: "Total Number of Individuals Reached (on Antiretroviral Treatment FY 2005–FY 2008)," in *Tables: Detailed PEPFAR Program Results*, The United States President's Emergency Plan for AIDS Relief, undated, http://www.pepfar.gov/about/tables/treatment/123461.htm (accessed July 9, 2009)

More Access to Treatment Is Needed

We cannot sustain a successful effort with HIV without prevention.... Of the projected 60 million infections that will occur by 2015, fully half of them are projected to be able to be prevented with already known and proven prevention methods.... [Before] we celebrate 26 years since the beginning of extraordinary accomplishments, we're actually going to be judged as a society in what we do in the next 20 to 20-plus years.

Anthony S. Fauci, director of the U.S. National Institute of Allergy and Infectious Diseases, July 2007

Ambitious Objectives

Government subsidies can and do provide relief. UNAIDS describes in *What Countries Need: Investments Needed for 2010 Targets* (February 2009, http://data.unaids.org/pub/Report/2009/JC1681_what_countries_need_en.pdf) the progress that has been made by many countries toward achieving universal access to HIV prevention, treatment, care, and support. Much of this progress has been financed by the Global Fund for AIDS, Tuberculosis, and Malaria (2009, http://www.theglobalfund.org/en/about/), a public-private partnership created in 2002 that provides 25% of all international financing for AIDS globally.

UNAIDS states that as of 2009, 111 countries were aiming to achieve universal access to reverse the course of the HIV/AIDS crisis. The objectives most countries hoped to meet include:

- Preventing perinatal transmission by providing antiretroviral treatment to 80% of HIV-infected pregnant women to prevent mother-to-child transmission of the virus.

- Ensuring access to and availability of prevention, treatment, and support services to key populations that are at increased risk for HIV exposure and infection, such as sex workers, MSM, and IDUs.

- Increasing support for orphans and vulnerable children.

- Strengthening health care delivery systems so that they are better able to deliver needed services.

- Instituting programs to prevent violence against women.

UNAIDS predicts that if each country achieves its objectives by 2010, 2.6 million new HIV infections and 1.3 million deaths will be prevented by the following programs and activities:

- 74.5 million pregnant women will be screened, and those in need will receive treatment to prevent mother-to-child HIV transmission

- 20.4 million MSM, 9.6 million IDUs, and 7.5 million sex workers will benefit from HIV prevention programs

- 8.2 billion condoms will be distributed

- 6.7 million people will receive antiretroviral treatment

- 6.7 million orphans will receive support

CHAPTER 10
KNOWLEDGE, AWARENESS, BEHAVIOR, AND OPINION

CONCERN ABOUT HIV/AIDS

During the first decade of the 21st century the U.S. public appeared less concerned about HIV/AIDS and its impact on health care than ever before. According to the Gallup Organization, in 2008 just 2% of Americans named AIDS as the most urgent health problem facing the country, compared with 68% of Americans in 1987, 41% in 1992, and 29% in 1997 who identified it as the most pressing health problem. (See Table 10.1.)

The 2001 Gallup poll marked the first time since 1987 that the percentage of Americans naming AIDS as the most urgent health problem facing the country dropped to a single digit. AIDS (7%) was fifth, trailing behind bioterrorism (22%), cancer (19%), heath care/insurance costs (14%), and access to health care (8%). By 2004 just 5% of Americans considered AIDS the most urgent health problem and by 2007 a scant 2% named AIDS as the most urgent health problem. (See Table 10.1 and Figure 10.1.)

Even though Americans no longer view HIV/AIDS as the most pressing health problem facing the United States, they appreciate that in the last decade gains have been made in combating the disease. Lydia Saad and Jeffrey M. Jones of the Gallup Organization note in *Gains under Bush Seen on AIDS, Race Relations, Little Else* (January 9, 2009, http://www.gall up.com/poll/113680/Gains-Under-Bush-Seen-AIDS-Race-Relations-Little-Else.aspx) that when Gallup researchers asked Americans in January 2009 to assess whether progress had been made on a variety of issues during the previous eight years—under the administration of the former president George W. Bush (1946–)—AIDS was the issue that most Americans credited the administration with effectively addressing. Thirty-eight percent of Americans said the country had made progress on AIDS, and 19% felt the United States had lost ground in the fight against AIDS. The "net progress made" of 19% was the highest of any issue considered in that Gallup poll (See Figure 10.2.) In contrast, a net of 15% of Americans said progress had been

made on race relations and just 3% thought progress had been made in addressing terrorism or in terms of national defense and the military.

Even Those at High-Risk Are Less Concerned

The Kaiser Family Foundation describes in *2009 Survey of Americans on HIV/AIDS: Summary of Findings on the Domestic Epidemic* (April 4, 2009, http://www.kff.org/ kaiserpolls/upload/7889.pdf) trends in public opinions, attitudes, knowledge, and awareness of HIV/AIDS and related issues. The 2009 survey was conducted less than a year after the Centers for Disease Control and Prevention (CDC) released new and revised data and estimates, which described the U.S. epidemic as larger than previously believed. The CDC revised statistics also underscored the fact that African-Americans and Hispanics are disproportionately affected—the rate of new HIV infections in African-Americans is seven times that of whites, and Hispanics had three times as many new infections as did whites. Because these groups are at increased risk, it would seem intuitively correct to assume that they would express more urgency and concern about the epidemic, or at least a heightened sense of personal risk. However, the Kaiser survey finds conflicting perceptions of personal concern about becoming infected, even among those at highest risk.

Consistent with the findings of the Gallup Organization, the Kaiser survey finds that the percent of Americans identifying HIV/AIDS as the "most urgent health problem facing the nation" plummeted from 44% in 1995 to 17% in 2006 and to 6% in 2009. African-Americans (40%) and Hispanics (35%) perceived HIV/AIDS as more urgent problems for their communities than did whites (10%). In 2009 fewer African-Americans and Hispanics named HIV/AIDS a more urgent problem, 40% and 35%, respectively, than in 2006, when nearly half of African-Americans (49%) and Hispanics (46%) felt it was an urgent concern.

TABLE 10.1

Public opinion on the most urgent health problem facing the country, selected years 1987–2008

WHAT WOULD YOU SAY IS THE MOST URGENT HEALTH PROBLEM FACING THIS COUNTRY AT THE PRESENT TIME?

[Open-ended]

	A.	B.	C.	D.	E.	F.	G.	H.	I.	J.	K.	L.	OT.	DK
	%	%	%	%	%	%	%	%	%	%	%	%	%	%
2008 Nov	30	25	12	11	2	2	2	1	1	*	—	—	4	10
2007 Nov	30	26	10	14	1	2	2	1	*	1	1	—	4	9
2006 Nov	22	29	8	14	3	6	1	1	*	1	1	*	6	8
2005 Nov	17	25	9	15	4	6	1	1	1	1	10	*	3	7
2004 Nov	29	29	7	9	2	5	*	1	*	*	2	*	8	8
2003 Nov	25	27	7	13	3	8	1	*	1	1	*	1	7	6
2002 Nov	14	25	7	21	5	8	1	1	2	*	1	1	5	9
2001 Nov	8	14	4	19	6	7	1	2	1	1	1	22	6	8
2000 Sep	13	25	3	20	3	18	1	1	1	2	—	—	6	7
1999 Feb	1	13	1	23	5	33	—	—	3	2	—	—	13	6
1997 Oct	13	9	*	15	3	29	—	—	2	6	—	—	18	5
1992 Mar	—	30	—	5	2	41	—	—	—	—	—	—	18	4
1991 Nov	—	20	—	6	2	55	—	—	—	—	—	—	14	3
1991 May	2	10	1	16	2	45	—	—	*	5	—	—	15	4
1987 Oct	—	1	3	14	7	68	—	—	1	4	—	—	8	3

*Less than 0.5%
Key: A = Access to healthcare. B = Healthcare/insurance costs. C = Obesity. D = Cancer. E = Heart disease. F = AIDS. G = Diabetes. H = Finding cures for diseases. I = Smoking.
J = Drug/alcohol abuse. K = Flu. L = Bioterrorism. OT = Other. DK = No opinion.

SOURCE: "What Would You Say Is the Most Urgent Health Problem Facing This Country at the Present Time?" in *Healthcare System*, The Gallup Organization, undated, http://www.gallup.com/poll/4708/Healthcare-System.aspx (accessed July 11, 2009). Copyright © 2009 by The Gallup Organization. Reproduced by permission of the Gallup Organization.

FIGURE 10.1

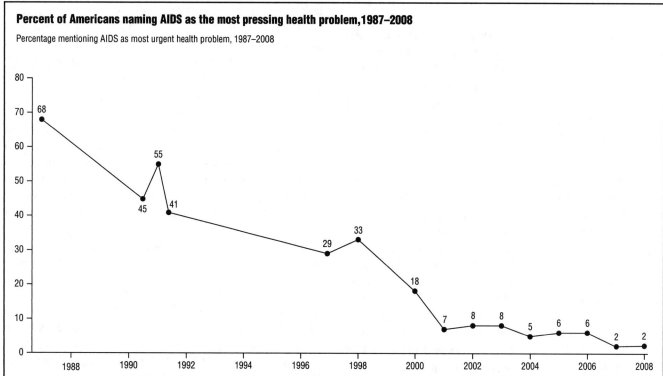

Percent of Americans naming AIDS as the most pressing health problem, 1987–2008

Percentage mentioning AIDS as most urgent health problem, 1987–2008

SOURCE: Jeffrey M. Jones, "Percentage Mentioning AIDS As Most Urgent Health Problem, 1987–2008," in *Healthcare Access, Cost Are Top Health Concerns*, The Gallup Organization, December 1, 2008, http://www.gallup.com/poll/112516/Healthcare-Access-Cost-Top-Health-Concerns.aspx (accessed July 11, 2009). Copyright © 2008 by The Gallup Organization. Reproduced by permission of the Gallup Organization.

FIGURE 10.2

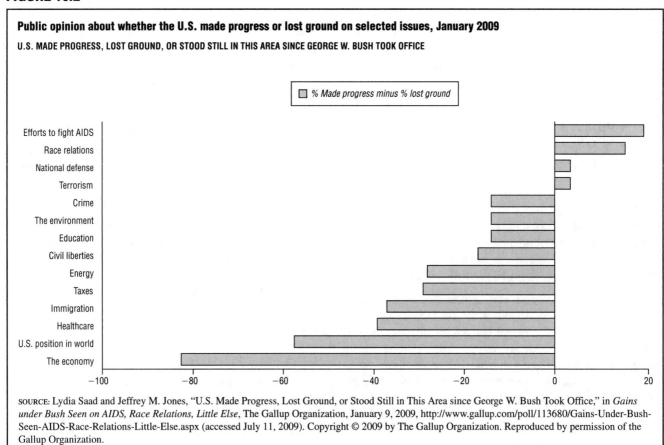

Public opinion about whether the U.S. made progress or lost ground on selected issues, January 2009

U.S. MADE PROGRESS, LOST GROUND, OR STOOD STILL IN THIS AREA SINCE GEORGE W. BUSH TOOK OFFICE

☐ *% Made progress minus % lost ground*

SOURCE: Lydia Saad and Jeffrey M. Jones, "U.S. Made Progress, Lost Ground, or Stood Still in This Area since George W. Bush Took Office," in *Gains under Bush Seen on AIDS, Race Relations, Little Else*, The Gallup Organization, January 9, 2009, http://www.gallup.com/poll/113680/Gains-Under-Bush-Seen-AIDS-Race-Relations-Little-Else.aspx (accessed July 11, 2009). Copyright © 2009 by The Gallup Organization. Reproduced by permission of the Gallup Organization.

Similarly, the percentage of young adults (aged 18 to 29) that expressed concern about becoming infected with HIV dropped from 30% in 1997 to 17% in 2009. African-Americans of the same age also expressed less concern about acquiring the virus—in 1997, 54% said they were personally concerned about infection; by 2009 only 40% expressed this concern.

Perhaps concern has diminished because media attention has waned or because other health messages predominate. The Kaiser survey participants reported seeing and hearing less about HIV/AIDS in the United States than they did just five years ago. The proportion claiming to have seen or heard "a lot" or "some" about the problem fell from seven out of 10 (70%) in 2004 to less than half (45%) in 2009. Even though African-Americans (65%) and Hispanics (54%) were more likely than whites (40%) to say they had seen or heard "a lot" or "some" about HIV/ AIDS in 2009, the percentages fell from 2004, when they were 83%, 74%, and 68%, respectively.

Despite the fact that they have seen or heard less about HIV/AIDS in recent years, Americans are aware that the U.S. epidemic has disproportionately affected African-Americans and Hispanics. More than half (56%) knew that the African-American community has been harder hit, and

more than two-thirds (68%) of the African-American community was aware of the impact of HIV/AIDS on them.

HIV Testing

The revised CDC guidelines in Bernard M. Branson et al.'s "Revised Recommendations for HIV Testing of Adults, Adolescents, and Pregnant Women in Health-Care Settings" (*Morbidity and Mortality Weekly Report*, vol. 55, RR-14, September 22, 2006) essentially changed HIV testing from an opt-in diagnostic test to an opt-out test that is a routine part of medical practice. Based on the findings of the 2009 Kaiser Family Foundation survey, this change has not, as might have been anticipated, translated into more people being tested for HIV.

Rates of testing have remained relatively unchanged since 2000. In 2009 almost half (47%) of adults said they have been tested for HIV, including 16% who reported testing within the 12 months before the survey. The majority (65%) of those tested said they chose to be tested because "it just seemed like a good idea." People aged 18 to 29 (30%) were the most likely to have been tested in the past 12 months.

In 2009 most (70%) survey respondents who had never been tested for HIV said they had not obtained testing because they did not believe they were at risk of contracting the virus. Thirty-three percent said their physicians had never recommended testing, 9% said they disliked needles or giving blood, 7% claimed they did not know where to obtain testing, and 4% said worries about confidentiality prevented them from getting tested.

KNOWLEDGE AND TOLERANCE GROW, BUT MISCONCEPTIONS PERSIST

During the more than two decades since HIV/AIDS was first identified, aggressive community health education and awareness programs have sought to increase the public's knowledge about the prevention, transmission, and treatment of HIV/AIDS. Based on the findings of the 2009 Kaiser Family Foundation survey, even though public understanding and awareness have improved in many areas, misconceptions about HIV/AIDS persist.

There is, however, an understanding that the U.S. HIV epidemic has had a profound effect on U.S. culture and society as well as on personal behaviors. Historically, the Kaiser Family Foundation surveys and other polling organizations have found that about half of Americans feel there has been considerable discrimination against people with AIDS. The results of the 2009 survey indicate that some of the stigma and discrimination associated with HIV/AIDS may be diminishing. Over four out of 10 (44%) Americans said they would feel comfortable working with someone with HIV/AIDS, up from 32% in 1997. More than two-thirds (69%, up from 62% in 2006) of adults opined that people they knew would not think differently about them if they discovered they had been tested for HIV. Just 16% (down from 21% in 2006) felt that people would think less of them if they found out they had been tested.

Some of these changing attitudes and declining stigma may be attributable to how widespread HIV/AIDS has become. More than four out of 10 (43%) Americans have had personal contact with HIV/AIDS—either they know someone infected with HIV, or someone who has AIDS, or someone who has died from the disease. The survey findings support the premise that familiarity reduces sigma. The overwhelming majority (83%) of people who said they know someone with HIV/AIDS said "they would be comfortable working with someone with HIV," compared with 65% of people who do not know anyone with HIV/AIDS.

Still, significant stigma persists. Almost a quarter (23%) of survey respondents felt they would be uncomfortable working with someone infected with HIV, 35% would be uncomfortable if their child's teacher was HIV positive, 42% would be uncomfortable if their roommate was HIV positive, and 51% would be uncomfortable having food prepared by someone who is HIV positive.

Knowledge of How HIV Is Spread Varies

Lingering stigma is likely the result of persisting ignorance and misconceptions. The Kaiser Family Foundation

survey finds that in 2009, 34% of Americans had at least one misconception about how HIV is transmitted. These misconceptions included not knowing that sharing a drinking glass with someone infected with HIV (27%), touching a toilet seat used by someone with HIV (17%), or swimming in a pool with someone who is HIV infected (14%) are not ways that the virus is transmitted. Older adults aged 65 and older (56%) were more likely to hold these misconceptions, but nearly one-third (32%) of young adults aged 18 to 29 also held one of these three erroneous beliefs. Worse still, despite ambitious public health education programs, the level of ignorance about HIV transmission is essentially unchanged from 1987.

Predictably, people who have misconceptions about how HIV is transmitted are more likely to feel uncomfortable working with someone who is HIV infected (43% versus 13% of people who understand how HIV is transmitted) and are more likely to be concerned about having someone who is HIV positive prepare food for them (71% versus 40%).

Beliefs about Prevention and Treatment

Along with misconceptions about how HIV is transmitted, many Americans are not well informed about HIV prevention measures and advances in treatment. For example, more than half (55%) of those surveyed were unaware of treatment to prevent mother-to-child transmission. More than a quarter (27%) believed that Magic Johnson (1959–) has been cured of AIDS, and a quarter (24%) thought there is a vaccine available to prevent people from becoming infected with HIV. Almost one out of five (18%) survey respondents did not know that there is no known cure for AIDS, and 12% were unaware that there are drug treatments that lengthen the lives of people infected with HIV.

The prevalence of misconceptions about HIV/AIDS varies by race and ethnicity. African-Americans were more likely to believe that Magic Johnson has been cured of AIDS (37%), that there is a vaccine to prevent HIV infection (36%), and that there are drugs that can cure HIV/AIDS (30%). By contrast, more African-Americans (58%) than whites (43%) or Hispanics (46%) were aware that drug treatment can help prevent the transmission of HIV from a pregnant mother to her child.

Furthermore, about two-thirds (62%) of the public credits the media (radio, television, newspapers, and the Internet) as its primary source of information about HIV/AIDS. Young adults and African-Americans are more likely than other groups to obtain information from other sources such as their doctors, schools, family, and friends.

Experiences Talking with Physicians about HIV/AIDS

Younger adults (those under the age of 50), African-Americans, and Hispanics are the most likely to have spoken with their physicians and/or partners about HIV/AIDS. The proportion of African-Americans that reported talking with physicians about HIV rose from about half (54%) in 2006 to two-thirds (67%) in 2009. In addition, more African-Americans (29%) and Hispanics (28%) said that a physician recommended that they be tested for HIV than did whites (14%).

Spending for HIV/AIDS in the United States

Since 1997, when the Kaiser Family Foundation began surveying Americans about HIV/AIDS, the majority of survey respondents have felt that too little money is devoted to combating HIV/AIDS domestically. In 2009 support for spending on prevention programs was strong, with nearly two-thirds (60%) of survey respondents indicating that prevention programs effectively slow the epidemic. In contrast, about half (48%) felt that spending on treatment will slow the epidemic and more than a third (38%) felt that spending on treatment will not make a difference in the course of the epidemic.

Although slightly diminished, the 2009 survey finds continued support for increased spending, which is somewhat surprising in view of the economic recession that began in 2008. Along with government spending for HIV/AIDS, the public is helping to foot the bill for HIV/AIDS research, prevention, and treatment. More than one-third (36%) of survey respondents reported donating money to an HIV or AIDS-related charity. Among African-Americans the rate was higher—nearly half (45%) said they had contributed.

HIV/AIDS AWARENESS EFFORTS

Many national and global initiatives and observances are conducted in an effort to inform the public, heighten awareness, and improve understanding of the HIV/AIDS pandemic. This section describes some of the activities, individuals, and groups involved in the ongoing effort to educate, motivate, and mobilize efforts to prevent the spread of HIV and assist people living with HIV/AIDS.

The U.S. Department of Health and Human Services (2009, http://www.hhs.gov/aidsawarenessdays/) designates the annual observation of HIV/AIDS Awareness Days. These include:

- February 7, National Black HIV/AIDS Awareness Day—this annual awareness day was created by a community-based coalition to raise awareness among African-Americans about HIV/AIDS and its disproportionate and devastating impact on African-American communities.

- March 10, National Women and Girls HIV/AIDS Awareness Day—this day aims to raise awareness of the increasing impact of HIV/AIDS on the lives of women and girls.

- March 20, National Native HIV/AIDS Awareness Day—this day was created to increase awareness of the impact of HIV/AIDS on Native Americans, Alaskan natives, and native Hawaiians.

- May 18, HIV Vaccine Awareness Day—this day recognizes and acknowledges the people who are working to help find an HIV preventive vaccine, such as the clinical trial volunteers, the nurses, the community educators/recruiters, and the researchers.

- May 19, National Asian and Pacific Islander HIV/AIDS Awareness Day—this awareness day intends to increase awareness among Asians and Pacific Islanders in the United States about the ruinous impact of HIV/AIDS.

- June 8, Caribbean American HIV/AIDS Awareness Day—this day is a national mobilization effort designed to encourage Caribbean-American and Caribbean-born individuals across the United States and its territories to become better informed and educated and to obtain testing and seek treatment.

- June 21, National Clinicians HIV/AIDS Testing and Awareness Day—this day asks clinicians to lead by example by taking an HIV test themselves to demonstrate that testing is easy and nonintrusive and to improve communication between health care clinicians and their patients about the wisdom and benefits of HIV/AIDS testing.

- June 27, National HIV Testing Day—this day aims to provide opportunities for testing, especially for those who have never been tested or who have engaged in high-risk behavior since their last test, and to help dispel the myths and stigmas associated with HIV.

- September 18, National HIV/AIDS Aging Awareness Day—this day aims to heighten awareness of the impact of HIV/AIDS on older adults. It intends to focus on HIV prevention, care, and treatment of people aged 50 and older.

- September 27, National Gay Men's HIV/AIDS Awareness Day—this day aims to regain and refocus the attention of a community that has been disproportionately affected by the HIV epidemic at a time when the United States confronts the simultaneous challenges of a resurgence of new HIV infections among gay men and growing complacency about HIV among gay men.

- October 15, National Latino AIDS Awareness Day—this awareness day marks an opportunity to communicate the devastating and disproportionate effects AIDS is having on the Hispanic community.

- December 1, World AIDS Day—started by the World Health Organization in 1988, this day serves to focus global attention on the HIV/AIDS pandemic. Observance of this day provides an opportunity for governments, national AIDS programs, churches, community organizations, and individuals to demonstrate the importance of the fight against HIV/AIDS.

The AIDS Memorial Quilt

The AIDS Memorial Quilt is not only an ongoing community art project that pays tribute to and commemorates the lives claimed by AIDS but also serves as a powerful visual way to inform, educate, and heighten awareness of the lives lost in this pandemic. The AIDS Memorial Quilt notes in "History of the Quilt" (2009, http://www.aidsquilt.org/history.htm) that the quilt consists of cloth panels designed and made by friends and families of people who died from AIDS. Cleve Jones, a San Francisco, California, gay rights activist, had the idea for the quilt in November 1985 and the quilt was "born" in June 1987, when Jones and a group of his friends in San Francisco decided to memorialize people who had died from AIDS-related illnesses.

The first public display of the quilt was at the National Mall in Washington, D.C., in October 1987. It contained 1,920 panels and was larger than a football field. The quilt, and enthusiasm for it, grew quickly. One year later the quilt had grown to 8,288 panels. Each time the quilt was displayed the names of those honored by it were read aloud by celebrities, politicians, families, and friends.

In "Quilt Facts" (2009, http://www.aidsquilt.org/quilt facts.htm), the AIDS Memorial Quilt states that over 18 million people have seen the nearly 1.3-million-square-foot (120,000-square-m) quilt, which weighs more than 54 tons (48.9 t) and contains over 91,000 names. The names on the quilt represent about 17.5% of all AIDS deaths in the United States. The quilt has traveled around the world, raising awareness and money (more than $4 million) for AIDS-related research and programs. It has been the subject of stories, papers, articles, and books and was nominated for a Nobel Peace Prize in 1989. That same year a feature-length documentary about it, *Common Threads: Stories from the Quilt*, won an Academy Award.

Shoes Provide Another Graphic Depiction of the Number of AIDS Deaths

In an effort to describe the number of lives claimed by the HIV/AIDS pandemic, some activists have staged "shoe demonstrations," in which each pair of shoes represents a life lost to AIDS. For example, Petula Dvorak reports in "AIDS Activists Walk, but the Shoes Talk" (*Washington Post*, May 6, 2005) that on May 5, 2005, an estimated 3,500 AIDS activists piled 8,000 pairs of shoes in front of the White House to graphically portray the number of deaths in the world each day that are attributable to AIDS-related illnesses.

AIDS Activists

AIDS activists have been credited with raising awareness and attracting money and media attention to the pandemic. Many groups, individuals, and celebrities have taken on the cause and become champions of HIV/AIDS research, prevention, and treatment. Others have agitated to change the course of national and government policy and to improve access to and availability of quality care, especially affordable drug treatment. Still others have defended the rights of people living with HIV and AIDS in an effort to counter stigmatization and discrimination. Using a variety of approaches—from fund-raising campaigns and political lobbying to protests and guerilla theater (dramatization of a social issue, often performed outdoors in a park or on the street)—AIDS activists have raised their voices and the consciousness of people around the world.

Even though there are many groups and organizations engaged in AIDS activism, the most effective and vibrant organization is probably the AIDS Coalition to Unleash Power (ACT UP). ACT UP (2009, http://www.actupny.org/) describes itself as "a diverse, non-partisan group of individuals united in anger and committed to direct action to end the AIDS crisis." It states, "We advise and inform. We demonstrate. We are not silent. Silence = Death." ACT UP has thousands of members in more than 70 chapters in the United States and worldwide. The organization advocates nonviolent direct action through vocal demonstrations and acts of civil disobedience that are intended to make the public aware of the crucial issues of the AIDS crisis. During a span of more than 20 years, ACT UP members have staged scores of protests and demonstrations and have often been arrested, usually for civil disobedience.

AIDS Action (2009, http://www.aidsaction.org/about-aids-action-mainmenu-187), another national organization, has as its slogan "Until It's Over," conveying the group's commitment to the development, cultivation, and support of effective and proactive policies and programs to address the HIV epidemic "until no one acquires HIV, until those living with HIV have the care and services they need, and until a cure is found." AIDS Action has played a key role in the development and implementation of public health policies to improve the quality of life for Americans who are HIV positive. It also works with the public health community to enhance HIV prevention programs and care and treatment services.

On June 29, 2009, AIDS Action participated in a White House LGBT (Lesbian, Gay, Bisexual, Transgender) Pride Month Reception. At this event President Barack Obama (1961–; http://www.whitehouse.gov/the_press_office/Rema rks-by-the-President-at-LGBT-Pride-Month-Reception/) reiterated his commitment to end discrimination against same-sex couples; to pass the Domestic Partners Benefits and Obligations Act, "which will guarantee the full range of benefits, including health care, to LGBT couples and their children"; and to put an end to the discriminatory ban on entry to the United States based on HIV status.

The AIDS Treatment Activists Coalition is also a national coalition of AIDS activists who work together to end the AIDS epidemic by advancing research on HIV/AIDS. The coalition's mission statement (2009, http://atac-usa.org/about/mission-goals.htm) describes its goals as:

- To encourage greater and more effective involvement of people with HIV/AIDS in the decisions that affect their lives by identifying, mentoring and empowering treatment activists in all communities affected by the epidemic.

- To develop within all communities affected by HIV/AIDS and related coinfections the leadership to provide the knowledge and skills needed to advocate for improved research, treatment and access to care.

- To enable treatment activists to speak with a united, powerful voice to provide meaningful input into issues concerning HIV disease and related complications and coinfections.

- To facilitate communications and set agenda items... between HIV/AIDS treatment activists and government, industry and academia in matters affecting research, treatment and access [and] among HIV/AIDS treatment activists and the larger HIV community in keeping up to date with the latest developments in research, treatment and access.

CELEBRITIES SHINE A SPOTLIGHT ON HIV/AIDS. When celebrities endorse or lend their name to charitable causes, the causes often benefit from increased media attention and visibility. When celebrities actively work to promote their chosen causes, the results can be even more dramatic. For example, the United Nations Children's Fund notes in "Business People, Celebrities, and Officials Join Forces to Raise Awareness about AIDS in China" (May 18, 2006, http://www.unicef.org/people/people_10165.html) that many celebrities, from the late Diana, Princess of Wales (1961–1997), the former U.S. president Bill Clinton (1946–), the business executive Ted Turner (1938–), and the Microsoft chairman Bill Gates (1955–), to the actors Elizabeth Taylor (1932–), Richard Gere (1949–), Sharon Stone (1958–), Catherine Deneuve (1943–), and Ashley Judd (1968–), and to the musician Elton John (1947–), have made outstanding contributions of time, energy, and money to combat the HIV/AIDS pandemic.

Bono (1960–), the Irish lead singer of the rock group U2, uses his celebrity to champion the fight against HIV/AIDS. In 2002 Bono formed the organization Debt AIDS Trade Africa (DATA), an advocacy organization dedicated to eradicating extreme poverty and AIDS in Africa.

In 2005 Bono was named *Time*'s Person of the Year along with Bill Gates and Melinda Gates (1964–). The following year he was nominated for a Nobel Peace Prize.

In *The DATA Report 2008* (http://www.one.org/report/en/index.html), DATA reports how its efforts to induce the G8 donor nations—the United States, the United Kingdom, Germany, France, Canada, Italy, Japan, and Russia—to provide $25 billion in additional assistance for Africa by 2010 and to ensure widespread access to AIDS and malaria treatment and prevention programs have already produced results. DATA asserts that "the promises that the G8 made, when delivered, will be put to use to achieve their intended outcome—saving lives, reducing extreme poverty. These successes should inspire us all to deliver fully that which has been pledged."

In January 2008 DATA merged with ONE, a global antipoverty organization (http://www.one.org/us/) that pursues high-level global advocacy in concert with grassroots mobilization efforts. Like DATA, ONE's (2009, http://www.one.org/c/us/faq/) mission is "fight extreme poverty and preventable disease in the poorest places on the planet, particularly in Africa." ONE (2009, http://www.one.org/us/partners/) partners with other global relief and HIV/AIDS initiatives, including CARE, Save the Children, Oxfam America, the Bill and Melinda Gates Foundation, United against Malaria, Bread for Life, and (RED).

(RED) (2009, http://www.joinred.com) involves the private and public sectors in a joint fund-raising initiative. Companies whose products carry the (RED) insignia pledge to contribute a significant percentage of their sales or a portion of their profits from those products to the Global Fund to finance AIDS programs in Africa, with an emphasis on the health of women and children. In 2009 American Express, Apple, Bugaboo, Converse, Dell, Emporio Armani, Gap, Hallmark, Microsoft, and Starbucks were participating in (RED). MySpace.com was the program's first media sponsor in the United Kingdom. In the press release "Lesotho Becomes Fourth Global Fund Country to Receive (RED) Funds" (April 3, 2008, http://www.theglobalfund.org/en/pressreleases/?pr=pr_080403), the Global Fund states that by April 2008 (RED) had raised more than $100 million for the Global Fund.

In May 2009 (RED) announced that it would sponsor a concert series, (Red)Nights (http://www.joinred.com/News/Articles/ArticleDetail/09-05-11/_RED_and_Live_Nation_Announce_RED_NIGHTS.aspx), to raise awareness of and funds for HIV/AIDS programs in Africa. The 26 live concerts, which were held at clubs and theaters throughout the country in 2009, featured a variety of artists, including Santigold, Gomez, O.A.R., Fall Out Boy, Lisa Hannigan, the Veronicas, and the All-American Rejects. In 2009 (Red) also launched (Red)Wire, a digital music service. The (Red)Nights artists joined the many high-profile (RED) artists who participate in (Red)Wire, including U2, Coldplay, the Killers, Jay-Z, Elvis Costello, John Legend, Sheryl Crow, Neko Case, Noel Gallagher, Conor Oberst, TV on the Radio, Death Cab for Cutie, and Michael Franti.

IMPORTANT NAMES
AND ADDRESSES

ACT UP/New York
332 Bleecker St., Ste. G5
New York, NY 10014
URL: http://www.actupny.org/

AIDS Action
1730 M St. NW, Ste. 611
Washington, DC 20036
(202) 530-8030
FAX: (202) 530-8031
URL: http://www.aidsaction.org/

**AIDS Treatment Activists
Coalition**
611 Broadway, Ste. 613
New York, NY 10012
(617) 267-0998
E-mail: etr@atac-usa.org
URL: http://www.atac-usa.org/

**American Foundation for
AIDS Research**
120 Wall St., 13th Floor
New York, NY 10005-3908
(212) 806-1600
FAX: (212) 806-1601
URL: http://www.amfar.org/

Center for Women Policy Studies
1776 Massachusetts Ave. NW, Ste. 450
Washington, DC 20036
(202) 872-1770
FAX: (202) 296-8962
E-mail: cwps@centerwomenpolicy.org
URL: http://www.centerwomenpolicy.org/

**Centers for Disease Control and
Prevention**
1600 Clifton Rd.
Atlanta, GA 30333
1-800-232-4636
URL: http://www.cdc.gov/

Human Rights Campaign
1640 Rhode Island Ave. NW
Washington, DC 20036-3278

(202) 628-4160
1-800-777-4723
FAX: (202) 347-5323
URL: http://www.hrc.org/

**Joint United Nations Program
on HIV/AIDS**
20 Ave. Appia
CH-1211 Geneva 27
Switzerland
(011-41-22) 791-3666
FAX: (011-41-22) 791-4187
URL: http://www.unaids.org/

Kaiser Family Foundation
2400 Sand Hill Rd.
Menlo Park, CA 94025
(650) 854-9400
FAX: (650) 854-4800
URL: http://www.kff.org/

National AIDS Fund
729 15th St. NW, Ninth Floor
Washington, DC 20005-1511
(202) 408-4848
FAX: (202) 408-1818
URL: http://www.aidsfund.org/naf

**National Association of People
with AIDS**
8401 Colesville Rd., Ste. 505
Silver Spring, MD 20910
(240) 247-0880
1-866-846-9366
FAX: (240) 247-0574
URL: http://www.napwa.org/

**National Association of Public Hospitals
and Health Systems**
1301 Pennsylvania Ave. NW, Ste. 950
Washington, DC 20004
(202) 585-0100
FAX: (202) 585-0101
URL: http://www.naph.org/

National Hemophilia Foundation
116 W. 32nd St., 11th Floor
New York, NY 10001
(212) 328-3700
1-800-424-2634
FAX: (212) 328-3777
E-mail: handi@hemophilia.org
URL: http://www.hemophilia.org/

**National Institute of Allergy
and Infectious Diseases**
6610 Rockledge Dr., MSC 6612
Bethesda, MD 20892-6612
(301) 496-5717
1-866-284-4107
FAX: (301) 402-3573
URL: http://www.niaid.nih.gov/

National Minority AIDS Council
1931 13th St. NW
Washington, DC 20009
(202) 483-6622
FAX: (202) 483-1135
URL: http://www.nmac.org/

**National Prevention Information
Network**
PO Box 6003
(404) 679-3860
Rockville, MD 20849-6003
1-800-458-5231
FAX: 1-888-282-7681
E-mail: info@cdcnpin.org
URL: http://www.cdcnpin.org/
scripts/index.asp

**National Women's Health
Network**
1413 K St. NW, Fourth Floor
Washington, DC 20005
(202) 682-2640
FAX: (202) 682-2648
URL: http://www.nwhn.org/

ONE
1400 Eye St. NW, Ste. 600
Washington, DC 20005
(202) 495-2700
URL: http://www.one.org/us/

Orphan Project
121 Avenue of the Americas, Sixth Floor
New York, NY 10013

(212) 925-5290
FAX: (212) 925-5675

**U.S. Department of Health and
Human Services AIDSinfo**
PO Box 6303
Rockville, MD 20849-6303
1-800-448-0440
FAX: (301) 315-2818

E-mail: contactus@aidsinfo.nih.gov
URL: http://aidsinfo.nih.gov/

**U.S. Food and Drug
Administration**
10903 New Hampshire Ave.
Silver Spring, MD 20993-0002
URL: http://www.fda.gov/cder
1-888-463-6332

RESOURCES

The Centers for Disease Control and Prevention (CDC) provides the most current accounting of the HIV/AIDS epidemic in the United States. Publications cited in this text include "Revised Recommendations for HIV Testing of Adults, Adolescents, and Pregnant Women in Health-Care Settings" (Bernard M. Branson et al., September 2006), "HIV/AIDS among Persons Aged 50 and Older" (February 2008), "New Estimates of U.S. HIV Prevalence, 2006" (October 2008), "Human Immunodeficiency Virus (HIV) Risk, Prevention, and Testing Behaviors—United States, National HIV Behavioral Surveillance System: Men Who Have Sex with Men, November 2003–April 2005" (Travis Sanchez et al., July 2006), "Recommendations for Preventing Transmission of Human Immunodeficiency Virus and Hepatitis B Virus to Patients during Exposure-Prone Invasive Procedures" (July 1991), "Updated U.S. Public Health Service Guidelines for the Management of Occupational Exposures to HBV, HCV, and HIV and Recommendations for Postexposure Prophylaxis" (June 2001), "Updated U.S. Public Health Service Guidelines for the Management of Occupational Exposures to HIV and Recommendations for Postexposure Prophylaxis" (Adelisa L. Panlilio et al., September 2005), *Patient Characteristics and the Use of Health Care Services by Persons with HIV* (Esther Hing and Christine Lucas, 2007), "Are Health Care Workers at Risk of Getting HIV on the Job?" (January 2007), "Investigation of Patients Treated by an HIV-Infected Cardiothoracic Surgeon—Israel, 2007" (Mitchell J. Schwaber, 2009), *Comprehensive HIV Prevention: Essential Components of a Comprehensive Strategy to Prevent Domestic HIV, 2006* (April 2006), and *Advancing HIV Prevention: New Strategies for a Changing Epidemic* (March 2007).

HIV/AIDS Surveillance Reports are prepared by the CDC and describe and quantify transmission categories, risk factor combinations, demographics, and people living with HIV/AIDS. Other CDC publications used to prepare this publication include "1994 Revised Classification System for Human Immunodeficiency Virus Infection in Children Less Than 13 Years of Age" (M. Blake Caldwell et al., September 1994), *STDs in Adolescents and Young Adults* (January 2009), "The Role of STD Detection and Treatment in HIV Prevention—CDC Fact Sheet" (April 2008), "HIV Testing Implementation Guidance for Correctional Settings" (January 2009), "Revised Surveillance Case Definitions for HIV Infection among Adults, Adolescents, and Children Aged <18 Months and for HIV Infection and AIDS among Children Aged 18 Months to <13 Years—United States, 2008" (Eileen Schneider et al., December 2008), and "Update: Syringe Exchange Programs—United States, 2005" (November 2007).

The CDC National Center for Health Statistics publishes findings from the *National Ambulatory Medical Care Survey*, the *Youth Risk Behavior* surveys, and the *National HIV Behavioral Surveillance System*, as well as the *National Vital Statistics Reports* and *Morbidity and Mortality Weekly Report*.

The U.S. Department of Justice's *HIV in Prisons, 2006* (Laura M. Maruschak, April 2008) provides information on HIV/AIDS in U.S. prisons and jails, inmate deaths from HIV/AIDS, and testing policies for the virus antibody by states.

Information about funds appropriated through the Ryan White Comprehensive AIDS Resources Emergency Act was published in *The Ryan White CARE Act: A Side-by-Side Comparison of Prior Law to the Newly Reauthorized CARE Act* (December 2006) by the Kaiser Family Foundation. The Kaiser Family Foundation report "U.S. Federal Funding for HIV/AIDS: The President's FY 2010 Budget Request" (May 2009) addresses government spending for HIV/AIDS care. The National Alliance of State and Territorial AIDS Directors describes in *National ADAP Monitoring Project Annual Report* (April 2009) spending for prescription drug treatment for HIV/AIDS.

Information about the worldwide effects of HIV/AIDS, as well as global projections, were provided by reports including the World Health Organization's *HIV Transmission through Breastfeeding: A Review of Available Evidence—An Update from 2001 to 2007* (2008), *Diagnostics for Tuberculosis: Global Demand and Market Potential* (2006), and *Children and AIDS: Second Stocktaking Report* (April 2008); *Scaling up Early Infant Diagnosis and Linkages to Care and Treatment* (January 2009) by the United Nations Children's Fund; and *Report on the Global AIDS Epidemic 2008* and *What Countries Need: Investments Needed for 2010 Targets* (February 2009) by the Joint United Nations Program on HIV/AIDS.

Medical and scientific journals provide a wealth of information about HIV and the AIDS pandemic. Articles cited in this publication were published in *AIDS, AIDS Research and Therapy, AIDS Reviews, American Journal of Medicine, American Journal of Men's Health, American Journal of Public Health, American Medical News, Annals of Emergency Medicine, Annals of Internal Medicine, Antiviral Chemistry and Chemotherapy, Archives of Internal Medicine, Brain, Behavior, and Immunity, British Medical Journal, Canadian Journal of Neurological Sciences, Changes in Health Care Financing and Organization, Clinical Infectious Diseases, Cochrane Database of Systematic Reviews, Current Opinions in Oncology, HIV/AIDS Prevention, Indian Journal of Experimental Biology, Indian Journal of Medical Research, Issues in Mental Health Nursing, Journal of Acquired Immune Deficiency Syndrome, Journal of the American Medical Association,* *Journal of Experimental Medicine, Journal of Medical Virology, Journal of Psychosocial Nursing, Journal of Urban Health, Journal of Virology, Lancet, Medical Care, Medical Decision Making, Medscape Medical News, Nature, Nature Medicine, New England Journal of Medicine, Pediatric Research, PLoS Medicine, PLoS ONE, Postgraduate Medical Journal, Science, Scientific American, Sexually Transmitted Diseases, Sexually Transmitted Infections, Social Science and Medicine, Southeast Asian Journal of Tropical Medicine and Public Health,* and *Substance Abuse Treatment, Prevention, and Policy.*

Timely information about many facets of HIV/AIDS may be found at the online site http://www.thebody.com. The National Coalition for the Homeless, the National AIDS Housing Coalition, and the U.S. Department of Housing and Urban Development provided information on housing opportunities for people with HIV/AIDS.

The Kaiser Family Foundation publications *2009 Survey of Americans on HIV/AIDS: Summary of Findings on the Domestic Epidemic* (April 2009) and "The Global HIV/AIDS Epidemic" (April 2009) were used to prepare this publication. The Kaiser Family Foundation also provides daily updates about a variety of issues related to HIV/AIDS at its online site (http://www.kff.org/).

We are grateful to the Gallup Organization for permitting us to present the results of its renowned opinion polls and graphics depicting Americans' feelings and concerns about HIV/AIDS.

INDEX

Page references in italics refer to photographs. References with the letter t *following them indicate the presence of a table. The letter* f *indicates a figure. If more than one table or figure appears on a particular page, the exact item number for the table or figure being referenced is provided.*

A

Abacavir, 68

Abstinence
    abstinence-only education, 111
    foreign policy aid tied to, 127
    HIV prevention and, 110
    PEPFAR funding, 128(*t*9.1)

"Access to AIDS Medicines Stumbles on Trade Rules" (WHO), 88

Acer, David J., 82, 83

ACOG (American College of Obstetrics and Gynecology) Committee on Obstetric Practice, 70

"ACOG Committee Opinion No. 418: Prenatal and Perinatal Human Immunodeficiency Virus Testing: Expanded Recommendations" (ACOG Committee on Obstetric Practice), 70

Acquired immunodeficiency syndrome (AIDS)
    case numbers, 29–31
    cases by transmission category, 23*t*
    cases, deaths, persons living with AIDS, 18*f*
    clinical categories of AIDS infection, 17*t*
    definition of, 1, 15
    diagnosis/symptoms of, 17–22
    progression from HIV to AIDS, 21–22
    surveillance case definition, 15–17
    trends in history of, 1–3
    See also Human immunodeficiency virus/acquired immunodeficiency syndrome

ACS (American College of Surgeons), 82

ACT UP (AIDS Coalition to Unleash Power), 136, 139

Activists, AIDS
    AIDS Memorial Quilt, 136
    criticism of prevention efforts, 109
    Elizabeth Glaser, 97
    Magic Johnson, 95
    Mary Fisher, 96
    work of, 136–137
    young people as, 74

Acyclovir, 89

"ADAP Emergency!" (AIDS Treatment Activists Coalition), 89

ADAPs (AIDS Drug Assistance Programs), 78

Addresses/names, 139–140

Adolescents/young adults
    as AIDS activists/organizations, 74
    condom use by, 111
    distribution of AIDS cases by age, 36
    estimated rates of adults/adolescents living with AIDS, 32*f*, 35*f*
    HIV infections among teens in Africa, 121
    HIV/AIDS cases among female adolescents/young adults, by transmission category, 73(*t*5.7)
    HIV/AIDS cases among male adolescents/young adults, by transmission category, 73(*t*5.6)
    MSM AIDS rates, 33
    patterns of HIV infection, 73
    reported AIDS cases for female adults/adolescents, by transmission, race/ethnicity, 45*t*
    reported AIDS cases for male adults/adolescents, by transmission, race/ethnicity, 44*t*
    sexual activity of, 73–74
    sexual behaviors of high school students, 75*t*
    sexual health education, 110–111

surviving into their teens, 71–73
talking with physicians about HIV/ AIDS, 134–135

Advancing HIV Prevention: New Strategies for a Changing Epidemic (CDC), 109–110

"Adverse Psychosocial Factors Predict Poorer Prognosis in HIV Disease: A Meta-analytic Review of Prospective Investigations" (Chida and Vedhara), 98

Africa
    AIDS activism for, 137
    effect of AIDS on death rates, 118
    HIV transmission in, 119–120
    HIV/AIDS in, 120–122
    nevirapine use in, 68
    orphans from AIDS in, 73
    sub-Saharan Africa, 117

African-Americans
    AIDS cases among, 37, 38–39
    AIDSvax vaccine trials and, 93
    CCR5 gene and, 69, 91
    children with HIV/AIDS, 69
    concern about HIV/AIDS, 131, 133
    female AIDS cases by race/ethnicity, 53–54
    HIV transmission via IDU for, 52
    HIV/AIDS cases from heterosexual contact, 49–50
    misconceptions about HIV/AIDS, 134
    MSM sexual contact, HIV transmission via, 56
    National Black HIV/AIDS Awareness Day, 135
    prevention services for, 112
    prisoners with HIV/AIDS, 59
    talking with physicians about HIV/ AIDS, 134–135

Age
    AIDS cases by, 97*t*
    distribution of AIDS cases by, 36

proportion of persons surviving, by number of months after AIDS diagnosis, 47f
See also Deaths
Moses, Lincoln E., 50
Mothers
children with HIV/AIDS and, 69
health problems of babies born to HIV-infected mothers, 63–64
maternal HIV testing among children with perinatally acquired AIDS, HIV exposure or infection, 71t
maternal transmission of HIV, 22, 54
perinatal infection, 65–68
pregnant women, testing for HIV, 70–71
racial disparity in HIV/AIDS from, 39
reported cases of HIV/AIDS in infants born to HIV-infected mothers, by year of report, 43(t3.9)
surveillance case definition for children and, 64
testing pregnant women/newborns, 107–108
See also Perinatal infection
"Mother-to-Child Transmission of HIV-1 Infection during Exclusive Breastfeeding in the First 6 Months of Life: An Intervention Cohort Study" (Coovadia et al.), 67
MSM. *See* Men who have sex with men
Mullins, Iris L., 81–82
"Multifactorial Nature of Human Immunodeficiency Virus Disease: Implications for Therapy" (Fauci et al.), 8
Murex Diagnostics Inc., 26
Mycobacterium avium complex, 10
Mycobacterium tuberculosis
TB caused by, 10
TB spread by, 11
worldwide cases of, 119

N

NAHC (National AIDS Housing Coalition), 100
Name reporting, 103
Names/addresses, 139–140
NASCAR (National Association of Stock Car Auto Racing), 96
NASEN (North American Syringe Exchange Network), 113–114
NAT test. *See* Nucleic acid test (NAT) system
National ADAP Monitoring Project Annual Report (National Alliance of State and Territorial AIDS Directors), 78
National Affordable Housing Act of 1990, 100
National AIDS Fund, 139
National AIDS Housing Coalition (NAHC), 100

National Alliance of State and Territorial AIDS Directors, 78
National Asian and Pacific Islander HIV/AIDS Awareness Day, 135
National Association of Health Underwriters, 86
National Association of People with AIDS
advocacy by, 74
contact information for, 139
National Association of Public Hospitals and Health Systems, 139
National Association of Stock Car Auto Racing (NASCAR), 96
National Black HIV/AIDS Awareness Day, 135
National Clinicians HIV/AIDS Testing and Awareness Day, 135
National Coalition for the Homeless (NCH), 100
"National Expansion of Antiretroviral Treatment in Thailand, 2000–2007: Program Scale-up and Patient Outcomes" (Chasombat et al.), 124
National Gay Men's HIV/AIDS Awareness Day, 135
National Hemophilia Foundation (NHF)
contact information for, 139
on infection through blood supply, 61
on payments to hemophiliacs, 62
National HIV Behavioral Surveillance System (NHBS), 104–105
National HIV Testing Day, 135
National HIV/AIDS Aging Awareness Day, 135
National Institute for Occupational Safety and Health, 83
National Institute of Allergy and Infectious Diseases (NIAID)
contact information for, 139
fusin discovery by, 8
on HIV in children, 63
on HIV vaccine cooperation, 92
on PCR test for children, 65
protein xCT identification by, 10
National Institute on Drug Abuse (NIDA), 114
National Institutes of Health (NIH)
AIDS research funding by institute/center, 87t
budget of, 87–88
on dementia and AIDS, 19
on funding for AIDS research, 86
nevirapine recommendation of, 68
Vaccine Research Center, 94
National Latino AIDS Awareness Day, 135
National Minority AIDS Council, 139
National Native HIV/AIDS Awareness Day, 135
"A National Physician Survey on Prescribing Syringes as an HIV Prevention Measure" (Macalino et al.), 115

National Prevention Information Network, 139
National Women and Girls HIV/AIDS Awareness Day, 135
National Women's Health Network, 139
National Youth Risk Behavior Survey, 73–74
Native Americans
AIDS cases among, 38, 39
HIV transmission via IDU for, 52
National Native HIV/AIDS Awareness Day, 135
Native Hawaiians/Other Pacific Islanders, 38
NCAIDS (Chinese National Center for AIDS Prevention and Control), 25
NCH (National Coalition for the Homeless), 100
Nduati, Ruth, 67
Needle exchange programs
in China, 125
funding for, 50
prisons and, 60, 61
supplies/services provided by syringe exchange programs, 114t
syringe exchange programs, 112–115
Needle use
among prisoners, 59–60
HIV transmission through IDU, 50–52
Needle-safety legislation, 83
Nelfinavir mesylate, 68, 89
Netherlands, 122
"NeuroAIDS: An Evolving Epidemic" (Power et al.), 19
Nevirapine, 68
New Jersey
HIV testing of pregnant women, newborns, 108
numbers of HIV-infected children in, 71
"New Study Is Easing Fears on AIDS and Mental Illness" (Altman), 18–19
New York
children with AIDS in, 69
mandatory testing of newborns, 108
numbers of HIV-infected children in, 71
prisoners with HIV/AIDS in, 58
New York Times, 123
Newborns, 107–108
See also Infants; Perinatal infection
NHBS (National HIV Behavioral Surveillance System), 104–105
NHF. *See* National Hemophilia Foundation
"NHF—Guardian of the Nation's Blood Supply" (NHF), 61
NIAID. *See* National Institute of Allergy and Infectious Diseases
NIDA (National Institute on Drug Abuse), 114
NIH. *See* National Institutes of Health
"1993 Revised Classification System for HIV Infection and Expanded

Russian Federation, HIV/AIDS in, 123

The Ryan White CARE Act: A Side-by-Side Comparison of Prior Law to the Newly Reauthorized CARE Act (Kaiser Family Foundation), 84–85

Ryan White Comprehensive AIDS Resources Emergency (CARE) Act
    description of, 84
    funding, 85*t*
    HIV/AIDS Stigma Program, 99
    mandatory testing of newborns, 108
    purpose of, 74

Ryan White HIV/AIDS Treatment Modernization Act, 84–85

Ryan White National Youth Conference on HIV and AIDS, 74

S

Saad, Lydia, 131

Salgado, María, 69

Saliva
    HIV transmission and, 22
    for home test, 107

San Francisco, California, 80

San Francisco Center for HIV Information, 92

Sanchez, Travis, 104

Saquinavir mesylate, 68, 89, 90

Sayer, Charlie, 92

Scaling up Early Infant Diagnosis and Linkages to Care and Treatment (United Nations Children's Fund), 69

Schackman, Bruce R.
    on cost of HIV health care, 77
    cost of treatment in developing countries, 126
    on life expectancy for HIV-infected people, 21

Scheid, Johannes F., 94

Schneider, Eileen, 64

Schwaber, Mitchell J., 108

Schwartz, Oliver, 91

Screening
    decline in AIDS due to blood transfusions, 35–36
    revised recommendations for HIV testing, 26, 28
    See also Testing

"Senate Passes Bill Requiring HIV Testing in Prisons" (Georgia Public Broadcasting News), 61

Senior citizens. *See* Older people

SEPs. *See* Syringe exchange programs

Severe immunodeficiency, 63

Severe immunosuppression, 15–16

"Sex and STI/HIV Education" (Guttmacher Institute), 111

"Sex, Drugs, Prisons, and HIV" (Okie), 60–61

Sex workers
    in Caribbean, 126

HIV transmission via, 120
HIV/AIDS in Europe and, 123
HIV/AIDS in Sudan from, 126
HIV/AIDS in Thailand and, 123–124
in India, 124

Sexual activity
    abstinence, foreign aid and, 127
    of adolescents, young adults, 73–74
    circumcision to slow HIV, 112
    distribution of HIV infection, 31
    global patterns of HIV infection, 119–120
    heterosexuals, increase in AIDS among, 49–50
    HIV prevention in Uganda, 122
    HIV transmission statistics, 39
    HIV transmission via, 22
    HIV transmission via IDU and, 52
    HIV/AIDS in Caribbean and, 126
    MSM sexual contact, 55–56
    postexposure treatment, 91–92
    sexual behaviors of high school students, trends in prevalence of, 75*t*
    See also Heterosexual contact; Men who have sex with men

Sexual health education, 110–111

Sexually transmitted diseases (STDs)
    among teenagers, 74
    condom use and, 111–112
    global patterns of HIV infection, 118
    HIV/AIDS designated as, 103
    interactions with HIV, 119
    prevention, identification, treatment of, 54–55

Shishana, Olive, 121

Shoe demonstrations, 136

Simian immunodeficiency virus (SIV), 4–5

Singer, Natasha, 88

Singh, Kumud K., 71

SIV (simian immunodeficiency virus), 4–5

Small towns, HIV/AIDS in women in, 54

"Smoke and Mirrors: HIV-Related Lung Cancer" (Bazoes, Bower, & Powles), 12

Social cognitive theory, 112

Sorrel, Amy Lynn, 78

South Africa
    children with HIV, TB in, 119
    death rates in, 118
    decline of infections in teens, 121
    number of people infected with HIV, 120

South African National HIV Prevalence, Incidence, Behaviour, and Communication Survey, 2008: A Turning Tide among Teenagers? (Shishana et al.), 121

Southeast Asia
    HIV transmission in, 120
    HIV/AIDS in, 123–124

Spain, HIV/AIDS in, 123

"Spain's War on AIDS Visits the Prado" (*New York Times*), 123

Specialists, 81

Spector, Stephen, 71

Spending. *See* Costs; Funding

"Starting HAART at Higher T-Cell Counts Improves Survival in Early-Stage HIV" (Hitt), 14

State prisons
    AIDS-related deaths among all deaths in state prisons and U.S. general population, 58(*t*4.6)
    AIDS-related deaths in, 59
    AIDS-related deaths in, rate of, 59(*t*4.7)
    HIV testing in, 108–109
    IDU in, 59–60
    inmate deaths in state prisons by gender, age, race/ethnicity, 59(*t*4.9)
    inmates in state/federal prisons, HIV/AIDS among, by gender, 60*t*
    prisoners, state/federal, percent of AIDS cases in general population and, 58(*t*4.5)
    prisoners with HIV/AIDS in, 56–57

States
    AIDS cases in children under 13 years old by, 70*f*
    AIDS rates for female adults/adolescents by, 56*f*
    estimated numbers of persons living with HIV/AIDS, 30*t*–31*t*
    estimated rates for adults/adolescents living with HIV/AIDS, 32*f*
    estimated rates of adults/adolescents living with AIDS, 35*f*
    estimated rates of children up to age 13 living with AIDS, 36*f*
    with greatest numbers of HIV-infected children, 71
    HIV/AIDS cases among prison inmates, 57*t*–58*t*
    reported AIDS cases/annual rates, by area of residence, 33*t*–34*t*
    reported cases of HIV infection, by area of residence, age, 104*t*–105*t*
    state programs to provide AIDS drugs, 78–79

Statistical information
    adults/adolescents living with AIDS, estimated rates of, 35*f*
    adults/adolescents living with HIV/AIDS, estimated rates for, 32*f*
    AIDS, estimated numbers of cases/rates of, by race/ethnicity, age, and gender, 43(*t*3.8)
    AIDS cases, deaths, and persons living with AIDS, 18*f*
    AIDS cases by age, 97*t*
    AIDS cases by transmission category, 23*t*
    AIDS cases by year of diagnosis, selected characteristics, estimated number of, 42*t*
    AIDS cases in children under 13 years old, by state, 70*f*

"A Systematic Review of HIV Partner Counseling and Referral Services: Client and Provider Attitudes, Preferences, Practices, and Experiences" (Passin et al.), 105–106

T

"Will I? Won't I? Why Do Men Who Have Sex with Men Present for Post-exposure Prophylaxis for Sexual Exposures?" (Sayer et al.), 92

Women
AIDS and, 53–55
AIDS surveillance case definition and, 15
heterosexual transmission of HIV, 49
with HIV/AIDS in Africa, 120
testing women/newborns, 107–108
See also Females; Mothers

World AIDS Day, 135–136

"A World First: Vaccine Helps Prevent HIV Infection" (Marchione and Casey), 94

World Health Organization (WHO)
AIDS vaccine and, 94
on circumcision, 112
on dementia and AIDS, 19
on HIV infection via blood, 24
on HIV prevention in prisons, 60
on HIV transmission through breastfeeding, 22
on reduction of perinatal infection, 67–68
on tuberculosis, 119
on XDR-TB, 119

World Trade Organization (WTO), 88, 126

Worldwide HIV/AIDS
Africa, 120–122
Asia, 123–125
Caribbean, 125–126
controversies, 126–129
Europe, 122–123
Latin America, 125
Middle East/North Africa, 126
patterns of HIV infection, 118–120
PEPFAR funding, 128(*t*9.1)
scope of problem, 117–118
U.S. government interventions, number of people receiving antiretroviral treatment supported by, 128(*t*9.2)

WTO (World Trade Organization), 88, 126

X

XDR-TB (extensively drug-resistant TB), 12, 119

Xu, Xiao, 112

Y

Young, Taryn, 91–92

Young adults. *See* Adolescents/young adults

Youth. *See* Adolescents/young adults

YRBSS: Youth Risk Behavior Surveillance System—National Trends in Risk Behaviors (National Youth Risk Behavior Survey), 73–74

Z

Zalcitabine, 68

ZDV. *See* Zidovudine

Zhang, Xinjian, 69

Zidovudine (ZDV)
decrease in HIV-infected babies from, 54
effects of, 88
for infants of HIV-infected mothers, 65
for PEP, 83
for perinatal infection treatment, 66–67
state programs to provide, 78
for treatment of children with HIV/AIDS, 68

Zimbabwe
HIV/AIDS drugs for, 88
HIV/AIDS in, 121
purchase of generic HIV/AIDS drugs, 126